COOKING FOR
Hormone Balance

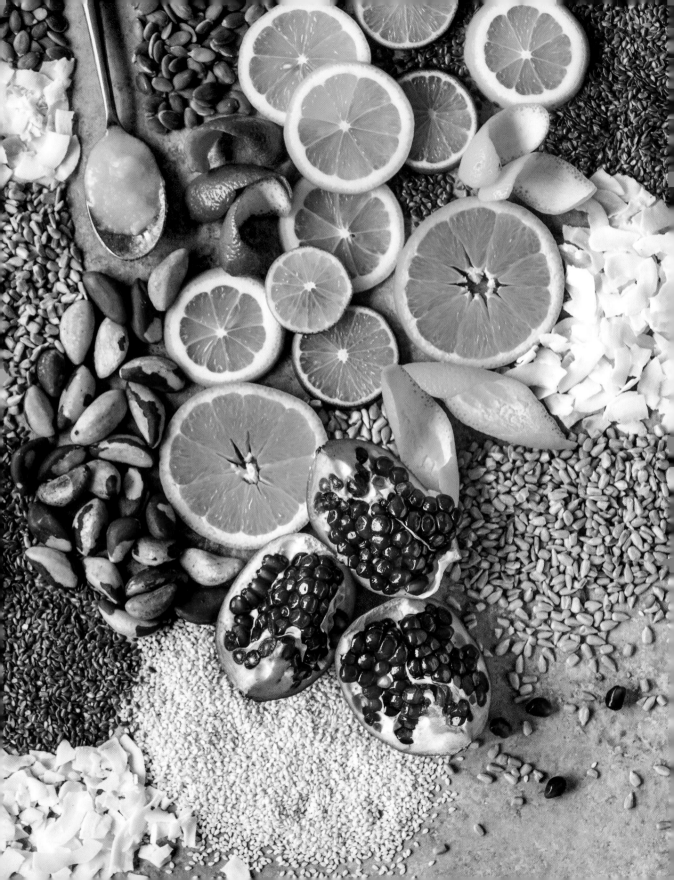

COOKING FOR
Hormone Balance

A Proven, Practical Program with Over 125 Easy, Delicious Recipes to Boost Energy and Mood, Lower Inflammation, Gain Strength, and Restore a Healthy Weight

Magdalena Wszelaki

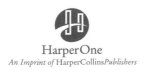

HarperOne
An Imprint of HarperCollinsPublishers

HarperOne

This book contains advice and information relating to health care. It should be used to supplement rather than replace the advice of your doctor or another trained health professional. If you know or suspect you have a health problem, it is recommended that you seek your physician's advice before embarking on any medical program or treatment. All efforts have been made to assure the accuracy of the information contained in this book as of the date of publication. This publisher and the author disclaim liability for any medical outcomes that may occur as a result of applying the methods suggested in this book.

FIRST EDITION

Designed by Kris Tobiassen of Matchbook Digital
All photographs by Gabriel Cabrera

Library of Congress Cataloging-in-Publication Data
Names: Wszelaki, Magdalena, author.
Title: Cooking for hormone balance : a proven, practical program with over 125 easy, delicious recipes to boost energy and mood, lower inflammation, gain strength, and restore a healthy weight / Magdalena Wszelaki.
Description: First edition. | New York, NY : HarperOne, [2018] | Includes bibliographical references and index.
Identifiers: LCCN 2017028154 (print) | LCCN 2017029732 (ebook) | ISBN 9780062643308 (e-book) | ISBN 9780062643131 (hardcover) | ISBN 9780062801449 (audio)
Subjects: LCSH: Functional foods. | Cooking—Psychological aspects. | Hormone therapy. | LCGFT: Cookbooks.
Classification: LCC QP144.F85 (ebook) | LCC QP144.F85 .W79 2018 (print) | DDC 641.3/02—dc23
LC record available at https://lccn.loc.gov/2017028154

18 19 20 21 22   LSC   10 9 8 7 6 5 4 3 2 1

Contents

PART THREE
Techniques for Life

PART FOUR
Recipes

Foreword

DR. IZABELLA WENTZ

Many of you probably have heard from a healthcare professional that the cause of your hormonal imbalances is your genes and that the only option you have to "manage" your hormones is to take a prescription medication. As a pharmacist who has dedicated my professional career to helping women with thyroid conditions get to the root cause of their health struggles, I have seen time and time again that genes are not our destiny, that we hold the power to recover our own health, and that there are often safer and more effective approaches to healing than a pill. While each person may have different symptoms, the fundamental way to heal the body is the same: support its ability to heal itself. Supporting your digestive process and your liver and balancing your sugar levels can give your body the boost it needs to repair and balance itself.

Every time you eat a meal, you choose to support or diminish your body's healing capabilities. I have seen that using food as medicine (or "food pharmacology," as I like to call it) can create profound transformations in a person's health. Food has the power to nourish, regulate hormones, improve digestion, and promote detoxification; yet the most common foods in our standard Western diet cause inflammation, digestive distress, and erratic blood sugar levels. If we continue to eat inflammatory foods, we will continue to be inflamed. To get our health back, we must break free from the conventional and take charge of our health destiny.

Magdalena Wszelaki is one of those rare people who has been where you are and has come out on the other side of healing. Fueled by her own health journey, she is a deeply passionate health coach with a special focus on using nutrition to balance hormones. Through her work with private clients and her popular hormone-balancing programs, she has helped thousands of women.

Magdalena and I met in 2013. I had been listening to her podcasts and was an avid reader of her blog. I was inspired by her empowering, can-do practical methods for helping women get their health back, and I thought to myself, "Wow, this woman is brilliant; I'd love to have her as a friend!" I reached out, and we've been close ever since. I've learned so much from Magda over the past few years, from practical kitchen tips like using a lemon squeezer to combining calf liver with broccoli to help iron absorption. We frequently share ideas and best practices on health, nutrition, and healing, and I've always been impressed with her ability to create approachable solutions for challenging health problems. In fact, I was the one who insisted she compile her knowledge into this very book.

I've also experienced the benefits of Magdalena's cooking, especially her Protein, Fat, and Fiber (PFF) breakfasts. When we attended a conference with a group of health experts, Magdalena generously offered to make us breakfast each morning. Every day we were treated to a healthy, creative, and mouthwatering dish. First, it was her Decadent Chocolate Cherry Smoothie, then the Farmer's Wife's Breakfast, and finally the Breakfast Casserole. We all looked forward to starting our day with her delicious meals, and everyone in the house reported that they felt calmer and more mentally clear and energetic throughout the day— and these were already very healthy people!

In *Cooking for Hormone Balance,* Magdalena shows you how to use food to awaken your healing capabilities. Whether you've been following a healthy diet for some time or are new to the world of nutrition, you will benefit from knowing how to avoid inflammatory foods, balance your blood sugar, and use nutrient-dense ingredients. You will feel vibrant and strong, and chronic conditions that you thought were "a part of your genetic makeup," "a result of getting older," or "normal"—such as mood swings, panic attacks, acne, menstrual cramps, digestive issues, and joint pain—may resolve. Most importantly, *Cooking for Hormone Balance* will help you identify the best dietary protocol for you on the basis of your unique symptoms. Whether you're struggling with estrogen dominance, PCOS, Hashimoto's disease, or adrenal dysfunction, this empowering and practical guide will provide you with a personalized plan to support your body.

I know that it can be difficult to change your diet—even if you know that doing so will help relieve your symptoms. Maybe, like many of my clients, you're afraid that eating a clean diet means eating boiled chicken and steamed vegetables for breakfast, lunch, and dinner. Fear not!

Celebrating everything she's learned living, dining, and cooking around the world, from Iceland, Poland, and Malaysia to California and now Colorado, Magdalena offers recipes in *Cooking for Hormone Balance* that are distinctive, flavorful, and healthy and will leave you nourished and satisfied while you're healing. You will not find a boring or unsatisfactory recipe here. Whether you're eating Coconut Kefir Chia Pudding for breakfast, enjoying Walnut Crusted Salmon for lunch, or having Raspberry and Green Tea Lime Melties as a dessert, you will never feel deprived. And because they're so delicious, Magdalena's recipes will please your whole family. They'll love this food and they won't even realize that it's good for them. You may even inspire your friends and family members to adopt a nutrient-dense, anti-inflammatory style of eating—and they will feel healthier and more balanced as a result.

While the recipes are showstoppers, *Cooking for Hormone Balance* also includes many of Magdalena's innovative, targeted protocols for specific conditions. You will love her hormone-balancing Seed Rotation Method. My clients who have followed it report better moods, fewer hormonal acne breakouts, and normalized menstrual cycles.

I am so grateful to Magdalena for putting her life's work and passions into this practical and beautiful guide. I know that utilizing the strategies in this book will bring you life-changing healing, many delicious meals, and lots of compliments from the people in your life.

To your health!

Izabella Wentz, PharmD, FASCP

#1 *New York Times* Bestselling Author
Hashimoto's Protocol

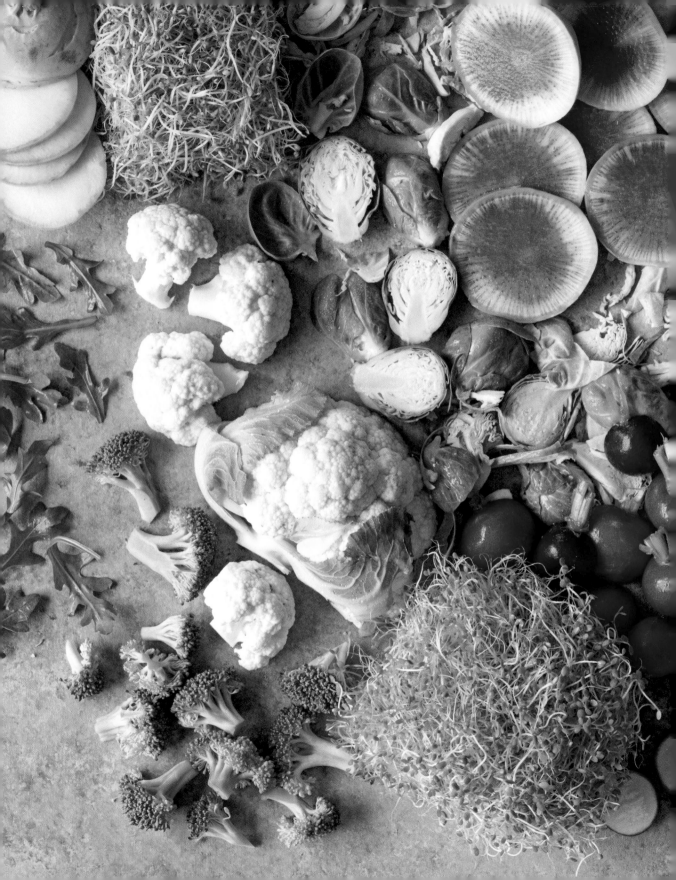

Before You Begin

I wrote this book because, just like you, I've suffered from many hormonal imbalances. At first, I bought into the belief that hormonal problems are genetic or the causes are "unknown." Some of you might have been told that there is little we can do about our hormones apart from taking birth control pills or supplementing our body's natural hormones. As much as this may be the case for some women, my inner wisdom was telling me that there must be more we, women, can do to help ourselves.

What I have discovered on this journey is that there are no magical foods or herbs that will immediately reverse hormonal imbalances. Instead, as the guardian of your sacred body, you can create an environment that is conducive to the hormones being produced, metabolized, and excreted in such a way that you enter that balance. Just as a gardener prepares the soil for a garden to bloom and thrive

so that she can later reap the benefits, so you can do the same with your body and hormonal balance.

I have found that hormonal balance requires a healthy digestion, stable sugar levels, and a well-functioning liver. I see these three things as the foundation of our hormonal health. Each represents one leg in the three-legged stool that is hormonal health. All three legs need to be stable for you to sit comfortably. Restoring your gut, sugar levels, and liver health will not only rebalance your hormones but will reverse many other, seemingly unconnected ailments that might have been plaguing you for years, such as seasonal allergies, hives, chronic pain, weight gain, depression, and anxiety.

I have been blessed with the opportunity to lead large online communities of women who have gone through my hormone-balancing diet, with life-changing results.

When I polled the community about the biggest change that this way of eating had created for them, I thought I was going to read replies pertaining to weight loss, better sleep, or better mental function. To my surprise, the biggest benefit the women reported was having learned to "listen" to their bodies.

This skill will set you free. What you will learn in this book might take away the frustration of dieting, counting calories or points, and the confusion of not knowing what is or is not healthy for you. The reason is simple: Many diets have been devised by people who got great results from a certain way of eating, so they passionately embark on getting the rest of the world to join them. As you might have found, some of these diets work for a while and others bomb; even though someone you know might have felt great on one of them, maybe you did not.

So what is different in this book? My approach to helping you find hormonal balance is based on the principles of functional medicine that emphasize uncovering the *root causes of disease* and treating a person from every aspect: from diet to sleep, genetics, infections, toxic exposure, and stress. On the diet front, I'm a firm believer in "bioindividuality" (one of the principals of functional medicine), which means that one person's food can be another person's poison. This could be due to many reasons, including genetics, current gut health, liver health, or the environment a person is living in. Certain truths are true for all; for instance, processed foods, excessive sugar, alcohol, drugs, and getting powered by coffee and stress will

harm anyone's health. But the rest is subjective and can depend on the complex biochemistry of an individual. Take sauerkraut, which is a vitamin C–packed, probiotic-rich food. Good for you, right? Maybe. A person with histamine issues, Candida yeast overgrowth, or a carbohydrate sensitivity will end up with hives, anxiety, vaginal itchiness, and a bloated tummy after eating sauerkraut. Not much of a health food for that person, is it? The same "unhealthy" reactions can occur with many other foods, such as nuts, seeds, grains, or even the healthiest of vegetables.

Often, I am asked what specific foods, supplements, or herbs to take to rebalance hormones. And quickly, too! This question comes from decades of conditioning by the medical establishment, which tells us that there is a medication and a pill for every pain and discomfort we experience. And these days, as a replacement for a pharmaceutical pill, some people seek instant relief from a few foods, supplements, and herbs. As much as I've created comprehensive guides, I didn't want to write a gimmicky book that promises a quick recovery with five magic foods or herbs—*because they don't exist.* Maca or black cohosh might bring some relief, but if your body is chronically inflamed from gut, sugar, and liver issues, the herbs might be only partially effective or work only temporarily. At the end of the day, food is the majority of what you put in your body—so change that first! Herbs and supplements will amplify healing when you are eating a clean diet.

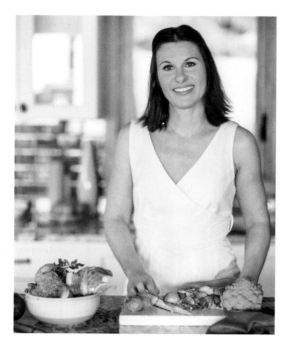

For some of you, it will be simple. Just eliminating gluten and dairy from your diet might resolve years of suffering. For others (and that's me), it takes some real tuning in (don't worry, I teach you how to do it) and figuring out what foods your body loves and what it rejects. By eating the "rejected" foods, you are in a constant state of inflammation that won't bring you to hormonal balance and bliss.

Apart from learning awesome, simple, yet nutritious recipes, my wish for you is to gain knowledge for life: eating not what is merely healthy, but what is *right for you*. This is no longer a "diet"; it's a way of eating that will nourish your body and soul for years to come, keeping you healthy and preventing future diseases so we can all meet up at age seventy-five to climb a mountain and pass the thirty-year-olds on the trail.

Come on this journey with me.

My mother hated to cook, and my grandmothers made food so bland that, as a kid, I would stuff my mouth with the food I disliked the most—spinach (cooked with heavy cream but no salt or lemon)—and run to the bathroom to spit it out. So no, I won't be telling you a story of having grown up under my grandmother or mother's table while she rolled, baked, pickled, and sizzled the freshest food straight from the garden. I learned to cook because I *had* to—to save my life and sanity.

At the time I'm writing this book, I'm forty-five years old. I've gone through having Graves' disease, Hashimoto's disease, adrenal fatigue stage II, estrogen dominance, and hypoglycemia. I've battled chronic Candida, heavy metal poisoning, bacterial infections (*H. pylori*), and parasitic infections (many times!), and I've had active Epstein-Barr virus (aka mononucleosis). Despite "eating well," I've suffered irritable bowel syndrome (IBS). For years, I dealt with an addiction to coffee and cigarettes. My brain neurotransmitters were so out of whack at one point that I became abusive to the one person I loved the most, which ended our many future plans and hopes. Having tested my genes, I was shocked to see how weak they are. I have a very high number of double mutations, so I like to joke that I'm an inferior human.

Yet despite all this, I came out on the other end. I'm in the best health today than I have been since I was twenty years old. Let me tell you how.

I was born in 1973 to a highly strung and anxious mother who smoked during her pregnancy. The birth was complicated and resulted in the doctor displacing my hips—something that resulted in my just going through bilateral hip replacement. I was never breast-fed because the milk powder companies bought the medical establishment, and nurses persuaded my mom that synthetic powdered milk was more nutritious than her own. During the first month of my life, I ended up at a hospital with pneumonia and a round of antibiotics. For the first year of my life, I cried relentlessly (an enduring family joke), probably because of digestive discomfort and hip pain. As you can tell, mine was a pretty rough start in life, with highly compromised gut health and a very weak immune system. Today, we know that children who are not breast-fed have low levels of healthy bifidobacterium in their guts, suffer from chronically low bacterial diversity (which is very important for achieving digestive health), and are more prone to developing autoimmune diseases.

As a young child, my arms were covered with eczema and I had chronic ear infections. I don't remember much when I was five years old, but I do remember being taken to the hospital for ear drainage every month. What Mom didn't know back then was that I had a high food intolerance to eggs, dairy, and gluten (staple foods in our home) that was probably caused by my weak gut microflora from birth. To add fuel to the fire, we lived through the Chernobyl nuclear disaster. What many people do not know is that Russian authorities hid the fiasco from the world, and by the time it was discovered by Sweden, the people of Ukraine and Poland, where we lived, were already contaminated. Eastern Europe still has the highest rates of thyroid diseases.

Since I didn't know about the connection between food sensitivities and my health, I continued eating foods that contribute to inflammation, and the symptoms evolved during my young adulthood (which is very common) into PMS; irregular periods; cystic acne on my face, back, and butt; daily migraines; sinus infections (and yes, as a young adult I took many antibiotics for that); vaginal infections; and energetic slumps that warranted mandatory afternoon naps.

Fed up with the cystic acne, since this was the one visible and annoying symptom that no twenty-five-year-old woman would want, I read online that gluten could be the cause. Mind you, back in 1997 such information was rare and revolutionary. Coupled with some food intolerance tests, I quit eating gluten, dairy, and eggs, and the majority of my symptoms went away. I was fascinated and encouraged.

I am often asked where I am from. I think this is partly because of my difficult-to-place accent. I was born to Polish parents. My father was a diplomat so we lived all over the world. I spent ages five to ten in windy Copenhagen, Denmark; ages fifteen to thirty-two I lived in Malaysia, a Southeast Asian paradise. My professional life took me to Hong Kong and Shanghai, China. It was an exhilarating and fast-paced four years of my life that I believe also triggered Hashimoto's disease, which is when your immune system attacks your thyroid. As a type A personality back then (I'm largely recovered now, I think), my career successes fueled my self-esteem, and I didn't know where to draw the line; I used to joke that sleep is for the dead. I would party until 1 A.M. and then get up early to hit the gym. My regional job in advertising as a strategic planner working on Fortune 100 brands required frequent traveling, which meant living between airports, eating crappy hotel food, and working late into the nights, even on weekends. I also used to smoke. I finally quit (for a while) because the air and water pollution in China were making me so ill.

In 2008 my health started collapsing. I was experiencing recurring anxiety attacks (for the first time in my life), memory loss, severe fatigue, insomnia, and foul mood swings. I became a person I did not recognize: bitter, impatient, snappy, and moody. I would cry for no reason. I was lucky to be quickly diagnosed with Hashimoto's, given my history of hyperthyroidism eight years earlier. But no resources were available to help me understand the cause, let alone learn about any treatment. My Western doctor looked at my file and announced: "Of course you're tired; you're now thirty-six years old." Since my thyroid markers were "normal" and only my antibodies were sky high (more than 1,000 IU/mL when they should be below 30 IU/mL), I was

sent home with no treatment options. I was in shock. A Venezuelan friend, the only other person I knew who had thyroid issues, had an integrative doctor, and I seriously contemplated taking a twenty-four-hour, $8,000 flight to crime-ridden Caracas to get some answers. That's how desperate I was. Instead, I started seeing a traditional Chinese medicine doctor in Shanghai who helped me get my antibodies down by half. However, she was not familiar with autoimmunity, so my recovery plateaued. I also had many of the symptoms of adrenal burnout and estrogen dominance, but I didn't know at that time what these conditions were.

On a deeper level, I also started questioning my life's purpose. Even though I worked on iconic brands in one of the largest markets in the world, I started feeling agitated that I was using my brains and talent to get people to buy stuff they didn't really need or want through the use of fear or unrealistic aspirations (start observing ads and you'll see that's what most of them are based on). What broke the camel's back was a brief from a client in which my job was to develop a marketing strategy to encourage young women to use skin-whitening products to boost their self-confidence and self-esteem. I was sickened and became determined to devote my intelligence and energy to better causes.

I moved to the United States and started nutrition school right away. Deep in my heart I knew I was going to recover and reverse my own body's attack on the thyroid; all I needed was organic food, clean air, less stress and travel, and more sleep. When I first quit my job, I slept for twelve to fourteen hours every day for three months straight. I didn't know what adrenal burnout was, but I had enough inner wisdom to just let my body do what it needed.

I started my nutrition practice in 2010, and by then I had regained much of my health. Everything I did to help myself can be found in the guides of this book. And I wish I could tell you that the rest is history. But I continue uncovering new issues and challenges even though I live the clean life I teach. The four years I spent in China most likely caused heavy metal toxicity, which makes clearing Candida really hard. I've recently discovered (after many tests) that the bacterium *H. pylori* has been causing low stomach acid my whole life and most likely my predisposition to being nutritionally depleted and getting parasites.

The latest testing technology has uncovered which pathogenic bacteria have been causing the gut dysbiosis (right after I took an unavoidable round of antiparasitic antibiotics) that are most likely the culprits behind a sudden oxalate sensitivity; food high in oxalates, such as chocolate, spinach, and nuts, cause severely sharp pain in my hips. Oxalates can also be the cause of kidney stones, pelvic pain, and painful urination, among other things. As always, I'm determined to get to the bottom of it.

What I have learned over the years is that our health is a journey, especially for those of us with difficult childhoods, past trauma, and undetected lingering infections. This journey can be highly frustrating and unrewarding at times; after all, I've committed my life resources to healing and I do not always get the results I hope for. Nevertheless, I've come

Your Hormonal Foundation, Phase I

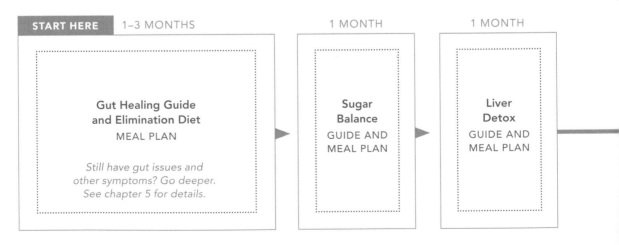

START HERE 1–3 MONTHS	1 MONTH	1 MONTH
Gut Healing Guide and Elimination Diet MEAL PLAN *Still have gut issues and other symptoms? Go deeper. See chapter 5 for details.*	**Sugar Balance** GUIDE AND MEAL PLAN	**Liver Detox** GUIDE AND MEAL PLAN

to appreciate this journey, as with every obstacle comes deep understanding and discovery that you, my reader, will learn and benefit from. What fascinates me equally is how this journey has armed me with the "soft" coping skills of patience and self-forgiveness. Without those, there will be no healing.

HOW TO GET THE MOST FROM THIS BOOK

This book is rich in content. As an author and content creator, I find it a challenge to strike a balance between delivering in-depth content that helps as many people as possible (including those with complex conditions) and presenting so much of it that it is overwhelming. The chart shows you where to start (but after you've read Chapter 1 for an overview of hor-

mones) and how to make the best use of the diets, guides, meal plans, and recipes to rebalance your hormones.

Start with Phase I, Your Hormonal Foundation

The Hormonal Foundation consists of three steps:

Step 1 is to heal your gut. Read Chapter 2 on the connection between the gut and hormonal balance, and print out and follow the Gut-Healing Guide and get familiar with the Elimination Diet. Then, begin the Elimination Diet Meal Plan. During the Elimination Diet, keep the Food Mood Poop Journal. If the Elimination Diet resolves most of your digestive issues, proceed to Step 2.

Your Hormonal Refinement, Phase II

THEN REFINE

Thyroid and Hashimoto's GUIDE AND MEAL PLAN	Adrenal Healing GUIDE AND MEAL PLAN
Estrogen Dominance and Low Progesterone GUIDE AND MEAL PLAN	Low Testosterone GUIDE AND MEAL PLAN
Low Estrogen and Menopause GUIDE AND MEAL PLAN	PCOS and High Testosterone GUIDE AND MEAL PLAN

If you are still suffering from digestive issues after you've finished the Elimination Diet, you may want to dive deeper and try one of the therapeutic diet protocols explained in Chapter 5, such as Paleo, the Autoimmune Protocol (AIP), anti-Candida, or low FODMAP, before proceeding to Step 2.

Step 2 is to balance your sugar levels. Having stable sugar levels is part of your Hormonal Foundation. Find out whether you have healthy sugar levels by reading Chapter 3. If you are hypoglycemic or hyperglycemic, print out and follow the Sugar-Balancing Guide and use the Sugar-Balancing Meal Plan for one month. Then proceed to Step 3.

Step 3 is to detox your liver. Since the liver is vital for metabolizing, converting, and excreting hormones, it will most likely need your support. Read Chapter 4, get familiar with the Liver Detox Guide, and then eat according to the Liver Detox Meal Plan for one month.

Phase I, the Hormonal Foundation, is now complete. ONLY when you have finished Phase I should you proceed to Phase II, your Hormonal Refinement. Do your best to create the strongest foundation you can for your hormonal balance.

Proceed to Phase II, Your Hormonal Refinement

Do you know what hormonal imbalance you might have? If not, take the Hormonal Imbalance Quiz on page 14 to get an indication. Then, refer to Chapter 6 for the specific guide and meal plan that support your imbalance.

If the quiz indicates that you may have several hormonal imbalances, please know it's quite common for women to concurrently experience, for example, low thyroid function (Hashimoto's), adrenal fatigue, and estrogen dominance. If you have multiple imbalances, I recommend you start with the Adrenal Healing Guide in Chapter 6. Fixing your adrenals can have a positive effect on all of your hormones. You'll experience results quickly, including better sleep and mood and a healthier weight.

I cannot emphasize enough how important it is to start with Phase I, the Hormonal Foundation, before you proceed, no matter how tempting it is, to Phase II, the Hormonal Refinement. It's very likely that you may not even need to implement much from the Phase II protocols because the Foundation will resolve most of your symptoms!

Chapter 1

The ABCs of Hormones

Your hormones are responsible for how you think, feel, and look. A woman with balanced hormones is sharp and upbeat, with a good memory. She feels energetic without caffeine during the day, falls asleep quickly, and wakes refreshed. She is blessed with a healthy appetite and maintains a desired weight with a good diet. Her hair and skin glow. She feels emotionally balanced and responds to stress with grace and reason. When menstruating, her menses comes and goes with no or little PMS. She has an active sex life. She can maintain a full-term pregnancy. When entering perimenopause or menopause, she slides into a new phase of life with ease.

If that doesn't describe you, your hormones are imbalanced. Don't despair. You are not alone. Millions of women experience hormonal imbalance. The good news is, you can rebalance your hormones naturally and resolve your symptoms.

Most conventionally trained doctors tell us that the only way to control our hormones is by taking birth control pills, undergoing hormone replacement therapy, applying creams, or even removing our organs, such as the uterus. I want you to know that these are not your only options. There are gentle and self-honoring methods for taking care of your body that will bring about the sacred balance you so deserve.

I know that your doctor has probably never explained the key role of the digestive tract, sugar balance, the liver, or food in rebalancing your hormones. The reasons are numerous, but still inexcusable. For one, doctors receive only a few hours of clinical training in nutrition and no education at all on the critical role of the gut in your overall health. Medical training also does not connect the dots from the health of the liver and sugar levels to overall hormonal balance. If that isn't disturbing enough, one of my colleagues, a Harvard-educated doctor, said that using food as medicine "isn't sexy enough" when compared to inventing the next celebrated drug. Given the medical establishment's perspective, it is high time we acknowledge that we have a personal responsibility to regain and maintain our health.

Whatever your reason for choosing this book, I'm so glad you are here. You are open-minded, proactive, smart, and resourceful. You refuse to see a pill as the only answer. I hope you share what you learn here with at least three other women you love and respect. She can be your mother, your daughter, your co-worker, or your friend. She can be someone you barely know but you can see she's struggling. Together, we can have an incredible impact on the healing of women everywhere. In this book, you'll learn how you can achieve this without pills, magic potions, or gimmicks.

WHAT ARE HORMONES?

Hormones are tiny chemical messengers produced by a network of endocrine glands, including the pituitary, adrenal, thyroid, and pineal glands; the pancreas; ovaries in women; and testes in men. Hormones are released directly into the bloodstream and carried to the organs and tissues of the body to perform their functions. Excess fat cells can also produce hormones such as estradiol or leptin.

Hormones do not exist in isolation. They work together like musicians in an orchestra.

When one hormone is out of sync, it throws off your other hormones and even other body systems.

For example, think of a time when you experienced a lot of stress. Your adrenals were busy releasing a lot of the hormone cortisol to help your body to deal with it. It's likely that your immune system became compromised by that excessive cortisol release and you came down with a nasty cold. And it's likely that weeks or months after that, you started showing symptoms of low thyroid function (such as hair loss, weight gain, or fatigue) or estrogen dominance (PMS, water retention, or miscarriages).

It may feel overwhelming to realize that many of your hormones could be out of balance, but the good news is that *all* of your hormones can be balanced to a large degree with a healthy gut, stable sugar levels, and a clean liver.

Key Hormone-Producing Glands

Thyroid Gland. This is your body's gas pedal. It produces hormones that are responsible for your metabolism, conversion of fat to energy, body temperature, mental functions, and hair and skin quality. Underactive thyroid (hypothyroid) conditions are more common than overactive thyroid (hyperactive) conditions. Ninety percent of cases of both conditions (in developed countries) result from autoimmune diseases: Hashimoto's disease causes hypothyroidism, and Graves' disease causes hyperthyroidism. Therefore, to treat any type of thyroid issue, it is essential to heal the immune system (to stop the immune system's attack on the thyroid) and not the thyroid alone.

Adrenal Glands. The adrenals are responsible for producing hormones that manage the stress response and regulate sugar levels, the immune system, water retention, and blood pressure. Cortisol is one of the main hormones produced by the adrenals. A person living in constant stress will eventually exhaust the adrenals so much so that the glands are unable to produce sufficient cortisol and aldosterone. This can cause you to get sick all the time (because of a weaker immune system), have sugar cravings, and experience low energy. Stressed adrenals also underproduce aldosterone, a hormone that stabilizes your blood pressure and causes water retention, making you feel light-headed and puffy.

Ovaries. These are our prime reproductive glands. They produce eggs for fertilization and the reproductive hormones estrogen and progesterone. In menopausal women, the ovaries stop producing the hormones. In menstruating women, a common problem is polycystic ovaries, an imbalance we discuss later in this chapter.

Steroid Hormone Production

As you can see, one hormone imbalance affects many others.

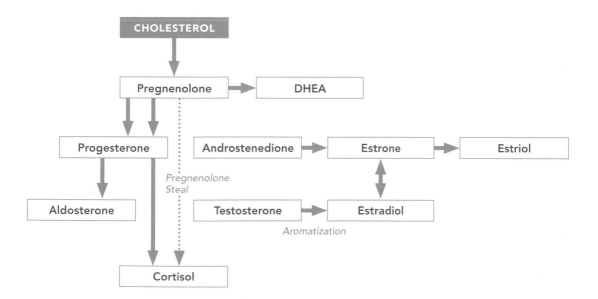

Let's take a closer look at the hormones that these glands produce and their interrelationships.

STEROID HORMONES

Steroid hormones are a type of hormone derived from cholesterol. This waxy, fatlike substance found in all cells of the body travels through your bloodstream in small packages called "lipoproteins." There are two kinds of lipoproteins: low-density lipoproteins (LDL) and high-density lipoproteins (HDL). LDL cholesterol is sometimes called "bad" cholesterol because a high LDL level can cause clogged arteries. HDL cholesterol, or "good" cholesterol, is vital to hormonal balance because this is what the steroid hormones are made of. Women with low HDL (less than 60 mg/dL) who follow a low-fat diet tend to develop hormonal problems.

Steroid hormones include the following:

Pregnenolone. A critically important steroid hormone produced in the adrenals, sex organs, brain, and spinal cord that is the source of progesterone, cortisol, dehydroepiandrosterone (DHEA), testosterone, and estrogen.

Progesterone. A steroid hormone produced by the corpus luteum of the ovary (and adrenals when the ovaries are missing). As the name implies, it's a pro-gestation hormone that allows women to get pregnant and maintain a full-term pregnancy. It is essential in nonpregnant women too because it helps you to stay calm, clear-headed, fall asleep easily, and feel balanced. Progesterone and estrogen are like two dance partners: A good balance between these two is vital.

Cortisol. A steroid hormone produced by the adrenals that influences many of the changes that occur in the body in response to emotional, physical, spiritual, or toxic stress. When you live in a state of chronic stress, your cortisol levels are constantly elevated, which can lead to adrenal fatigue.

DHEA (dehydroepiandrosterone). A steroid hormone produced by the adrenals. It is the precursor hormone to testosterone and all of the estrogens. DHEA levels in the body begin to decrease after age thirty and decrease more quickly in women. DHEA is often touted as the "antiaging" hormone because both testosterone and estrogen are critical for women to feel physically strong and mentally sharp, and to have their joints and vaginas lubricated. Women with adrenal fatigue often experience low DHEA (hence symptoms of low estrogen and testosterone), so it is vital in the case of low DHEA to support the adrenals.

Testosterone. A steroid hormone and the primary male sex hormone. In women it is produced in the ovaries and adrenal glands. As much as testosterone is associated with being the "male" or "aggressive" hormone, women need it in smaller amounts to feel and look good. Testosterone gets converted to all three estrogens, so adequate amounts of this hormone are necessary to maintain optimal estrogens levels.

Estrogens. A group of steroid hormones and the primary female sex hormones that give us boobs, butts, and periods. Produced largely by the ovaries, some estrogens can also be produced by visceral fat or the adrenals (this is especially the case when the ovaries have been removed). There are three forms of estrogens that play very different roles:

Estrone (E1) is the "weaker" estrogen that is higher in pregnant and menopausal women.

Estradiol (E2) is often called the "antagonistic estrogen," and many women tend to have an excess of it. The synthetic version is found in skincare and house-cleaning products. It is highest in premenopausal women and is the leading cause of estrogenic breast, ovarian, uterine, thyroid, and lung (in nonsmokers) cancers.

Estriol (E3) is the "protective" estrogen, contributing to healthy and youthful skin, keeping the vagina moist and lubricated, and preventing hot flashes and night sweats. Estriol also has an anticarcinogenic role.

NONSTEROID HORMONES

These are a few of the most important nonsteroid hormones:

Thyroxine (T4) and triiodothyronine (T3). The T4 produced by the thyroid can't be directly used by the body until it's converted to the active T3 hormone because the conversion happens mainly in the gut and liver. The amount of energy you have, your body fat, mental alertness, and the quality of your hair, skin, and nails depend on the availability of the T3 hormone.

Insulin. A hormone made by the pancreas, insulin sweeps sugar from the blood and delivers it to cells. When a person eats a daily diet full of sugar and processed carbohydrates (such as flours, cereals, and packaged foods), the insulin receptors in the cells eventually shut down and won't accept insulin. This is called "insulin resistance" (IR), and nearly half of the U.S. population suffers from it. People with prediabetes and diabetes suffer from IR. Women with high testosterone and polycystic ovary syndrome (PCOS) often have IR.

Leptin. A hormone produced by the body's fat cells that signals to the brain that you have just eaten, you are full, and it's time to stop eating. People with leptin resistance don't get that signal delivered, resulting in obesity or years of unsuccessful dieting.

The Hormonal Imbalance Quiz
Which Hormonal Imbalance Do You Have?

Your doctor might have told you, on the basis of your lab test results, that you don't have hormonal issues. This is a common problem, especially when the steroid hormones were tested using blood, a highly misleading and inaccurate method. Testing urine or saliva is a much more accurate way to identify hormonal imbalances.

It's really important that you listen to the internal voice telling you that you are not balanced. Do not ignore it or silence it. When you tune in to your symptoms, you will get an accurate picture of which hormones might need attention.

To help you, I've created the following quiz. Check each question that is a "yes." (This quiz is only for women.)

Part 1

- ☑ Are you running from task to task?

- ☑ Do you feel jittery, unfocused, or moody when hungry?

- ☑ Are you tired and wired?

- ☑ Do you have sugar cravings (dinner feels incomplete without something sweet)?

- ☐ Do you experience indigestion, acid reflux, or ulcers?

- ☑ Do you struggle to calm down and slow down?

- ☐ Do you have pink or purple stretch marks on your belly or back?

- ☑ Are you quick to get angry?

- ☐ Have you experienced infertility or miscarriages?

- ☐ Do you have a hard time getting over adversity or diseases?

- ☑ Do you experience hair loss?

- ☑ Is it hard for you to fall asleep and/or stay asleep?

- ☑ Do you retain water (puffy face, fingers, or feet)?

- ☑ Do you have memory lapses, especially when emotional?

- ☑ Do you get frequent colds and flus?

- ☐ Do you experience heart palpitations?

- ☑ Do you have muffin top (a roll of body fat around your waistline)?

- ☐ Do you have skin conditions such as eczema or thinning skin?

- ☐ Do you have bone loss (osteopenia or osteoporosis)?

Part 2

- ☑ Do you experience fatigue or burnout (do you have to use coffee to keep going)?

- ☑ Do you crave salt?

- ☑ Do you have low blood pressure?

- ○ Do you feel dizzy after getting up from a seated or lying position?
- ○ Do you see life and people in a negative way?
- ☑ Do you cry for no good reason or become easily emotional?
- ☑ Do you lose stamina, especially in the afternoon and evening?
- ☑ Do have a hard time getting out of bed, or do you need two cups of coffee to wake up?
- ○ Have your problem-solving skills decreased?
- ○ Has your tolerance to stress decreased?
- ○ Do you struggle to get over a simple cold, the flu, or infections?
- ☑ Are your blood sugar levels low or unstable?
- ○ Is your sex drive lower?
- ○ Do you feel mildly depressed?

Part 3

- ☑ Do you have headaches, especially around your period?
- ☑ Have you had ovarian cysts, breast cysts, or endometriosis?
- ○ Are your legs itchy or restless, especially at night?
- ○ Have you had any miscarriages during the first trimester?
- ○ Have you experienced infertility or subfertility (you can't hold on to a pregnancy)?

- ☑ Do you have heavy or painful periods?
- ☑ Do you experience bloating, especially in the belly and ankle area, and/or water retention?
- ○ Are your breasts ever painful and/or swollen?
- ○ Have you had irregular periods and/or cycles that have become more frequent as you age?
- ○ Do you have hot flashes?
- ☑ Are you irritable or anxious?
- ☑ Do you have difficulty falling and/or staying asleep?
- ☑ Do you have dry skin or skin that has lost its fullness?
- ○ Do you experience spotting in the middle of your menstrual cycle?

Part 4

- ○ Do you have spider or varicose veins?
- ☑ Do you have any cellulite?
- ☑ Are your periods heavy?
- ☑ Have you had breast or ovarian fibroids?
- ☑ Do you experience irritability, mood swings, or anxiety?
- ☑ Do you get headaches or migraines, particularly before your period?
- ○ Are you fat around your hips?
- ○ Do you use birth control pills?
- ○ Have you experienced heavy bleeding or postmenopausal bleeding?

- ☑ Do you experience bloating, puffiness, or water retention?
- ○ Are your breasts ever enlarged or do they feel tender?
- ○ Do you have endometriosis or painful periods?
- ☑ Do you have PMS and/or depression?
- ○ Do you sometimes cry for no good reason?
- ☑ Do you have trouble falling asleep?
- ○ Do you have gallbladder problems, or has your gallbladder been removed?

Part 5

- ☑ Is your memory ever poor ("Why did I walk into this room?")?
- ○ Do you have night sweats and/or hot flashes?
- ○ Is your bladder leaky or overactive?
- ○ Do you feel emotionally fragile, especially when compared to years ago?
- ☑ Do you experience depression, anxiety, and/or lethargy (loss of enthusiasm)?
- ☑ Do you have trouble falling and staying asleep?
- ☑ Do your joints ache?
- ☑ Have you lost interest in exercise?
- ○ Do you have bone loss or osteoporosis?
- ○ Have you experienced vaginal dryness, irritation, or loss of feeling?
- ☑ Are your eyes, skin, and/or vagina dry?

- ○ Do you have a low sex drive?
- ○ Is sex painful?
- ○ Is your skin dry and saggy?
- ☑ Is your skin thinning?
- ○ Are your breasts shrinking and sagging?
- ○ Have you experienced menopause?
- ○ Do you have "love handles" or fat gain around your abdomen?

Part 6

- ○ Do you have acne?
- ☑ Do you have oily skin and/or hair?
- ○ Have you lost hair on your scalp?
- ☑ Do you have hair growth on your chin, upper lip, breasts, or stomach?
- ○ Have you experienced infertility?
- ○ Are your breasts shrinking and saggy?
- ☑ Do you experience irritability or aggression or get easily agitated?
- ○ Have you gained fat around your belly?
- ○ Do you crave sweets and/or carbohydrates?
- ○ Do you have fatty liver?
- ☑ Are your armpits discolored (darker and thicker skin than normal)?
- ○ Are you hypoglycemic or hyperglycemic (low or high blood sugar levels)?
- ○ Do you experience depression and/or anxiety?
- ○ Do you have ovarian cysts or PCOS?

○ Do you experience pain in the middle of your menstrual cycle?

☑ Are you constantly hungry and/or has your appetite increased?

Part 7

☑ Have you experienced muscle loss?

☑ Have you experienced muscle weakness?

☑ Have you gained weight, especially "soft fat" around the waist?

☑ Has your ratio of fat to muscle moved toward fat?

○ Do you lack confidence compared with previously?

○ Do you lack drive and assertiveness?

○ Is your libido low?

☑ Are you tired?

☑ Do you experience mood swings, depression, and/or low mood?

☑ Do you have difficulty concentrating?

○ Do you have bone loss or osteoporosis?

○ Does your skin sag?

☑ Have you experienced hair loss?

Part 8

☑ Have you lost any hair on your scalp?

○ Have you lost any hair from your eyebrows and/or eyelashes?

☑ Have you gained weight despite a healthy diet and exercise?

☑ Do you experience depression, anxiety, and/or lethargy?

○ Do your eyelids flicker?

☑ Are your hair, nails, and skin brittle or thinning?

☑ Is your skin dry?

○ Do you have high LDL cholesterol levels?

○ Do you experience muscle or joint pains and aches?

○ Are you constipated?

○ Do you feel tingling in your hands and/or feet?

○ Are your hands and/or feet cold?

☑ Are you tired?

☑ Do you experience "foggy brain" (slow thoughts, difficulty focusing)?

○ Have you experienced infertility?

○ Is your sex drive lower than it was previously?

○ Is your thyroid enlarged?

☑ Do you have a family history of thyroid problems?

○ Do you have hives?

○ Are there indents on the sides of your tongue when you stick it out?

Part 9

☑ Do you still feel hungry even after a full meal?

☑ Are you tired after a meal?

- ⊘ Do you crave sweets and carbohydrates all the time?
- ⊘ Are you tired throughout the day?
- ⊘ Do you experience extreme thirst or hunger?
- ◯ Do you experience frequent or increased urination?
- ◯ Do you feel tingling sensations in your hands or feet?
- ◯ Do you have dark patches on the back of your neck, groin, and/or armpits (acanthosis nigricans)?
- ◯ Have you been diagnosed with type 2 prediabetes or diabetes?
- ◯ Do you have cardiovascular problems?

- ◯ Have you experienced vision changes and/or have you had cataracts?
- ◯ Have you experienced infertility or irregular periods?
- ⊘ Have you experienced hair growth above the mouth or on the chin or nipples?
- ◯ Do you have high LDL cholesterol, high triglycerides, or high blood pressure?
- ◯ Have you been diagnosed with fatty liver?
- ◯ Is your hemoglobin A1c (HA1c) sugar marker higher than 5.4 percent?
- ◯ Is your insulin level higher than 15 IU/mL?
- ◯ Is your fasting glucose level higher than 90 mg/dL?

READING YOUR QUIZ RESULTS

If you answered "yes" to more than three questions in any part of the quiz, there is a good chance that you are experiencing the hormonal imbalance listed below:

Part 1: High cortisol
Part 2: Low cortisol
Part 3: Low progesterone
Part 4: High estrogen (estrogen dominance)
Part 5: Low estrogen
Part 6: High testosterone (androgen dominance) and/or PCOS
Part 7: Low testosterone
Part 8: Underactive thyroid (hypothyroidism and/or Hashimoto's disease)
Part 9: Insulin resistance or leptin resistance and/or PCOS

Is it possible to have high and low cortisol levels at the same time?
Yes! It's not unusual to experience low cortisol levels in the morning (this is why you need two cups of coffee to get you going) and high cortisol at night, which can interfere with your sleep, as you may be feeling wired and tired.

Can you have high and low estrogen at the same time?

Yes! It is completely possible to have estrogen dominance (high estrogen, specifically estradiol) and also experience symptoms of low estrogen. Here are two possible scenarios. In the first, even though you have overall low levels of estrogen (hence the symptoms), you might also have too much of estradiol, the "antagonistic estrogen," compared with estriol, the "protective" estrogen—and this could be causing the symptoms of estrogen dominance. In the second scenario, even though you might have overall low levels of all estrogens, estradiol might be too high compared with progesterone, causing the symptoms of estrogen dominance.

KEY STRATEGIES FOR EACH HORMONAL IMBALANCE

Part 1: High Cortisol

You are in a state of chronic stress and your adrenals are working extra hard. Family issues, poor relationships, job problems, finances, overexercising, and past trauma and abuse could be causes, as well as chronic digestive issues or infections. Create a list of all of the things, people, places, actions, and situations that deplete and stress you, and then make a plan to reduce or eliminate them: What can you avoid? What can you change? Can you change the emotion around a situation or trigger that causes a stress response (also called "reframing")? For example, one of my clients told me that she was driving on the highway when an erratic and dangerous driver cut her off. Instead of allowing herself to feel rage, she told herself a different story: "He's driving like crazy because he's rushing a critically sick child to the hospital." Reframing the situation like that immediately changed her feelings and stress levels around the event. Some triggers you can't change immediately (such as an abusive marriage or a bad boss), but you *can* change "the story" and how you feel about the triggers. Your adrenals will love that.

First, implement the protocols outlined in the next three chapters to establish the Hormonal Foundation for healthy adrenals. Then, proceed to the Adrenal Healing Guide in Chapter 6.

Part 2: Low Cortisol

If you have low cortisol levels, you have had high cortisol levels for a while now and your adrenals are therefore too tired to produce sufficient cortisol. To confirm whether you do have low cortisol levels, it's important to get a diagnosis from a qualified functional physician and get a urine or saliva test four times a day.

While waiting for the diagnosis (or perhaps you already have it), implement the protocols outlined in the next three chapters to establish the Hormonal Foundation for healthy adrenals. Then, proceed to the Adrenal Healing Guide in Chapter 6.

Part 3: Low Progesterone

Low progesterone can be caused by excess cortisol levels (from chronic stress) or excess estradiol, the antagonistic estrogen produced in your body or introduced externally as synthetic estrogens (known as "xenoestrogens") from skincare and house-cleaning products. High cortisol levels are inflammatory and can block progesterone receptors, inhibiting progesterone from doing its work. This is why women who become so stressed out trying to become pregnant are finally able to conceive once their stress lessens (because they have decided to stop trying and adopt a child, for example) and their cortisol levels go down.

High cortisol levels also can cause "pregnenolone steal" (see page 110), whereby the body diverts (or "steals") the majority of the available pregnenolone toward cortisol production to help us cope with excessive stress, rather than channeling it for progesterone production. The end result: When stressed, we end up with less progesterone.

Symptoms of low progesterone can also occur when there is excess estradiol caused by poor liver function (the liver is not detoxifying this antagonistic estrogen), poor digestive health, use of birth control pills, or use of commercial skincare and house-cleaning products.

Women who take synthetic progesterone in the form of progestin (also found in birth control pills) also end up producing less of their own progesterone as the body thinks it does not need to produce its own hormones. Progestin does not work the same as your own progesterone and can suppress ovulation.

First, implement the protocols outlined in the next three chapters to establish the Hormonal Foundation for producing sufficient progesterone. Then, proceed to the Reversing Estrogen Dominance and Boosting Progesterone guides in Chapter 6.

Part 4: High Estrogen (Estrogen Dominance)

This condition can manifest in a few ways. You could have more estradiol (E2), the antagonistic estrogen, compared with estriol (E3) and estrone (E1), which often happens when many xenoestrogens, or synthetic estrogens, are present in your life. Second, you might have insufficient progesterone to oppose estradiol (even if your estradiol levels are within range). Estrogen dominance can also happen when there are more antagonistic estrogen metabolites (which are the by-products of estrogen metabolism). Visceral fat also produces estradiol.

Women with high testosterone levels (and often PCOS) can suffer from estrogen dominance, too. This is because testosterone gets converted to estradiol in the aromatization process (see page 105). Inhibiting this process can break the cycle of estrogen production and relieve symptoms of estrogen dominance. Estrogen dominance is the leading cause of estrogenic cancers such as thyroid, breast, ovarian, and uterine cancers in women; lung cancer (in nonsmokers); and prostate cancer in men.

First, implement the protocols outlined in the next three chapters to establish the Hormonal Foundation for producing and metabolizing the various estrogens. Then, proceed to the Reversing Estrogen Dominance and Boosting Progesterone guides in Chapter 6.

Part 5: Low Estrogen

Declining estrogen levels typically happen to women going into perimenopause and menopause, but I have seen young women suffering from stress and toxic lifestyles experience this too. The ovaries are producing less estrogen because of aging, stress (and high cortisol levels), or toxicity.

First, implement the protocols outlined in the next three chapters to establish a Hormonal Foundation for producing sufficient estrogens. Then, proceed to the Reversing Estrogen Dominance and Easing the Transition into Peri/Menopause guides in Chapter 6.

Part 6: High Testosterone (Androgen Dominance)

You likely have elevated DHEA and/or testosterone levels, which is called "androgen dominance." The leading cause is high sugar

levels. Polycystic ovarian syndrome is commonly caused by androgen dominance. If you are overweight, the great news is this: Just a 5 percent drop in weight may normalize your blood sugar levels and reverse androgen dominance.

First, implement the protocols outlined in the next three chapters to establish a Hormonal Foundation for balancing your sugar levels. The Sugar-Balancing Guide will be especially important for you. Then, proceed to the Lowering High Testosterone Levels and Treating PCOS Guide in Chapter 6.

While making dietary changes, get a formal diagnosis of PCOS and high testosterone level.

Part 7: Low Testosterone

Most often, when the adrenals are exhausted, they also underproduce testosterone, causing the symptoms you are currently suffering.

First, implement the protocols outlined in the next three chapters to establish a Hormonal Foundation to strengthen your adrenals. Then, proceed to the Adrenal Healing Guide in Chapter 6.

Part 8: Underactive Thyroid (Hypothyroidism and/or Hashimoto's Disease)

Sadly, too many thyroid conditions go undiagnosed because of incomplete tests and wrong lab ranges that conventional doctors use. The consensus among functional practitioners is that 30 percent of the population experiences subclinical hypothyroidism (this means the symptoms are subtle). This could be an underestimate. One study in Japan found 38 percent of the healthy subjects to have elevated thyroid antibodies (indicating the body's immune system attacking the thyroid). Another study reports that 50 percent of patients, mostly women, have thyroid nodules. If you are showing many of the thyroid symptoms, insist on getting a complete range of tests or order them yourself online. If you have been diagnosed with hypothyroidism, it was most likely caused by Hashimoto's disease, an autoimmune condition. When you put out the fire in your gut and the immune system, you will see your thyroid health improve and symptoms subside or go away.

First, implement the protocols outlined in the next three chapters to establish a Hormonal Foundation to strengthen your immune system. Then, proceed to the Restoring Thyroid Health and Treating Hashimoto's Guide in Chapter 6.

Part 9: Insulin Resistance or Leptin Resistance

If you eat processed carbohydrates (including cereals, puffy rice, breads, bagels, pasta, cakes, and cookies), sugar (found in incredibly high amounts in most packaged foods),

or processed proteins (such as protein shakes), it's likely you have a problem with sugar. It first manifests with high and/or low blood sugar levels (you feel cranky, unfocused, light-headed, and tired when hungry) and ends up with a full metabolic disorder such as insulin or leptin resistance. Women suffering from high testosterone or PCOS tend to have elevated sugar levels or insulin or leptin resistance. The good news is this: These conditions are completely reversible with diet, exercise, detoxification, and stress management.

First, implement the protocols outlined in the next three chapters to establish the Hormonal Foundation for hormonal balance and stable sugar levels. Then, depending on what other hormonal imbalance you have, proceed to the relevant guide in Chapter 6.

The key to balance is not too much or too little of any hormone.

YOUR BODY FAT DISTRIBUTION REVEALS YOUR HORMONE IMBALANCES

Where fat is stored in your body can tell a bigger picture—one of a hormonal imbalance. Take a look at the illustration to determine which hormone could be causing your weight gain.

Body Fat Distribution Reveals Hormone Imbalances

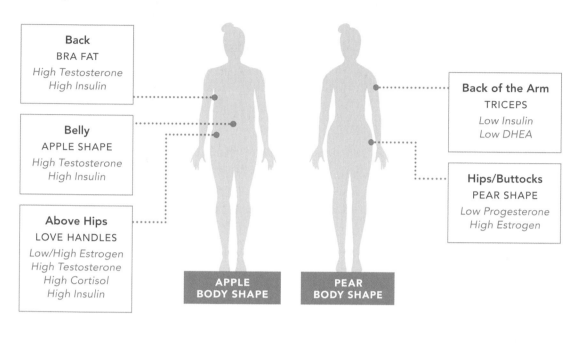

Back
BRA FAT
High Testosterone
High Insulin

Belly
APPLE SHAPE
High Testosterone
High Insulin

Above Hips
LOVE HANDLES
Low/High Estrogen
High Testosterone
High Cortisol
High Insulin

Back of the Arm
TRICEPS
Low Insulin
Low DHEA

Hips/Buttocks
PEAR SHAPE
Low Progesterone
High Estrogen

APPLE
BODY SHAPE

PEAR
BODY SHAPE

WHEN TO TAKE HORMONES AND WHEN NOT TO

To be clear: Some women and men need to take hormones to live and function, period. If, for example, your thyroid has been removed or you suffer from Addison's disease, you must take natural or synthetic thyroid or cortisol to live. Some women have so many medical conditions that hormonal support is necessary. If you are going through a very difficult menopause and suffer from cardiovascular problems, dementia, or advanced osteoporo-

sis, do talk to your doctor about bioidentical hormone therapy.

For everyone else, avoid getting caught up in the "pill-popping" and quick-fix mentality, replacing one pill (such as medications) with another, such as cocktails of supplements or hormones.

I am a big proponent of having a short-term and a long-term strategy when it comes to your hormonal health. In the short term, you might need an estrogen or progesterone cream, thyroid medications, or DHEA cream to regain energy, strength, and mental clarity to help you develop a nutritional and lifestyle plan that will move you forward. As a long-term plan for life, strive to rebalance your body and your hormones naturally using resources like this book so you depend on supplemental hormones at the very minimum or not at all.

Why? Because taking supplemental hormones masks all of the other imbalances in your body that could manifest later with a vengeance. For example, on the basis of a diagnosis of low estrogen, progesterone, or testosterone, and under your doctor's advice or pressure, you might be taking these hormones. But they are masking the root causes of these imbalances. What role did your poor gut health, sluggish liver, chronic stress, and toxicity play? Working with clients over many years, I have met numerous women who ignored these early signs and developed autoimmune diseases like lupus, fibromyalgia, and multiple sclerosis, which today we are beginning to understand are connected to compromised gut health and toxicity.

Why not just remove your uterus because of fibroids and "be done with it"?

 Find out at
www.HormonesBalance.com/book.

WHAT CAUSES HORMONAL IMBALANCES?

I lived in and traveled extensively through Asia for twenty-two years. During that time I visited "underdeveloped" yet well-nourished communities, and in those areas, it was unusual to find women struggling with issues related to weight, fertility, hair loss, depression, and anxiety. Like researcher Weston A. Price, I noticed the connection between an avoidance of "modern" processed foods and improved overall health.

Many of the factors that contribute to hormonal imbalance reflect the impact of modern life. Consider the following:

1. Poor Nutrition

Our food choices have a tremendous effect on the health of the digestive tract, including the microbiome, the liver, and blood sugar levels, which directly affect your hormonal balance. In the next chapter, I explain which foods to remove from or add to your diet to support your hormonal health.

2. Birth Control Pills, Hormones, and Antibiotics

To quote one naturopathic doctor I overheard at a conference, "Antibiotics and birth control pills are the two worst things Western medicine has given women." Birth control pills are known to be vitamin and mineral muggers, depleting women of zinc; vitamins B2, B6, B12, and C; magnesium; selenium; and folate. They distort the bacterial balance in the gut microbiome, causing many women to suffer from estrogen dominance, the leading cause of estrogenic cancers like those of the breast, uterus, thyroid, and ovaries.

There is an ongoing debate on the safety of synthetic steroid hormones. Synthetic estrogen, like Premarin and progestin, have been linked to breast cancer.

3. Toxins in Skincare and House-Cleaning Products

You start the day by drinking a glass of tap or filtered water. You jump in the shower, lathering your body with a shower gel and then washing your hair with a shampoo, followed by a conditioner. You slather on some body lotion and put on clothes you washed a few days ago in a washing powder and a softener. You apply expensive perfume to the bottom of your neck, just where the thyroid is. On the way to work, you stop by a coffee shop and grab a cup of joe, which you sip through a plastic lid. The office carpet has just been cleaned, and you wonder why by the afternoon you develop a headache. Lunch must be short, so you grab a soup in a Styrofoam cup from the local deli. A few colleagues pop plastic-wrapped lunch boxes in the microwave. In the effort to prevent flu, you wash your hands with an antibacterial soap provided by the office. When you are back home, you light a scented candle to relax. Before bed, you brush your teeth with toothpaste that promises no cavities, and you gargle with mouthwash.

You get the picture. Each one of the items mentioned above, if manufactured by a traditional mass consumer brand, carries a high toxic load. Many of these products are loaded with xenoestrogens, synthetic estrogens that disrupt hormonal balance. Some are well-documented carcinogens. Others disrupt the gut microbiome, which affects your metabolic, cardiovascular, autoimmune, and neurological systems. That is a lot of toxins for your body to process every day. I share the leading toxins to avoid in Chapter 4, and how to substitute them with safe and clean alternatives.

4. Chronic Stress and Lack of Self-Care (please don't skip this part)

One of the most underestimated triggers of hormonal and health issues in women is stress. There are four types of stress: emotional (past trauma, abuse, unresolved shame, guilt), physical (viral or bacterial infections, over-exercising, accidents, giving birth), digestive (IBS, food intolerances, frequent use of antibiotics), and chemical (toxic exposure and mold at home or work). All these forms of stress, especially when present on an ongoing basis, can cause excess cortisol release. And as we've seen, high cortisol levels can pull down all the other hormones—just like that one bad musician in an orchestra.

When I meet women who have been eating a clean diet and living a toxin-free life, but still feel sick and unbalanced, I divert the conversation to their emotional issues. I have seen women clear years of digestive issues, psoriasis, and body pains and aches by doing the "emotional work." Have you noticed that some symptoms get worse during times of stress, during unpleasant events, or when old traumatic memories resurface? I encourage you not to ignore stress in your life from now on (yes, diet is important, but it might not be enough) and look for a qualified practitioner to help you address your emotional well-being proactively through any of various modalities, such as eye movement desensitization and reprocessing (EMDR), neurofeedback, the emotional freedom technique (EFT), or shamanism, on the more liberal spectrum.

When it comes to physical stress, it is the fitness-obsessed women who hit the gym five times a week no matter how tired they are who suffer from adrenal exhaustion. Knowing when to stop is key. If you feel tired after exercising or need two days to recover, your body is telling you that you need to back off. If you have done many things to address fatigue or weight gain with poor results, ask your functional doctor to run a set of urine or saliva labs to test your adrenals.

When I polled my online community about the one piece of health advice they would give themselves a few years ago, an overwhelming number of women responded with one of these three comments: "Take better care of myself and listen to my body," "Put my health first before everyone else," and "Get more sleep."

If there is one piece of health advice you could give yourself a few years ago, what would it be? Share with us at www.facebook.com /hormonesbalance.

---

5. Lack of Sleep

It is hard to tell whether your hormones cause poor sleep or your poor sleep habits cause hormonal issues. It can be both or either. What we know for certain is that sleep is a very powerful and overlooked tool in hormonal rebalancing, especially when it comes to adrenal fatigue.

According to Dr. Michael Breus, the "Sleep Doctor," because of estrogen and progesterone fluctuations, women tend to have more problems with sleep than men. Menopause and perimenopause bring their own set of hormone-related sleep challenges; insomnia is a common and often overlooked problem for women experiencing menopause.

Hormonal imbalances that cause sleep disturbances including insomnia and nighttime awakening are low and high cortisol levels, high thyroid hormones (including Graves' disease), high blood sugar levels, low progesterone, low serotonin, low melatonin, low dopamine, or low gamma-aminobutyric acid

(GABA). It is common for women in the follicular phase, the first half of their menstrual cycle, to experience insomnia because of rising estrogen levels. With the progesterone rising in the luteal phase, which starts after ovulation, women tend to feel sleepy and want to go to bed earlier but also wake up earlier.

In addition, many women experience poor sleep because of food intolerances; overdependence on caffeine, sugar, and alcohol; chronic worrying; unstable sugar levels; eating sugary snacks before bedtime; and gut issues (which impair serotonin, the precursor for melatonin, the sleep hormone). According to traditional Chinese medicine, nighttime awakening can also be due to poor liver function.

How is sleep a healer? I do not need to persuade you that you feel so much better after an undisturbed eight-hour sleep versus a disrupted four-hour sleep. This is because cell regeneration happens during sleep. Your liver does most detoxification at night. Research shows that sleep-deprived people crave more carbohydrates, sugar, and coffee, which explains why losing weight is hard when you are sleep deprived.

If I have trouble falling asleep or don't sleep well, why not just take melatonin or sleeping pills?

 Find out at
www.HormonesBalance.com/book.

---

6. Genetic Predispositions

Your genes can shine a lot of light on your body's unique behavior. I, for example, discovered by testing my genes that I'm a "dopamine junkie" and I therefore have addictive tendencies and look for constant stimulation. I also have the MTHFR, COMT, and CBS genetic mutations, which make me a slow liver and estrogen and sulfur detoxifier.

But your genes are not your destiny. We now know that your lifestyle—what you eat, how much you exercise, the quality of your sleep, and your exposure to environmental and synthetic hormones (including birth control pills)—can affect whether or not your genes "turn on," or express themselves. So, do not ever feel that your genetics are your health sentence. You have more control over your health than you know!

I hope this chapter has helped you understand what hormonal imbalances you might be dealing with and what might have caused them. Do not feel discouraged if you struggle with many hormonal issues or if you have been experiencing them for a long time. With this book, you'll be able to change your health. Turn to the next page to begin balancing your hormones and building a strong Hormonal Foundation.

Part One

Phase I: Your Hormonal Foundation

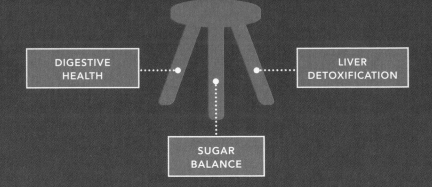

DIGESTIVE HEALTH

LIVER DETOXIFICATION

SUGAR BALANCE

If you've ever tried to sit on a three-legged stool, you know that only when each of the three legs is even and firmly in place can you sit down comfortably and confidently. If one leg is weak or shorter than the others or goes missing, you'll lose your balance and fall, right? Your hormonal health relies on three legs as well: your **digestive health,** your **blood sugar levels (sugar balance),** and your **liver health (liver detoxification).** If one of these legs is compromised, you'll experience a hormonal imbalance. Chapters 2, 3, and 4 explain how each of these legs form the Foundation of your hormonal health and show you how to support them so that they can support you.

"WHERE SHOULD I BEGIN?"

I'm often asked, "Where should I begin? Should I start by focusing on my digestive health, my blood sugar levels, or my liver? Do I need to heal them all at once? Can I proceed in any order?" My answer is this: Always start by healing your digestion first. It is the center of your health and I have yet to meet a person who suffers from digestive issues and is in good health. Most women with hormonal issues experience gas, bloating, tummy ache or burping after eating, acid reflux, constipation, or loose stool. Maybe these issues have been plaguing you for so long that you might not even realize they are happening to you. Please read "How to Get the Most from This Book" in the Introduction for guidance on how to proceed.

Chapter 2
Healing Your Digestion for Hormonal Balance

Optimal digestive health is vital for hormone balance (and much more). If you frequently experience any digestive issues, even if they seem benign, resolving them is the first step in rebalancing your hormones. I know it's tempting to think, "Well, I'm going through menopause," or "I've got thyroid issues," so "I just want to know what food will help these conditions." Bear with me, and you will find that your gut health is far more important than cherry-picking which foods to eat for a specific hormone imbalance (which won't give you lasting results anyway).

WHY YOUR DIGESTION IS SUCH A MESS (AND WHY YOU MIGHT NOT REALIZE IT)

In the words of the renowned gastronome Jean Anthelme Brillat-Savarin, "Tell me what you eat, and I will tell you what you are." Even Aristotle, the father of Western medicine, believed that all physical afflictions begin in the gut, and this holds true when it comes to hormones, too.

⚠ Do you experience any of these symptoms?

- Constipation
- Diarrhea or loose stool
- Bloating
- Abdominal pain
- Gas
- Acid reflux, or gastroesophageal reflux disease (GERD)
- Burping

These are all signs of a digestive system in distress. Sadly, so many of us are suffering from chronic digestive issues that we assume these symptoms are normal. Let me assure you: They are not.

Once you recognize that you are experiencing digestive distress and determine the causes, you can restore your gut health. It may take time, but with patience, determination, and the protocols and recipes in this book, it is possible. Repairing your digestive system is the first step in rebalancing your hormones.

Causes of Digestive Distress

- Poor digestive health of your mother
- Soy milk or cow's milk fed at birth instead of breast milk
- Overuse of antibiotics, especially early in life
- Birth control pills
- Processed food
- Chronic stress
- Food intolerance such as to gluten, dairy, eggs, and grains
- Low stomach acid
- Parasites and yeast, such as Candida
- Intestinal infections such as small intestine bacterial overgrowth (SIBO)
- Heavy metals such as mercury and lead
- Overuse of drugs such as steroids, antacids, hormones, and anti-inflammatories (such as ibuprofen [Advil])
- Zinc deficiency

THE GUT AND HORMONE CONNECTION

Digestive problems lead to five major hormone-disrupting issues: lack of micronutrient absorption, imbalanced gut bacteria responsible for metabolizing estrogen, elevated cortisol levels, chronic inflammation of hormone receptors, and compromised serotonin production.

Lack of Micronutrient Absorption

A lack of micronutrient absorption starves hormone-producing glands such as the thyroid, ovaries, and adrenals that need sufficient nutrients to function properly. For example, the thyroid needs sufficient amounts of selenium, iron, and vitamin B12 to convert the inactive T4 hormone into the active T3 hormone, a hormone essential for proper cell function. These nutrients can be found in food or supplements. Most of what you eat gets absorbed in the small intestine, which is 70 feet (21 meters) long, enough to cover the length of a tennis court when stretched. The inside of this tube has a carpetlike lining called the "villi." These tiny protrusions are responsible for the absorption of food's micronutrients. People who suffer from chronic digestive issues often have compromised villi, and that can prevent nutrients from being absorbed into the body. This explains why, despite taking so many supplements, many individuals are still nutrient-deficient and feel depleted.

Imbalanced Gut Bacteria Responsible for Metabolizing Estrogens

The subset of gut bacteria responsible for metabolizing estrogens are known as the "estrobolome." The latest medical research connects the health of these little bugs in your intestine to the state of your hormones. When there are imbalances in the estrobolome, estrogen isn't metabolized properly, resulting in elevated estrogen levels. Too much estrogen or too much of the harmful estrogen metabolites (or "by-products") has been linked by researchers and doctors to the development of cancers in the breasts, ovaries, uterus, thyroid, and even lungs in nonsmokers. High estrogen levels can also be the cause of breast and thyroid lumps, fibroids, and ovarian cysts.

For me, taking care of my gut health was essential in regaining hormonal balance. Since the age of forty, I experienced severe and debilitating PMS symptoms, including rage, which was damaging my marriage. I also struggled to get pregnant and had three miscarriages. After following the gut-healing protocol (and adding bone broths, fermented foods, and nutrient-dense foods to my diet), I immediately started feeling the difference in my hormones and I'm delighted to report that at age forty-four I conceived naturally!

—CARRIE ANN SCHEMENAUER

Elevated Cortisol Levels

Our bodies perceive digestive difficulties as a form of stress. They do not differentiate between stresses caused by emotional, physical, or digestive triggers like food intolerances. Stress is stress, regardless of the source. Eating foods that you are unable to digest causes inflammation that you may experience as bloating or indigestion. In response, our adrenals release cortisol to cope with the stress. Elevated cortisol levels contribute to adrenal fatigue, which can have a cascading effect on your thyroid hormones and your levels of progesterone.

Chronic Inflammation of Hormone Receptors

Chronic digestive distress leads to chronic inflammation. Under normal circumstances, inflammation is temporary and helps the body rebound from injury, such as a wound or twisted ankle, or fight off infections, such as a sore throat. Chronic inflammation is long-lasting and has been linked to an increased risk of various conditions, including diabetes, heart disease, and hormonal imbalances. One way this happens is by desensitizing hormone receptors. (A hormone receptor is a molecule in the cell that allows the hormone to attach itself and let the cell perform a set of tasks.) For example, you may be producing sufficient levels of progesterone, but chronic inflammation can desensitize (or shut down) the hormone receptor, preventing progesterone from entering the cells and causing many related symptoms, such as insomnia, infertility, or anxiety.

Compromised Serotonin Production

Serotonin is mainly produced in the gastrointestinal tract, not in the brain. People with digestive issues often experience low serotonin levels that can affect bowel movement and therefore the detoxification of various harmful hormonal metabolites. Low serotonin levels will cause low melatonin (serotonin is the precursor for melatonin) and severely disrupt your sleep. Good sleep is essential to facilitate detoxification and curb food cravings.

As you can see, your digestive health has a tremendous impact on your hormones. Now that you know how important the gut is for balanced hormones, I hope you feel empowered and motivated to heal it.

HOW TO HEAL YOUR DIGESTIVE SYSTEM

Let's dive deeper into a few of the worst causes of digestive problems in women and how to address them. These include

- Food intolerances

- Low stomach acid

- Candida yeast overgrowth

- SIBO

- Parasites

Addressing Food Intolerances

Most adults experience some form of food intolerance in their lifetimes. You can certainly see that in health stores: products free of gluten, wheat, dairy, soy, or nuts are now offered by countless small and big brands alike. And

I found two lumps in my right breast and one in the left. Breast cancer runs in my family, so this diagnosis was the most alarming, eye-opening (but also frustrating) event in my life. I was a healthy eater, and I exercised regularly. One of the first things I did was look at my diet after reading about the role of the gut bacteria that can affect my estrogen levels. I did have chronic digestive issues, like constipation (which I thought was normal) and signs of Candida. After adding 2 cups of fermented food per day and a good-quality probiotic to my diet, my breast lumps reduced and stopped hurting. I then added 2 tablespoons of ground flaxseed per day, and within a month the breast lumps completely disappeared. I realize now that I had estrogen dominance, which was probably due to chronic constipation and Candida issues that affected the estrobolome and my estrogen levels. I feel empowered to know things my doctors never told me, and, most importantly, not to fear cancer. —ELLA

for good reason: There is a growing awareness among consumers who see their health returning when they avoid trigger foods.

What's the difference between allergies and food intolerances?

These two terms are used interchangeably, but they mean two different things. Allergies cause an immediate reaction (within three seconds to thirty minutes) and symptoms such as swelling, rash, itch, or runny nose. They can be determined with an IgE allergy panel. Food intolerances cause delayed reactions that can take from thirty minutes to three days to manifest. They can be identified with IgG tests, which are often inaccurate and show false negatives (your problem foods don't show up). Because of the delayed response of the immune system and poor testing options, the most reliable method of identifying your food intolerances is by committing to the Elimination Diet, described later in this chapter.

For the health of your hormones, it is important to get rid of both allergies and intolerances as they both cause an inflammatory response in the body.

THE TOP FOOD INTOLERANCES

The following foods are the most common causes of digestive distress:

The Big 7 are gluten, dairy, eggs, soy, corn, peanuts, and nightshades (includes tomatoes, potatoes, eggplant, peppers, chili peppers, and goji berries). More people tend to have a problem with these foods.

The Small 7 are nuts, seeds, chocolate, beef, coffee, sugar, and bananas. Fewer people have trouble with these foods, but they can still be an issue for many.

Many other foods not listed here may cause you problems, too. My client Brandie, for example, developed digestive issues from chicken and certain foods high in FODMAPs (Fermentable Oligosaccharides, Disaccharides, Monosaccharides, and Polyols) such as onions, garlic, and beets. I've worked with women who found that "healthy" foods such as quinoa, strawberries, and cinnamon were creating havoc in their digestive systems.

DISCOVERING YOUR FOOD INTOLERANCES

I completely understand if right now you're thinking, "So what should I eat now? I eat all the foods on that list of food intolerances!" I hear you. But that's exactly why you should take the time to determine your specific food intolerances. Foods don't affect everyone in the same way. You may find that eggs don't cause you any trouble while sugar triggers a negative response.

The best way to discover your food intolerances is to do the Elimination Diet (see page 44). You'll eliminate certain foods from your diet for a period of time and monitor your symptoms to see whether any resolve. If they do, that's an indication that you may have an intolerance to that food. I've made the Elimination Diet as easy for you to follow as possible, walking you through the process step-by-step and providing an abundance of delicious food options. *All of the recipes in this book are free of the Big 7 food intolerances (gluten, dairy, eggs, soy, corn, peanuts, and nightshades), and many are free of the Small 7, especially sugar.*

Can't I just get tested for food intolerance?

Various labs test between ninety-eight and three hundred different food items. Most holistic/integrative doctors and naturopaths can run these food intolerance tests for you. I have found that many food items do not show up on the tests, resulting in a "false negative." I use such tests with clients who have multiple food intolerances and already are on highly restricted diets. Otherwise, I recommend doing the Elimination Diet, because your body never lies.

Please note that IgA tests show allergies and not intolerances, and many allergists lead their patients to believe that allergies are the only thing they need to test for. You now know, that is not the case.

I encourage you to identify your food intolerances because they damage your digestive system, and, as we've seen, a damaged digestive system causes a cascade of hormone imbalances and inflammation in the body. Eating foods that support your digestive health is an important step in achieving optimal hormonal health.

If you are dealing with multiple food sensitivities, allergies, and ongoing digestive problems despite having implemented the Elimination Diet, I recommend that you seek out a skilled functional doctor who will take your concerns seriously with his or her full attention. Such conditions can be caused by chronic gut infections or parasites that make you overreact to many foods.

In my nutrition practice, I've found that addressing potential food intolerances is the first step to rebalancing my clients' hormones. Quite simply, no one can achieve hormonal bliss while eating trigger foods that keep them in a constant state of inflammation.

Addressing Low Stomach Acid

Low stomach acid also affects hormonal balance, and it is often overlooked as a factor in ensuring that the digestive system functions properly. Believe it or not, despite what most conventional doctors believe (while they're recommending antacids), acid reflux is a sign of low stomach acid, not excessive stomach acid. Dr. Jonathan V. Wright of the Tahoma Clinic, in his book *Why Stomach Acid Is Good for You* (written with Lane Lenard), asserts: "When we carefully test people over age forty who're having heartburn, indigestion and gas, over 90 percent of the time we find inadequate acid production by the stomach."

Stomach acid is essential to the breakdown of vital nutrients. It allows for the digestion and absorption of trace minerals that are vital for good health, such as zinc, iron, copper, magnesium, calcium, selenium, and vitamins B3 and B12. We need certain trace minerals and vitamins for our glands to produce hormones. Sufficient stomach acid helps absorb these nutrients. Stomach acid also triggers the pancreas to produce the bile and enzymes needed to digest and absorb proteins, carbohydrates, and fats. An inability to digest fats well can lead to low cholesterol levels, and that in turn can cause an imbalance in sex hormone levels, such as estrogen, progesterone, cortisol, DHEA, and testosterone.

Stomach acid also sterilizes the stomach, which helps kill off pathogens found in food and prevents the overgrowth of yeast, fungus, and bacteria. If you have low acid levels, it may lead to chronic bacterial or yeast infections, and you are more likely to become a host for parasites.

A vast majority of the women I work with begin by saying, "I eat really well," and they probably do. But when we dive into details, I often discover that most have low stomach acid levels, which is often one of the reasons they do not absorb the food they eat, they are nutritionally deficient, and many struggle with Candida yeast overgrowth.

✔ Determining Whether You Have Low Stomach Acid

You can do a simple test at home to determine whether you have sufficient stomach acid. Purchase Betaine HCl with pepsin, which helps increase the level of hydrochloric acid in your stomach needed for proper digestion (any brand will do, such as NOW, TwinLab, or Thorne). Prepare a high-protein meal of at least 6 ounces meat. In the middle of eating the meal, take one Betaine HCl pill. Finish your meal. There are two possible outcomes. One is that you won't notice any change. This means it is likely you have low stomach acid levels. The second is that you experience stomach distress, such as heaviness, burning, or hotness. This means you have sufficient stomach acid and do not need to add any more HCl pills.

If you felt nothing after one pill, keep increasing the dose; at the next meal, take two pills. If you get no reaction, keep dosing up by one pill at each meal until you feel a burning sensation or discomfort. Once you experience a reaction, you'll need to take one pill less at each meal to have sufficient stomach acid and well-functioning digestion. For example, if you need four HCl pills to feel discomfort, you'll take three pills at each meal. Some individuals with very low stomach acid need to take as many as five to eight HCl pills before feeling a burning sensation.

A consistent dosing of HCl pills and a change in diet (for example, eliminating food intolerances) may help increase stomach acid naturally. Once your stomach acid returns to normal, maintain it by drinking 1 to 2 tablespoons apple cider vinegar, lemon juice, or lime juice before meals. If your stomach acid stays consistently low despite the changes, ask your doctor for an *H. pylori* stool test.

Addressing Candida Yeast Overgrowth

Candida albicans is a common and highly opportunistic yeast that shows up in the digestive tract, on the skin (especially the feet), in the mouth, and in the reproductive organs. About 70 percent of women I work with suffer from varying degrees of Candida overgrowth at some point in their lives. It's normal to have Candida strains in the body, but too much Candida can result in symptoms ranging from cravings for sweets and digestive problems to brain fog.

SYMPTOMS OF CANDIDA

Keep in mind that many of these symptoms can be caused by other conditions. The ones marked with an asterisk tend to be most often related to Candida.

- Generally not feeling well. Craving sugar and alcohol,* feeling that a meal is incomplete without dessert,* brain fog.

- Digestion problems. Feeling tipsy after drinking kombucha,* mucus in the stool,* ongoing digestive issues (especially bloating), many food sensitivities, itchy anus.

- Skin problems. Athlete's foot,* fungal infections of the nails and skin, body odor.

- Mouth problems. Thrush (white coating on the tongue),* swollen lower lip, metallic taste in the mouth, bad breath.

- Respiratory problems. Sinus congestion,* persistent cough, mucus in the throat, chronic postnasal drip, flulike symptoms, sinusitis.

- Eye and ear problems. Ringing in the ears,* ear infections,* eye pain, itchy eyes, sensitivity to light, blurred vision.

- Genitourinary system problems. Recurring vaginal yeast infections,* vaginal discharge,* recurring urinary tract infections,* cystitis (inflammation of the bladder).

- Weight problems. Inability to lose weight, water retention, unexplained weight loss.

Many women are surprised to find they're susceptible to Candida yeast overgrowth. When I suggest it as a potential problem, they say, "But I don't eat that much sugar." You don't need to be a sugar junkie to experience Candida overgrowth. Yes, it is a condition that can develop in women who live on diets rich in sugar (which can include fruit), processed carbohydrates (which include flour products, even if gluten free, such as breads and pastas), and alcohol (which most people don't realize is just liquid sugar). If you were prescribed multiple rounds of antibiotics in the past, or if you use antacids, birth control pills, hormone replacement therapy, steroids, or anti-inflammatory drugs, your chance of developing Candida is much higher as well. Estrogen dominance (including birth control pills) can also fuel Candida's growth. On the other hand, Candida can mimic estrogen (and create estrogen dominance), contribute to systemic inflammation, and cause digestive distress. In other words: It's bad news altogether.

You are also susceptible if your immune system is compromised. A healthy immune system can eradicate extra Candida, but if you eat foods that your body has trouble digesting (such as gluten, dairy, or eggs) or experience a stressful time in your life, your overburdened immune system will be unable to clear the Candida. Parasites and heavy metals can also inhibit your body's ability to kick Candida.

TESTING FOR CANDIDA

Candida is infamously hard to diagnose because it can be masked as many different conditions for years. Testing for Candida can be tricky and often returns a false negative, so it is therefore important to recognize your symptoms, especially the ones marked with an asterisk in the symptoms list above. Your doctor can test for IgG, IgA, and IgM Candida antibodies in your blood or stool.

I've found one test, however, that's surprisingly accurate, and you can easily complete it at home. It's called the "Candida Saliva Test" and here's how it works: Do not eat any dairy products for two days before administering the test. Place a glass of water next to your bed before you go to sleep. Upon waking, and before you drink, eat, or brush your teeth, build up a nice ball of saliva in your mouth

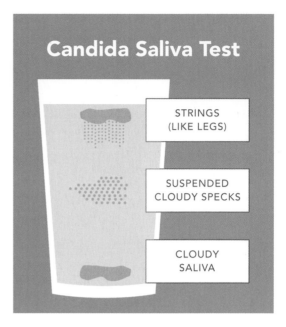

Candida Saliva Test

STRINGS (LIKE LEGS)

SUSPENDED CLOUDY SPECKS

CLOUDY SALIVA

and spit it into the glass. Wait about twenty minutes. What do you see? If your saliva develops "legs," suspends cloudy specks, or sinks to the bottom of the glass, you might have Candida. If it floats on top with no legs, you most likely do not have Candida. The longer the legs and the faster the saliva sinks, the higher the amount of yeast in your body.

TREATING CANDIDA

The key strategy for treating Candida is to starve it by eliminating the foods it feeds on, such as *any* form of sugar, processed grains (and initially all grains), fruit (with the exception of small amounts of berries), root vegetables, fermented foods, and mushrooms. The secondary strategy is to support your gut, the immune system, and your liver in clearing the Candida. Start with the Elimination Diet and add the anti-Candida diet (see page 81) to get the best results.

If you are still experiencing stubborn Candida symptoms, look for other underlying causes such as estrogen dominance, parasites, and heavy metals.

Addressing SIBO

Small intestine bacterial overgrowth (SIBO) occurs when bacteria escape the large intestine and migrate to the small intestine, causing digestive havoc that manifests as chronic abdominal bloating and gas (no matter what you eat), belching, abdominal pain, food sensitivities, and fatty stool (steatorrhea).

SIBO is a vast topic of its own. If you suspect you have it, look up Dr. Allison Siebecker, a leading expert on SIBO, who runs an informative website, www.SIBOinfo.com. Find the right diagnosis using the practitioners and tests she recommends.

Some of the most difficult cases I have worked with are caused by undiagnosed gut infections like SIBO. One way to identify whether you could potentially be afflicted with SIBO is to try the low-FODMAP diet (see page 86) to see whether your digestive issues improve. If they do, it could be a good incentive for you to find a SIBO-skilled practitioner to test and treat you with herbal or pharmaceutical antibiotics. Individuals with SIBO make little recovery progress through diet alone.

 Addressing Parasites

Parasites are often the most overlooked cause of digestive and hormonal problems, and they are far more common than you think. According to the parasitologist Dr. Omar M. Amin, 30 percent of us are hosts to parasites. If you suffer from chronic digestive, skin, and mental issues that won't go away, get the full scoop on diagnosing and treating parasites on my website at www.HormonesBalance.com/book.

MANAGE YOUR DIGESTIVE HEALTH BY STUDYING YOUR POOP

In traditional Chinese medicine, the health of the gut is partly assessed by a stool analysis. Western medicine has caught up, and in 1997, the Bristol Stool Chart was created. Most Western functional practitioners use it to assess the health of the digestive tract.

Types 1 and 2 indicate constipation and a long transit time through the gut, which is toxic to the body. This could be due to low thyroid function, food intolerances, lack of soluble and insoluble fiber, magnesium deficiency, low stomach acid, or low bile output.

Types 3 and 4 are what you want. A perfect poop is when the end sinks to the bottom and the top is afloat.

Types 5, 6, and 7 indicate that your body is trying to eliminate the food as quickly as possible, most likely because of food sensitivities or allergies (gluten and dairy are common causes), overconsumption of caffeine or alcohol, over-active thyroid, IBS, or medications. These stool types cause malabsorption of nutrients, which leads to vitamin and mineral deficiencies.

Oscillating between types 1 or 2 and types 5 to 7 can be an indication of advanced IBS, bacterial infections (such as SIBO), or parasites.

You should not see food particles (such as undigested vegetables) in your poop; this indicates poor digestion that could be caused by low stomach acid or low bile production. The poop color should be dark brown, and the poop should not smell foul (a sign of overfermentation).

Once you heal your gut, you will be seeing types 3 and 4 on a regular basis.

GUT-HEALING GUIDE

As you can see, maintaining or restoring digestive health is an important "leg" of your Hormonal Foundation. If you are just beginning this journey, you might feel like you have a steep mountain to climb, and that may be so. For some women, just a few simple changes like going gluten free or reducing dairy and caffeine can do the trick; their hormones bounce back as their digestion improves and inflammation subsides. Others, like me, must do some deep investigative work. Don't fret if you are a complicated case. You are learning how to listen to and observe your body like never before.

To get started, do the Elimination Diet (see page 44) and keep a Food Mood Poop Journal (see page 49), the best investigative tool you will ever use. You will discover what your body

What Does Healthy Poop Look Like?

TYPE 1
Separate peanut- to walnut-size pieces. Hard to pass. Indicates constipation.

TYPE 2
Banana-shaped but very lumpy. Can be hard to pass. Indicates slight constipation.

TYPE 3
Size of a thick sausage, comes out easily and bowels feel emptied. Indicates a good bowel movement.

TYPE 4
Size of a banana, easy to evacuate and bowels feel emptied. Indicates a good bowel movement.

TYPE 5
Stool falls apart easily, visible food particles, comes out easily. Indicates slight diarrhea.

TYPE 6
Mushy stool that has no shape. Indicates diarrhea.

TYPE 7
Watery stool. Indicates diarrhea.

loves and what it rejects (even if the food is cited as "healthy"). Once you tune in to your body, it will tell you loud and clear which foods serve you well and which do not. If your digestive symptoms are erratic and persistent no matter what you do, work with a functional doctor to look more deeply into the possibilities of parasites, bacterial infections, or heavy metals that could be undermining your digestive health. Getting your gut to function optimally will be the most rewarding act of kindness to yourself.

To make it easy for you, I have consolidated all the gut-healing options into this Gut-Healing Guide. Download a PDF version of it from my website at www.HormonesBalance .com/book and print it out to hang in your kitchen as a convenient way to help you develop and maintain a new routine.

ADD (+)

Start with the Elimination Diet (see page 44) to start healing your gut and reducing inflammation.

Bone broth (page 157). Use bones from beef, lamb, or chicken and/or chicken feet. Bone broth provides collagen, proline, glycine, glutamine, phosphorus, silicon, and sulfur.

Consume a minimum of 1 cup per day. As a vegetarian alternative, try the Mineral Vegetable Broth (page 160) (but it won't offer the same healing benefits).

Cooked food. Cooked food is easier to digest than raw food. Soups, stews, and braised meats are exceptionally healing.

Vitamin A–rich food. Vitamin A rebuilds the intestinal lining. Found in liver, sweet potato, fish oils, and carrots. Consume a minimum of 1 serving per day.

Good fats. Good fats rebuild the intestinal lining. Use coconut oil, ghee, avocado, or duck fat at a minimum of 3 tablespoons per day, or eat fatty fish like wild salmon, 3 servings per week.

Probiotic-rich foods. A probiotic supplement is not enough. Create a healing environment for the gut by adding fermented vegetables, coconut yogurt, soy-free miso, or non-GMO soy miso (if you can tolerate soy), and kvass. Aim for 2 to 3 servings per day.

Stomach acid. Stomach acid aids digestion and enzymatic activity for maximum nutrient absorption. Take 2 tablespoons lemon juice, lime juice, apple cider vinegar, or sauerkraut juice before breakfast or before each meal, if stomach acid is low. If you need more, use HCl pills.

Fiber. Fiber helps food move along in the gut and aids liver function. Great sources are ground flaxseeds, chia seeds, nuts, and other seeds. Take 30 grams (2 tablespoons) per day.

Sprouts. Sprouts help enzymatic activity in the gut. Take 1 serving per day.

Bitter greens. Bitter greens aid in the production of bile, a digestive aid. Found in radishes, dandelion leaves, and artichokes. Eat a minimum of 1 serving per day.

Probiotic supplement. Choose a high-quality probiotic with eight to twelve strains consisting of several types of bifidobacterium and lactobacillus. It should have no fillers and be hypoallergenic. My favorite probiotics are Equilibrium, Custom Probiotic, and the spore-based MegaSporeBiotic.

REMOVE (–)

Food intolerances. Gluten, dairy, eggs, soy, corn, sugar, nightshades, yeast, citrus, nuts, and seeds are common culprits in creating digestive issues.

Artificial sweeteners. Avoid artificial sweeteners at all costs, as they have been shown to cause neurological damage and disrupt the gut microbiome.

Sugar. Sugar changes the intestinal pH and feeds pathogens such as Candida. Do not eat more than 20 grams (5 teaspoons) per day. Pay attention to product labels: 4 grams sugar = 1 teaspoon.

Processed and packaged foods. Avoid white flour, white sugar, additives, and preservatives, including protein shakes and powders, quick oats, and rice or quinoa puffs.

Coffee. Coffee creates intestinal inflammation and slows healing. It also makes your system more acidic.

Alcohol. Avoid alcohol, as it is highly inflammatory for the intestinal lining and feeds pathogenic bacteria.

Medications. Some medications destroy intestinal lining and bacterial microflora. These include, but are not limited to, antibiotics, antacids, birth control pills, nonsteroidal anti-inflammatory drugs (NSAIDS) (aspirin, acetaminophen, ibuprofen), and steroids (such as corticosteroids).

Kombucha. Its wild yeast content can create an autoimmune response and a yeast infection flare-up.

Stress. The brain-gut connection can cause digestive issues and lower stomach acid production. Stress can be emotional, physical, or chemical.

Pathogens and infections. If you are suffering from ongoing digestive issues despite trying various nutritional approaches, test for Candida yeast overgrowth, bacterial infections such as SIBO, *H. pylori* and parasites.

BALANCE

Based on your unique bioindividuality.

Good food, but not right for you. Some people react poorly to "good" food, for example, chicken, beef, legumes, onions, or pineapple. Listen to your body to learn what does not agree with you. Set up and stick to the Food Mood Poop Journal (see page 49) to tune in to your body's signals and reactions.

Supplements. Most people take too many supplements. If they do not improve your overall well-being, talk to your doctor about cutting them down to the bare minimum. Consider the Gut Restore Kit on Hormone BalanceNutritionals.com.

Movement. Low-intensity exercise such as yoga, Pilates, tai chi, or dancing is best. Avoid excessive exercise, as most individuals who suffer from chronic digestive problems also have weak adrenals. Excessive exercise like running, mountain biking, CrossFit, and other cardio workouts can further weaken the adrenals.

THE ELIMINATION DIET

You now know so much about the role of food in balancing hormones. How can you use all of this information to create daily eating habits that work best for you?

Certainly, eating a whole-food diet and an abundance of green leafy vegetables while reducing the amount of processed foods, sugar, and alcohol in your diet is a good place to start for good health. But there is no one-size-fits-all diet plan or nutritional protocol that will work for every single woman. You have probably noticed that the same food affects you and a family member or friend differently. Perhaps your best friend can't stop talking about how great quinoa is, but you find it upsets your stomach. Or, you love fermented vegetables as a good source of pro-biotics, but your colleague can't tolerate them, breaking out in hives and feeling itchy and anxious after just a bite. One person's health food can be another person's poison.

The only way to find a diet that supports your health is to respect your body and lis-ten to what it tells you about which foods are friends and which are foes. The Elimination Diet will help you hear what your body is saying.

Is it possible to restore hormone balance with a vegan or vegetarian diet?

Because I respect the ethical decision to eat as a vegan or vegetarian, I wish my answer could be "yes," but I have found that not to be the case for most people. In my practice, I've seen only a small percentage of people enjoy good long-term health eating a vegan or vegetarian diet. Often, they feel great for the first year or two but then find them-selves sliding into general fatigue, depres-sion, Candida yeast overgrowth, frequent colds, and feeling cold. Many of my clients, especially those who embarked on a soy-rich diet, developed problems with low thyroid function.

Hormones are made of proteins, and some specific amino acids, vitamins, and minerals are not present in plant-based pro-teins. So many women suffer from digestive issues, and relying on plant-based proteins such as beans, legumes, nuts, and seeds upsets their digestion even more and leads to various health conditions. These foods are high in oxalates, leading to oxalate sen-sitivity. Overall, I've seen clients experience significant health improvement after adding even small amounts of animal proteins back into their diets.

I don't promote eating bacon all day long. I advocate for a 70 percent to 80 per-cent plant-based diet and eating only meats from pasture-raised, responsibly raised, and responsibly slaughtered animals—never meats from factory farms. Honoring that we are all different and have unique dietary needs will set you free to find what works for you.

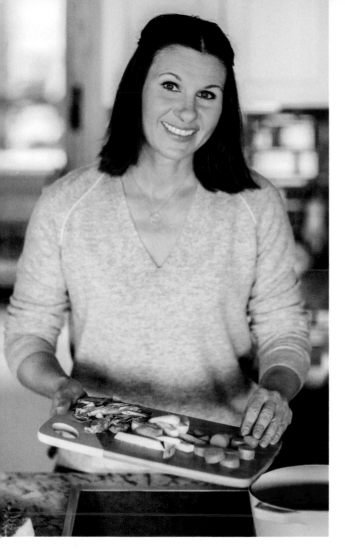

you to eat delicious, satisfying meals, snacks, and drinks even during the Elimination Diet.

The Elimination Diet is transformative. Here is a list of benefits I've found people experience after having gone through the Elimination Diet and figured out which foods hamper their gut health:

WEIGHT LOSS

- Stubborn weight starts going away
- No more yo-yo weight gain
- No puffy hands and legs from water retention
- Belly fat is reduced

CALMER GUT

- Elimination or reduction of bloating, constipation, acid reflux, gas, loose stool, tummy pain, and cramping
- Healing of IBS
- Healing of autoimmune conditions
- Better bacterial microflora
- Fewer pathogenic microbes such as Candida

LESS OR NO PAIN; ELIMINATION OR REDUCTION OF

- Arthritic pain
- Unexplained muscle and joint pain
- Back pain
- Carpal tunnel pain
- Headaches and migraines

By first removing the most inflammatory foods from your diet, the Elimination Diet reduces inflammation throughout your body and promotes the Hormonal Foundation of gut healing, sugar balance, and gentle liver detoxification. Then, as you reintroduce foods, you'll be able to determine which ones support your health and which ones you are sensitive to.

All of the recipes in this book can be part of the Elimination Diet, so it will be very easy for

BETTER MENTAL FUNCTIONS; ELIMINATION OR REDUCTION OF

- Brain fog
- Forgetfulness
- Difficulty concentrating
- Depression
- Anxiety

MORE ENERGY

- Easier to get up in the morning
- Less sleep needed
- Less reliance on stimulants like coffee

BETTER BREATHING; ELIMINATION OR REDUCTION OF

- Asthma
- Sinus infections
- Stuffy nose

FEWER ALLERGIES; ELIMINATION OR REDUCTION OF

- Seasonal allergies
- Chronic allergies (such as to cats and dogs)

BETTER SLEEP

- Easier to fall asleep
- Deeper and higher-quality sleep
- Waking rested
- Less or no reliance on sleeping pills and supplements

CLEARER SKIN; ELIMINATION OR REDUCTION OF

- Eczema
- Acne
- Psoriasis
- Unexplained rash
- Hives

HORMONAL BALANCE; ELIMINATION OR REDUCTION OF

- PMS
- Hot flashes
- Irregular periods
- No periods
- Adrenal fatigue

How to Do the Elimination Diet

There are two versions of the Elimination Diet. The basic version removes the Big 7, that is, the top inflammatory foods. The comprehensive version also removes the Small 7, the foods less likely to cause inflammation. It's up to you which version you follow. Listen to your intuition. Even though the basic version does not remove all sugar, by following the recipes in this book you will significantly reduce your sugar intake. All of the recipes are low in sugar. However, if you suspect you have a sensitivity to one of the Small 7, such as sugar, it's best to try the comprehensive version.

Let's review the Big 7 and Small 7:

THE BIG 7

1. Gluten (a protein found in grains such as wheat, spelt, rye, couscous, and barley; also found in many soups, sauces, and processed and packaged foods)

2. Dairy (includes milk, cheese, butter, and yogurt)

3. Eggs (found in baked goods, mayonnaise, pastas, and puddings)

4. Soy (found in tofu, soy milk, soy sauce, and some supplements as a filler)

5. Corn (found in corn syrup, tortilla chips, salads; also found in sauces, soups, and supplements as a filler)

6. Peanuts

7. Nightshade vegetables (includes tomatoes, potatoes, eggplants, peppers, chili peppers, and goji berries)

THE SMALL 7

1. Nuts (almond intolerance is the most common)

2. Seeds (includes quinoa, sunflower seeds, and flaxseeds)

3. Chocolate (with cacao content, not white chocolate)

4. Beef (includes beef bone broth)

5. Coffee (includes decaf)

6. Sugar (especially processed, white sugar and high-fructose sugar such as agave)

7. Bananas

Remember, it is up to you to decide whether you start with eliminating the Big 7 only or both the Big 7 and Small 7. If you are feeling overwhelmed by the idea of cutting out fourteen foods all at once, then start with the Big 7 first. Keeping the Food Mood Poop Journal (see page 49) will help you identify whether you are reacting to any other foods (such as the Small 7 or others).

How to Do the Elimination Diet

ELIMINATION PHASE (2 to 4 weeks)

Gentle: Remove only the Big 7—gluten, dairy, eggs, corn, soy, peanuts, and nightshades
Deep: Also remove the Small 7—nuts, seeds, chocolate, beef, coffee, sugar, and bananas

CHALLENGE PHASE (3 to 8 weeks)

1	2	3	4	5	6	7	8	9	10	11	12	13	14

Reintroduce each food over 3 days. Recommended sequence: 1) gluten, 2) dairy, 3) eggs, 4) corn, 5) soy, 6) peanuts, 7) nightshades, 8) nuts, 9) seeds, 10) chocolate, 11) beef, 12) coffee, 13) sugar, and 14) bananas

Step 1: The Elimination Phase

During this phase, if you've decided to follow the basic diet, you will completely avoid the Big 7: gluten, dairy, eggs, corn, soy, peanuts, and nightshades.

Or, if you are following the more comprehensive version, you will completely avoid the Big 7 and the Small 7, which includes nuts, seeds, chocolate, beef, sugar, and bananas.

Additionally, if you know you have food sensitivities, cut out those foods as well.

To see results, you should stay on the Elimination Diet for at least two weeks, but I recommend committing to four weeks. Many people experience a reduction of symptoms during the first few days, while others need four to eight weeks to feel relief.

The Elimination Diet changed my life by reducing inflammation and pain and helping me to put my Hashimoto's thyroiditis into remission. Yes, REMISSION, with the right food from the kitchen! I suffered for years with depression, digestive issues, excess mucus, Hashimoto's thyroiditis, stomach bloating, cystic acne, dry eyes, PMS, migraine headaches, joint pain, and hair falling out. And the simplest, cheapest answer was the Elimination Diet. Many of my ailments improved or disappeared after I was on the diet for just a few weeks. I feel healthier, happier, and more energized now than I did in my younger years.

—LISA GARCIA

It is not unusual to experience detoxification symptoms, such as a white coating on the tongue, fatigue, mood swings, rashes, weird dreams, or sleep problems. But they should go away within days.

PRACTICAL TIPS

Be gentle with yourself. This is a big step! And it isn't easy giving up what are probably staple foods for you. Don't be hard on yourself if you find it difficult. Use this time to learn more about yourself. The harder it is to give up a certain food, the more of a sign it is that you might have a problem with that food. Also, we now know that gluten and dairy contain peptides that mimic the effects of opiate drugs like heroin and morphine. They numb our pain in a way no carrot or hummus ever could! No wonder it is hard to give them up. The good news is that once you do give them up and start feeling better, you will have a hard time going back to them. You won't want to feel bloated, fatigued, depressed, or anxious again.

Change the mindset. This is an exciting time when you are trying new things that heal you. This diet is not forever. You are doing it only for a few weeks, and later you will most likely be able to eat some of the foods you are currently avoiding. Remind yourself *why* you want to feel better. What will you be able to do when you get healthy that you are unable to do now because you feel sick all the time?

Clean out your kitchen. Get rid of the foods that you will be temporarily avoiding. It'll be easier for you to follow the diet without any temptations around.

Surround yourself with alternatives. Look at the recipes in this book and prepare a list of substitutes closest to the foods you think you will miss the most. Have them on hand when you need them.

Print out a food list of what you can eat. Create a food list from the Elimination Diet sample meal plan on pages 52–55, print it out, and hang it in the kitchen. There are so many delicious and nourishing foods you *can* have.

Timing. Choose a low-stress time to do the diet. Do not do it when you are traveling, on vacation, or during holidays or a major family event. If you have terrible PMS, don't start the diet during that week.

⚠ KEEP A FOOD MOOD POOP JOURNAL

I strongly recommend that you keep a journal to track the foods you eat; how you feel physically and emotionally, including how you are sleeping; and your bowel movements. See the sample for one way to approach it. Some of my clients are reluctant to keep this journal at first, but let me assure you that the benefits far outweigh any initial inconvenience.

By keeping a journal, you will start spotting patterns. For example, you might note that each time you eat chicken, you feel fatigued two hours later. The journal will help you connect the dots between certain foods and your reaction to them. Many clients have told me that the journal helped them realize that they were eating the same things over and over (eating a variety of foods is important!) or that they binge eat when stressed, depressed, or in pain. Some realized they were eating a lot more sugar than they had thought.

A Food Mood Poop journal is a powerful detective tool for spotting your food triggers and your good and bad habits.

Carol has stopped eating the Big 7 during her Elimination Diet but is still eating the Small 7. She starts her day with a cup of coffee rather than water or apple cider vinegar. She reports a tummy ache and bloating after the chia pudding. It could be that seeds or coconut do not agree with her. Her poop shows food particles, a sign of low stomach acid and/or poor enzyme production. Carol drinks only 32 ounces of water; for her weight, she should double her water intake. She's feeling exhausted after having the coconut ice cream, a common reaction to sugar.

Keeping the Food Mood Poop Journal is a great detective tool for spotting food triggers but also your good and bad habits.

 All of the recipes in this cookbook are free of the Big 7: gluten, dairy, eggs, soy, corn, peanuts, and nightshades.

You can find and download a sample of a blank Food Mood Poop Journal at www.HormonesBalance.com/book.

Carol's Food Mood Poop Journal (Sample)

Time	Food	Drink	How you feel (mood, gut, sleep)	Poop
8:00 A.M.	Coconut kefir chia pudding	Coffee with coconut creamer	Didn't sleep too well	See food particles, not fully emptied, constipated
9:30 A.M.			Tummy ache, slightly bloated	
11:30 A.M.	Turkey sandwich on gluten-free bread, sweet potato chips, apple	16 ounces water		
12:00 P.M.			Feel slightly better: less moody, headache gone, still tired	
3:00 P.M.	Small bag of trail mix			
6:30 P.M.	Roast chicken, 1 bowl vegetable soup, salad (lettuce, cucumber, tomato, carrot, Italian dressing)			
7:00 P.M.		16 ounces water	Feel much better after dinner	
9:00 P.M.	Bowl of vanilla coconut ice cream			
9:20 P.M.			Feel exhausted just want to go to sleep	

THE GLUTEN-FREE TRAP

Today, a lot of packaged gluten-free foods are available on grocery store shelves to make going gluten free easier. But read labels! Many of these products are just gluten-free junk food, loaded with sugar, preservatives, additives, and stabilizers. Eat naturally gluten-free foods or follow the recipes in this book to make wholesome gluten-free options.

Step 2: The Challenge Phase (Reintroduction)

During the challenge phase of the Elimination Diet, you will observe how you respond when you reintroduce into your diet the foods you eliminated. Use your Food Mood Poop Journal to track your emotional and physical reactions. When you reintroduce a suspect food, do it at each meal on that day. It is best to start off with a food that you suspect is not a problem for you and reintroduce commonly problematic foods such as dairy and gluten only at the end.

Let's say you start by reintroducing corn on Monday. The process is simple: Eat a generous amount of corn for breakfast, lunch, and dinner. It can be in any form; frozen, fresh corn kernels or corn tortillas. Tune in to your body right away. There are two possible outcomes: You start feeling some changes (digestive issues, brain fog, fatigue, headaches, anxiety, just feeling "off") within thirty minutes to two days later, or you get no reaction at all.

If you develop no symptoms on the first day, continue eating the food you are testing on the second day as well. Sometimes the food reaction manifests after the first day. Even if no symptoms occur immediately on the second day, wait two more days and observe whether you get any reactions. (For a complete list of possible reactions, refer to the beginning of this chapter.) If you do not react, it is a sign that you have no problem with that food.

Weight gain can be a common sign of food intolerance as well. Measure your weight toward the end of the Elimination Diet, first thing in the morning. Let's say you are ready to reintroduce gluten on a Monday. Jot down your weight on Monday morning before you start eating it. Weigh yourself on Tuesday morning; if your weight shot up more than 2 pounds in one day, there is a high likelihood that this food is a suspect.

One of my clients, a senior executive at a top Silicon Valley tech company, came to me complaining of severe mood swings and aggression directed at her co-workers and her husband. Her behavior had gotten so bad that her husband had started divorce proceedings. As you can imagine, her career was on the rocks as well. We discussed the Elimination Diet as the first step on her healing journey, but she was reluctant to give up dairy products. She was a vegetarian (for religious reasons), and dairy was her main source of protein. But she gave it up anyway, and to her great surprise, removing all dairy products helped her become a totally different person, one who was calm and kind. She said she didn't even know she could ever be such a person. As you can see, food can have a huge impact on our lives!

A NOTE ON REINTRODUCING DAIRY

Even though I advise eliminating all dairy products from your diet, I know that it can be difficult to do. Therefore, when reintroducing dairy, test four different categories:

- Cow's milk and cheese

- Cow's yogurt, kefir, or cottage cheese

- Goat or sheep cheese

- Goat or sheep yogurt

You may find it easier to digest fermented dairy products or dairy from a goat or sheep.

Even if you find that you can tolerate some dairy (such as goat cheese or fermented dairy like yogurt), I advise that you treat dairy as an occasional indulgence and not an everyday food.

Step 3: Completion of the Elimination Diet

After reintroducing all of the foods you have eliminated, you will know your food intolerances. Remove these foods from your diet to heal your digestion and reduce inflammation, which is essential for regaining hormonal balance and overall well-being.

If you had a mild reaction to a food, you may be able to keep it in your diet, but eat it less than once a week. Eating a food too often can result in a food sensitivity. For example, replacing dairy with almond-based products such as almond milk and yogurt may result in an almond intolerance or allergy.

By the time you complete the Elimination Diet, you should see a decrease in the number and intensity of your symptoms. Continue to use your Food Mood Poop Journal to monitor what you eat, and always listen to your body's signals—they are there to tell you what bothers it.

 ALTERNATIVES TO THE ELIMINATION DIET

In case the Elimination Diet does not produce concrete results, you can also try IgG testing, the heart rate method, or kinesiology (also known as "muscle testing"). Get the full scoop at www.HormonesBalance.com/book.

Elimination Diet 14-Day Sample Meal Plan for Two

For warm lemon water: Add 2 tablespoons freshly squeezed lemon juice to 8 to 16 ounces warm water. Lime juice or apple cider vinegar can also be used.

Bone broth: Sip 1 to 2 cups broth per day with a dash of coconut milk, freshly grated ginger, lemon juice, and sea salt.

Abbreviations
[NR] No recipe
[LO] Leftovers
[MA] Made ahead; full recipe or parts of
[DB] Double the recipe
EVOO Extra virgin olive oil

WEEK 1

Morning ritual/ breakfast	Snack (optional)	Lunch	Dinner	Bedtime ritual (optional)
Day 1				
Warm lemon water Healing Bone Broth [MA] (page 162) Farmer's Wife's Breakfast [DB] (page 182)	Salmon and Avocado in Nori Sheets [DB] (page 298)	Quick Salads— Four Ways, pick one (page 254)	Creamy Rosemary Chicken [DB] (page 249) Creamy Celeriac and Cauliflower Mash (page 267) Steamed or sautéed greens or broccolini with EVOO and sea salt [NR]	Everyday Nourishing Tea (page 306) Raspberry Melties [DB] (page 338)
Day 2				
Warm lemon water Healing Bone Broth [LO] Farmer's Wife's Breakfast [LO]	Salmon and Avocado in Nori Sheets [DB]	Nutritious Quick Bowls, pick one (page 232)	Creamy Rosemary Chicken [LO] Creamy Celeriac and Cauliflower Mash [LO] Steamed or sautéed greens or broccolini with EVOO and sea salt [LO]	Liver Cleanser Tea (page 307) Raspberry Melties [LO]
Day 3				
Warm lemon water Ginger Beet Kvass [MA] (page 317) Breakfast Casserole One: Salmon and Broccoli (page 189)	Decadent Chocolate Cherry Smoothie (page 207)	Quick Salads— Four Ways, pick one Healing Bone Broth [LO]	Fennel and Coriander Crusted Liver (page 246) Creamy Celeriac and Cauliflower Mash [LO]	Nourishing Lattes, pick one (page 309) Raspberry Melties [LO]
Day 4				
Daily Balancer Tea (page 306) Teff and Cherry Porridge (page 198)	Ginger Beet Kvass [LO]	Fennel and Coriander Crusted Liver [LO] Sautéed greens with EVOO, lemon, and sea salt [NR]	Seriously Mushroom Soup (page 216)	Healing Bone Broth [LO] Raspberry Melties [LO]

Morning ritual/ breakfast	Snack (optional)	Lunch	Dinner	Bedtime ritual (optional)
Day 5				
Warm lemon water Ginger Beet Kvass [LO] Teff and Cherry Porridge [LO]	Energizing Matcha Lime Smoothie [DB] (page 191)	Seriously Mushroom Soup [LO] Raspberry Melties [LO]	Quick Salads—Four Ways, pick one (page 254) Healing Bone Broth [LO]	Nourishing Lattes, pick one (page 309)
Day 6				
Warm lemon water Ginger Beet Kvass [LO] Farmer's Wife's Breakfast [DB]	Carrot and Beet Smoothie (page 203)	Nutritious Quick Bowls, pick one [DB] Healing Bone Broth [LO]	Porcini Mushroom Beef Stew (page 224) Side salad of mixed bitter greens with lemon, EVOO, and sea salt [NR]	Sugar Balancer Tea (page 308) Raspberry Melties [LO]
Day 7				
Warm lemon water Healing Bone Broth [LO] Farmer's Wife's Breakfast [LO]	Better Than Coffee Latte (page 313)	Porcini Mushroom Beef Stew [LO] Ginger Beet Kvass [LO]	Japanese Seaweed and Cucumber Salad (page 273)	Liver Cleanser Tea Raspberry Melties [LO]

WEEK 2

Morning ritual/ breakfast	Snack (optional)	Lunch	Dinner	Bedtime ritual (optional)
Day 8				
Warm lemon water Porcini Mushroom Beef Stew [LO]	Decadent Chocolate Cherry Smoothie	Japanese Seaweed and Cucumber Salad [LO]	Bacon, Oysters, and Collard Greens Stir Fry [DB] (page 204)	Immune-Boosting Chicken Broth (page 158)
Day 9				
Warm lemon water Breakfast Casserole Two: Pork Chops and Apples (page 195) Fresh greens, lemon, EVOO, and sea salt [NR]	Matcha Frappe (page 299)	Bacon, Oysters, and Collard Greens Stir Fry [LO]	Seriously Mushroom Soup	Liver Cleanser Tea Raspberry Melties [LO]

Morning ritual/ breakfast	Snack (optional)	Lunch	Dinner	Bedtime ritual (optional)
Day 10				
Warm lemon water Seriously Mushroom Soup [LO]	Easy French Pate [MA] (page 290) with vegetable sticks [NR] or Flaxseed Crackers [MA] (page 327)	Quick Salads—Four Ways, pick one	Walnut Crusted Salmon [DB] (page 244) Detoxing Beet and Carrot Salad (page 252)	Immune-Boosting Chicken Broth [LO]
Day 11				
Warm lemon water Adrenal Love Tea (page 305) Teff and Cherry Porridge	Easy French Pate [LO] with vegetable sticks [NR] or Flaxseed Crackers [LO]	Walnut Crusted Salmon [LO] Detoxing Beet and Carrot Salad [LO]; add Life-Giving Sprouts [MA] [DB] (page 163)	Seriously Mushroom Soup [LO]	Immune Booster Tea (page 303) Raspberry Melties [LO]
Day 12				
Warm lemon water Teff and Cherry Porridge [LO]	Immune-Boosting Chicken Broth [LO] Raspberry Melties [LO]	Steam 'n Toss Veggies and Proteins on the Run (page 260)	Nomad's Kebabs (page 239) Detoxing Beet and Carrot Salad; add Life-Giving Sprouts [LO]	Nourishing Lattes
Day 13				
Warm lemon water Adrenal Love Tea Sweet Potato and Sage Pancakes (page 179)	Rosemary Pear Muffin (page 335)	Nomad's Kebabs [LO] Detoxing Beet and Carrot Salad [LO]; add Life-Giving Sprouts [LO]	Nutritious Quick Bowls, pick one [DB] Immune-Boosting Chicken Broth [LO]	Immune Booster Tea Raspberry Melties [LO]
Day 14				
Warm lemon water Coconut Kefir Chia Pudding (page 185)	Rosemary Pear Muffin [LO]	Sweet Potato and Sage Pancakes [LO] Fresh greens with Life-Giving Sprouts [LO], EVOO, lemon, and sea salt [NR] Ginger Beet Kvass [LO]	Steam 'n Toss Veggies and Proteins on the Run	Immune-Boosting Chicken Broth [LO]

Chapter 3

Balancing Sugar Levels for Hormonal Health

The second leg of the three-legged stool of hormonal balance, which is often wobbling and making the whole "sitting on the stool" experience a real challenge, is your blood sugar level leg. Balanced sugar levels are essential for your hormonal health. Sugar addiction, sugar cravings, and high or low sugar levels can undermine your efforts to rebalance your hormones. Among my friends, colleagues, clients, and community, I find that any mention of sugar prompts a variety of emotions: from denial ("I just need it after dinner, but I'm not addicted") and excuses ("I've always had a sweet tooth") to shame and guilt ("I'm so angry with myself for having that cupcake"). Roughly three out of four women I work with have a less-than-healthy relationship with sugar. They are either suffering from hypoglycemia (low blood sugar levels), hyperglycemia (high blood sugar levels), sugar cravings, or feeling controlled by

sugar. This is hardly surprising. One of the first things I distinctly remember about moving to the United States is how sweet everything tasted, how many names sugar had, and how much of it was hiding everywhere, including in savory foods like soups, in salad dressings, in almost all snacks, and in condiments such as ketchup.

More sugar is in our food than ever before. In 2006, the *Chicago Tribune* published an investigative article stating that Kraft Foods Inc. hired scientists from Philip Morris USA, the tobacco company, to develop foods that encourage addiction (or "loyalty," as the industry calls it) to their products with the use of sugar, salt, and fat. If you grew up in the United States eating the standard American diet (SAD), you were most likely fed sugar-loaded food right from the start, without your parents even realizing it. Mother's milk is sweet, so it's no surprise we are attracted to sugary foods from the time we are babies, and food manufacturers work on getting us to want sugar even more from the day we start eating solid foods. Most of the leading baby food makers, even the organic brands, contain no less than 10 grams sugar per pouch of pureed food. That's 2½ teaspoons per serving for an infant. (For an easy reference: 1 teaspoon sugar is equivalent to almost 4 grams [3.8 grams, to be exact]).

Furthermore, during the time that governmental agencies encouraged a low-fat diet, which was supposed to lead to better health but did not, companies added more sugar to their products to compensate for the poor flavor that resulted once the fat was removed. According to the Centers for Disease Control and Prevention, this resulted in the average American consuming 17 teaspoons sugar a day—more than three times what I recommend.

If you recognize any of the symptoms of hypoglycemia or hyperglycemia, you have some work to do to balance your sugar levels. Many women with hypoglycemia use sugar "to bring back their sugar levels," which is a

Signs and Symptoms of High and Low Sugar Levels

HYPOGLYCEMIA (LOW BLOOD SUGAR LEVELS)

Having to eat every few hours
    to avoid crashing
Needing sugar to "bring the sugar levels up"
Shakiness
Nervousness or anxiety
Moodiness and feeling unfocused
Sweating, chills, and clamminess
Irritability or impatience
Confusion, including delirium
Rapid/fast heartbeat
Light-headedness or dizziness

HYPERGLYCEMIA (HIGH BLOOD SUGAR LEVELS)

Blood glucose level greater than
    90 mg/dL (even though labs/doctors
    say 99 mg/dL is acceptable)*
HA1c greater than 5.4 (even though labs/
    doctors say 5.6 is acceptable)
Insulin greater than 15 IU/mL (even though
    labs/doctors say 24.9 IU/mL is acceptable)
Blurry vision
Difficulty concentrating
Frequent urination
Constant thirst
Constant hunger
Fatigue after eating
Stubborn belly fat

*Use functional medicine ranges that are more stringent than lab ranges, which, in some markers, such as glucose and HA1c, are derived from the average values of tested patients. Given how sick people are, some of these ranges are not considered "healthy" by functional medicine practitioners.

harmful misconception. Most people start with hypoglycemia and progress to developing hyperglycemia, insulin resistance, leptin resistance, and type 2 diabetes. The good news is that you can reverse these conditions by applying the solutions presented in this chapter. Whether you have hypoglycemia or hyperglycemia, you most likely have an unhealthy relationship with sugar, that is, you crave it, can't focus without it, and feel tired and sick when you eat it. Know that this is not your fault. Craving sugar and feeling that uncontrollable need for a cupcake or three is not about a lack of willpower. Our desire for sugar is based on a chemical reaction in the gut and the brain, and besides, sugar is highly addictive.

UNDERSTANDING SUGAR ADDICTION

Scientists have found that sugar stimulates the same pleasure centers of the brain as cocaine and heroin. Neuroscientists at Connecticut College found that "rats formed an equally strong association between the pleasurable effects of eating Oreos and a specific environment as they did between cocaine or morphine and a specific environment. They also found that eating cookies activated more neurons in the brain's 'pleasure center' than exposure to drugs of abuse." It should come as no surprise, then, that giving up sugar can be as hard as giving up any other addictive drug.

To know how to break this addiction, it's important to understand that sugar cravings are driven by emotional and physiological triggers.

Emotional triggers: Let's go back to your childhood for just a second. Did your parents deprive you of treats? Did they bribe or reward you with sugar? Were you raised by critical, abusive, or emotionally unavailable parents? Was sugar your best friend—something you could always turn to, to make you feel better? Did you have low self-esteem as a child and young adult? Did you feel like sugar would make you feel better? Do you see the same patterns of reaching for sugar to make you feel better in your adult life?

If your cravings stem from emotional triggers, I recommend working with a skilled therapist to resolve your past or present issues and to find feel-good foods other than those that contain sugar (try the desserts in this book). Only when you address these emotional triggers will you be free from sugar, guilt, and shame. And only then will you truly be able to eat well and heal.

Physiological triggers: When you were a child, were cakes, cookies, sodas, and treats always around your house? Did you take antibiotics as a child or young adult with no probiotic treatments afterward? Did you live on processed foods during college? Have you had a "sweet tooth" your whole life? Has sugar been your go-to source of energy?

If you are nodding yes to any of these questions, there is a chance that these past food habits and choices, combined with the possibility of Candida overgrowth, are at play here. Most of the women I work with have a problem with Candida, a leading cause of uncontrollable sugar cravings. Eliminating Candida will help reduce sugar cravings.

In addition, the more sugar you eat, the more your body will crave it. It takes higher and higher amounts of sugar to achieve a dopamine "sugar" high.

THE IMPACT OF SUGAR ON YOUR HORMONES AND OVERALL HEALTH

Sugar has been labeled as "white death," and this label is in no way sensational.

Sugar and inflammation. Chronic inflammation can shut down hormone receptors, making them unresponsive to hormone molecules entering the cells and doing their job. Sugar, alongside gut issues, chronic stress, and lack of sleep, is a major contributor to inflammation in the body.

High testosterone levels. High blood sugar levels are the leading cause of high testosterone in women (and low testosterone in men). High blood sugar levels suppress the sex hormone binding globulin (SHBG), a hormone responsible for, as the name implies, binding and regulating excess sex hormones such as testosterone. One of the diagnostic criteria for PCOS is high blood sugar levels (glucose, HA1c, and insulin) and high testosterone levels. Therefore, the first recommended dietary step for women

with PCOS is to lower their blood sugar levels to sensitize their insulin receptors.

Estrogen dominance. High blood sugar levels can also cause or contribute to estrogen dominance. Estrogen is made from testosterone, so if you suffer from high blood sugar levels, which cause high testosterone levels, you may also be experiencing estrogen dominance.

Adrenal fatigue. Experiencing hyperglycemia or hypoglycemia is stressful to the body because the adrenals are responsible for balancing the sugar highs and lows. Sugar is a stimulant, and eating it when your adrenals are exhausted adds fuel to the fire, exhausting them even further.

Insulin resistance. According to researchers at the University of Washington in Seattle, 32 percent of the American population is insulin resistant. Insulin's job is to "sweep up" glucose from the blood and let the glucose into cells. Insulin resistance happens when the body cells do not let the insulin in (hence "resistance"). This can happen because of a diet overloaded with sugar, and especially fructose; processed carbohydrates; and systemic body inflammation. Symptoms include high blood sugar levels, fatigue, resistance to weight loss, belly fat, depression, prediabetes, and type 2 diabetes.

Leptin resistance (and why you can't stop eating). If you are overweight and never feel full after a meal, another physiological factor

Not All Sugars Are the Same

[!] "Sugar" is a general term for sweet, short-chain, soluble carbohydrates. Knowing the difference between two types of sugar, glucose and fructose, will help you to understand the impact sugar has on hormonal health.

Glucose, an important energy source for our cells and organs, comes from the food we eat. Carbohydrates such as fruit, bread, pasta, and cereals are common sources of glucose. Our stomachs break these foods down into glucose, which is then absorbed into the bloodstream. Glucose in our bloodstream is called "blood sugar." Higher glucose in the blood prompts the pancreas to release insulin, a hormone that facilitates the entry of glucose into cells.

Fructose is a form of sugar found naturally in many fruits, vegetables, and sweeteners such as agave, honey, and brown rice syrup. Since fructose is 73 percent sweeter than glucose and acts as a preservative, it is very popular with processed food manufacturers and often is added to packaged foods and beverages such as soda and fruit-flavored drinks. Fructose is not a preferred energy source for the cells in our body and is more fat-producing than glucose. It is also metabolized in the body very differently than glucose. *Only the liver can break down fructose,* and fructose does not stimulate the release of insulin. Since fructose has no effect on blood sugar levels, sweeteners such as agave have been declared "the better and healthier sweeteners." But this overlooks the negative impact on the liver of too much fructose. Give the liver enough fructose and tiny fat droplets begin to accumulate in liver cells—just like what happens to the livers of people who consume too much alcohol. In this case, it is called "nonalcoholic fatty liver disease." Too much fructose in the liver also results in increased belly fat, elevated triglycerides (a form of fat), increased LDL (the so-called bad cholesterol), increased production of free radicals (energetic compounds that can damage DNA and cells), and increased production of uric acid (linked to hypertension and kidney failure), not to mention a sluggish liver.

Today, numerous scientific studies show that a diet high in fructose is responsible for both insulin resistance and leptin resistance.

---

may be leptin resistance. Leptin is a hormone produced in the fat cells of the body that tells the brain when you have had enough to eat and it's time to stop. For someone with a lot of body fat, leptin levels are high. Too much leptin will cause the leptin receptors in the brain to shut down, and the brain will be unable to "hear" the message. Even though the signal to stop eating has been sent, it is not being received and the brain erroneously thinks the body is starving, compelling you to eat more and conserve energy (hence storing fat).

As you can see, calorie counting, dieting, exercise, willpower, or ignorance (a common accusation directed at overweight people) have very little to do with losing weight if a person is suffering from insulin or leptin resistance.

Can you reverse them? Absolutely! Is it easy? There is no magic pill, but you can certainly do it with the diet changes I outline in the Sugar-Balancing Guide. If you are willing to put in the effort like the women I have worked with, you will succeed as well!

Sugar affects your mood and self-esteem. When we eat sugar, our brain rewards us by releasing mood-enhancing neurotransmitters such as serotonin (a mood balancer), dopamine (which mediates a sense of reward and pleasure in the brain), and beta-endorphins (natural pain killers), resulting in a short-lived high. It is no surprise, then, that many former drug, gambling, and sex addicts and alcoholics recover from their addictions only to become sugar addicts. A diet high in sugar has been linked to poor mental health, including an increased risk of depression, worsened anxiety symptoms, compromised cognitive abilities such as learning and memory, and low self-esteem.

Empty calories and a nutrient robber. Sugar provides "empty calories," that is, it is a food with no nutrients. But what's worse, it robs us of key vitamins and minerals. Fructose, according to research, inhibits the absorption of calcium, magnesium, and vitamin D, which are all critical in bone health. Sugar depletes vitamin B1, which is essential in energy production and liver detoxification, and vitamin C,

which can lead to a weakened immune system. Sugar also lowers stomach acid production and pulls our body's pH in the acidic direction.

Sugar and cancer. Sugar feeds cancer cells. Researchers at the Stanford University School of Medicine have found that glucose deprivation can kill cancer cells. It is not a surprise to learn that women with high sugar levels are more prone to developing breast cancer.

What does a craving for chocolate mean?

✅ If you are craving chocolate, chances are that your body is not calling for sugar, but for magnesium. Check out the Hot Chocolate with Pink Roses recipe on page 314 for inspiration.

HOW TO BALANCE YOUR SUGAR LEVELS

Now that you know how bad sugar is for your health and hormones, I hope you are inspired to kick the sugar habit and balance your sugar levels. The good news is that once you do that, your taste buds will recalibrate and you will find that sugary things taste disgustingly sweet. That margarita will taste awful. That apple juice will need juice from vegetables such as celery, cucumber, or fennel bulb to feel nourishing. That fruit smoothie will taste like a sugar bomb. You will naturally ignore what the front of a product label says and turn to the ingredients list to check how much sugar the product contains. Your power bar brands will change. And you won't spend any more time searching for a sugar "pick me up" to beat a 3 P.M. slump.

Limit the Amount of Sugar You Consume

How much sugar is okay? The U.S. dietary recommendation is a maximum of 32 grams sugar (8 teaspoons) per day. In my practice, I recommend keeping sugar intake to a maximum of 20 grams (5 teaspoons) per day. That includes sugar found naturally in food (such as in carrots and sweet potatoes) and added sugar. If you are doing the anti-Candida diet or are working on reversing insulin resistance and PCOS, I would bring that number down even lower, to no more than 2 teaspoons per day.

Become a sugar detective. According to the U.S. Census Bureau, each American consumes 136 pounds of sugar per year. That is 35 teaspoons per day! You must be thinking, "That's most certainly not me! I don't drink soda and eat junk." Even if that's the case, you can still overload on sugar easily. One of the biggest steps you can take toward self-healing is to bring a great sense of self-awareness to the amount of sugar you consume daily.

And let me tell you, it might be a shocker.

First, take stock of what you have in your refrigerator and pantry. Look at the backs of packages for nutritional information rather than the often empty promises on the fronts of packages. Examine the sugar content of every product. And remember:

4 grams sugar = 1 teaspoon sugar

Take a look at *everything*, including canned soups, snacks, juices, cereals, cookies, kombucha, ketchup, almond milk, milkshakes, bottled coffee drinks, and ice cream. One of the biggest surprises is how much of a sugar bomb coffee drinks can be. For instance, a 16-ounce Starbucks Caffe Vanilla Frappuccino Blended Coffee with nonfat milk and whipped cream contains 69 grams sugar, or more than 17 teaspoons. Can you imagine eating 17 teaspoons of pure sugar? Yet that's just what you are doing when you drink the entire thing. Energy and snack bars are another surprising source of sugar: Clif Bars contain between 20 and 22 grams sugar (more than 5 teaspoons), a Larabar Cherry Pie bar has 23 grams, and an Almond and Apricot Kind bar contains 10 grams.*

✔️ **Sauerkraut Curbs Your Sugar Cravings**

Many of my clients report having fewer sugar cravings when they add probiotic-rich foods such as sauerkraut, dill pickles, coconut yogurt, and kimchi to their diets.

---

* All product sugar levels are correct at the time of publication and are subject to change. For the most up-to-date information, read the product labels.

Eat a Protein, Fat, and Fiber (PFF) Breakfast

I have received hundreds of emails from women claiming that eating a breakfast rich in protein, fat, and fiber—and not carbohydrates such as cereals, pancakes, toast and jam, and oatmeal—has changed their lives. They report craving no sugar and coffee, having more energy, and sleeping more deeply. It makes perfect sense—a PFF breakfast helps stabilize your sugar levels right from the start of the day.

PFF breakfasts have been a game changer. My blood sugar is now balanced first thing in the morning, setting me up for more energy, better mood, and balanced hormones, and I am satiated for hours without dips in my blood sugar throughout the day. I no longer crave sugar and caffeine or need to snack throughout the day. My sleep has improved and my athletic performance is stronger. And PFF breakfasts have also been a great way to invite more creativity into the kitchen. — JONLYN ZYDENBOS

In addition to reading the labels of packaged goods for sugar content, examine the labels of widely popular juices (for example, juices from Jamba Juice range from the Great Greens containing 17 grams sugar, or more than 4 teaspoons, to Kale Orange Power containing a surprising 33 grams, or more than 8 teaspoons*), probiotic-rich health drinks, lattes, and smoothies. Even though these may not be highly processed foods, they can still contribute significantly to your sugar highs and lows.

The bottom line: Always check the sugar content in your food, and limit your intake accordingly. Better yet, make food and beverages from scratch so that you can control the amount of sugar they contain.

Watch out for the serving size. Often, a product we typically consume in one sitting reads "2 servings," creating the illusion of a lower sugar content. For example, a bottle of kombucha states "1 serving contains 8 grams" (that's 2 teaspoons) and there are two servings per bottle. "Not bad," you think. But if you drink the whole bottle in one sitting, like most people, you will actually ingest 16 grams sugar, or 4 teaspoons.

Choose Healthier Sweeteners

What is the best sugar and sweetener? My favorites are coconut syrup, blackstrap molasses, honey, and maple syrup. For a complete list of sugars and sweeteners, see page 138.

How to Make Food Taste Sweeter

Add a pinch of sea salt to juices and smoothies as well as muffin, cake, and cookie batters to amplify their sweetness.

Why you shouldn't use artificial sweeteners. Artificial sweeteners are far more toxic than you imagine. Studies have linked artificial sweeteners to changes in the gut microflora, obesity, cardiovascular diseases, inflammation and depression, and ironically, insulin resistance.

 You will find a list of healthy low-sugar power and protein bars, cereals, juices, smoothies, lattes, and kombuchas and my advice on "new" sweeteners such as stevia, xylitol, monk fruit, and erythritol at www.HormonesBalance.com/book.

Choose Low-Sugar Foods

I am often asked, "Should I stop eating all fruit to avoid fructose?" The answer is no. Instead, cut out all processed forms of fructose, and be mindful of how much fruit you consume and how it affects you.

SUGAR-BALANCING GUIDE

As with any addiction or highly ingrained habit, the first step is for you to acknowledge that you have a problem, and then you have to want to fix it. You do not need to go cold turkey or try every change I suggest all at once. You may find that doing one thing at a time and seeing small improvements encourages you enough to keep going and make additional changes. Or you may find that cold turkey is best for you. There is no right or wrong

way to part from sugar. Honor your desire to make this change by finding a way that works for you.

Use this guide to help you put the content of this chapter plus additional strategies into action by following these simple suggestions. To download a digital version of this guide, go to www.HormonesBalance.com/book. Print it out and hang it in the kitchen to help you make this new routine easy to follow.

ADD (+)

PFF Breakfast. Breakfast rich in proteins, fat, and fiber, within one hour of rising. Refer to breakfast recipes in this book.

Protein-rich foods and snacks. Some examples are soaked nuts and seeds, jerky, kale chips, and bacon bits. Eat high-protein small meals if you feel your blood sugar levels dropping.

Fat. Fat slows down sugar absorption and helps regulate blood sugar levels. Refer to the Fats and Oils Guide (page 139) to pick the right fats. Add 2 to 3 tablespoons per day.

Fiber. Helps to slow down the metabolism of sugar (a good thing!). Great sources are ground flaxseeds, chia seeds, and other nuts and seeds. Add 30 grams or 2 tablespoons per day.

Low glycemic index/glycemic load. Focus on foods that are low on the glycemic index/glycemic load (GI/GL) scale, especially in the morning. (See www.glycemicindex.com.) Foods high on the GI/GL scale deregulate blood sugar levels.

Sugar selection. Refer to Sugars and Sweeteners for details (page 138).

Fenugreek. Regulates glucose, HA1c, insulin, and LDL cholesterol levels. Make my Sugar Balancer Tea (page 308) and sip it daily.

Probiotic-rich food and probiotics. Fermented food helps reduce sugar cravings. Add 1 to 2 servings per day. Also add top-quality probiotics like MegaSporeBiotic, Equilibrium, or Custom Probiotic.

Supplements. Consider the Sugar Balance Kit on HormoneBalanceNutritionals.com.

Detox. Make time and space for a detox once a year in spring or fall; it's a good way to reset your body and reverse sugar cravings.

REMOVE (–)

Artificial sweeteners. Avoid them. Artificial sweeteners can cause neurological damage, gut dysbiosis, and increased inflammation.

Sugar high in fructose. Fructose gets metabolized in the liver, creating additional stress on the liver. Refer to Sugars and Sweeteners (page 138) for more details.

Processed and packaged foods. These include white flour, white sugar, refined grains, additives, and preservatives, as well as cereals, rice puffs, quinoa puffs, and protein shakes and powders.

Coffee. Coffee increases sugar levels. Get off caffeine, or, if you must consume it, do so with meals and never on an empty stomach.

Alcohol. Alcohol is sugar, too. If you must drink, limit to two to three drinks per week, always with or after food. Avoid drinking late at night as this may disturb your sleep and create additional load on the liver. Avoid drink mixers as they contain high-fructose corn syrup.

Late-night desserts and snacks. Eating sugar before bedtime is a recipe for a poor night's sleep and additional strain on the liver. If you must snack, have nuts, seeds, kale chips, or jerky.

Food intolerances. Gluten, dairy, eggs, soy, corn, nightshades, yeast, sometimes grains, and of course sugar can contribute to fluctuating sugar levels. Do the Elimination Diet to find out what your sensitivities are.

Stress. Chronic stress depletes us of serotonin and dopamine; sugar creates an illusion of a quick fix, but instead it is dangerous. Learn to respond to stress differently or avoid it, if you can.

BALANCE

Tune in to your body. "Good" food, such as grains, might not be good for you. For some people with insulin resistance, hypoglycemia, or type 1 diabetes, even gluten-free grains can be triggers and cause leptin resistance.

Use supplements strategically, as most people take too many of them. Chromium picolinate and magnesium (in malate or glycinate form) can help reduce glucose and insulin levels. Take them in conjunction with dietary changes to get the best results. Studies show that berberine has the same efficacy as metformin but without the side effects.

Maintain a regular movement routine. Weight training improves insulin sensitivity. Having more muscle increases the surface area for insulin to do its work. Avoid excessive exercise if suffering from adrenal dysfunction.

Sugar-Balancing 14-Day Sample Meal Plan for Two

This meal plan will also lower testosterone and treat PCOS.

For warm lemon water: Add 2 tablespoons freshly squeezed lemon juice to 8 to 16 ounces warm water. Lime juice or apple cider vinegar can also be used.

Bone broth: Sip 1 to 2 cups per day with a dash of coconut milk, freshly grated ginger, lemon juice, and sea salt.

Add 1 to 2 tablespoons collagen powder to smoothies, teas, soups, and stews at least once per day.

Abbreviations
[NR] No recipe
[LO] Leftovers
[MA] Made ahead; full recipe or parts of
[DB] Double the recipe
EVOO Extra virgin olive oil

WEEK 1

Morning ritual/ breakfast	Snack (optional)	Lunch	Dinner	Bedtime ritual (optional)
Day 1				
Warm lemon water	Nourishing Lattes, pick one (page 309)	Nutritious Quick Bowls, pick one [DB] (page 232)	Icelandic Fish Stew (page 214)	Immune-Boosting Chicken Broth [MA] (page 158), freeze half for next week
Sugar Balancer Tea (page 308)				
Farmer's Wife's Breakfast [DB] (page 182)				Raspberry Melties [DB] (page 338)
Day 2				
Warm lemon water	Energizing Matcha Lime Smoothie [DB] (page 191)	Nutritious Quick Bowls, pick one [LO]	Icelandic Fish Stew [LO]	Easy Digestion Tea (page 305)
Sugar Balancer Tea				
Farmer's Wife's Breakfast [LO]				Kudzu Calming Pudding (page 348)
Zucchini Olive Muffin (page 205)				

Morning ritual/ breakfast	Snack (optional)	Lunch	Dinner	Bedtime ritual (optional)
Day 3				
Warm lemon water Sugar Balancer Tea Breakfast Casserole One: Salmon and Broccoli (page 189)	Zucchini Olive Muffin [LO] Raspberry Melties [LO]	Icelandic Fish Stew [LO]	Fennel and Coriander Crusted Liver (page 246) Creamy Celeriac and Cauliflower Mash (page 267)	Easy Digestion Tea Kudzu Calming Pudding [LO]
Day 4				
Warm lemon water Sugar Balancer Tea Bacon, Oysters, and Collard Greens Stir Fry (page 204)	Immune-Boosting Chicken Broth [LO] Zucchini Olive Muffin [LO]	Fennel and Coriander Crusted Liver [LO] Creamy Celeriac and Cauliflower Mash [LO]	Sticky Spare Ribs Casserole (page 242) Side salad of mixed bitter greens with lemon, EVOO, and sea salt [NR]	Easy Digestion Tea Raspberry Melties [LO]
Day 5				
Warm lemon water Sugar Balancer Tea Coconut Kefir Chia Pudding [LO]	Better Than Coffee Latte (page 313) Zucchini Olive Muffin [LO]	Sticky Spare Ribs Casserole [LO] Creamy Celeriac and Cauliflower Mash [LO]	Quick Detoxifying Soup (page 218)	Nourishing Lattes, pick one (page 309) Raspberry Melties [LO]
Day 6				
Warm lemon water Sugar Balancer Tea Breakfast Casserole Two: Pork Chops and Apples (page 195)	Creamy Lime Pudding (page 342)	Quick Detoxifying Soup [LO] Flaxseed Crackers [MA] (page 327)	Steam 'n Toss Veggies and Proteins on the Run (page 260)	Immune-Boosting Chicken Broth [LO] Zucchini Olive Muffin [LO]
Day 7				
Warm lemon water Sugar Balancer Tea Parsnip Dill Pancake with Arugula and Smoked Salmon (page 199)	Decadent Chocolate Cherry Smoothie (page 207)	Quick Detoxifying Soup [LO] Flaxseed Crackers [LO]	Easy Chicken Curry Stew (page 212) Side salad of mixed bitter greens with lemon, EVOO, and sea salt [NR]	Nourishing Lattes, pick one Creamy Lime Pudding [LO]

WEEK 2

Morning ritual/ breakfast	Snack (optional)	Lunch	Dinner	Bedtime ritual (optional)
Day 8				
Warm lemon water Sugar Balancer Tea Breakfast Casserole One: Salmon and Broccoli	Creamy Lime Pudding [LO]	Nutritious Quick Bowls, pick one [DB] Flaxseed Crackers [LO]	Easy Chicken Curry Stew [LO] Side salad of mixed bitter greens with lemon, EVOO, and sea salt [NR]	Immune-Boosting Chicken Broth [LO] Raspberry Melties [LO]
Day 9				
Warm lemon water Sugar Balancer Tea Teff and Cherry Porridge (page 198)	Easy French Pate [MA] (page 290) Flaxseed Crackers [LO] Strawberry Ginger Ale [MA] (ferment takes 1 to 3 days) (page 318)	Steam 'n Toss Veggies and Proteins on the Run	Nomad's Kebabs (page 239) Jicama and Pomegranate Slaw (page 268)	Nourishing Lattes, pick one Raspberry Melties [LO]
Day 10				
Warm lemon water Sugar Balancer Tea Teff and Cherry Porridge [LO]	Easy French Pate [LO] Flaxseed Crackers [LO]	Quick Salads— Four Ways, pick one (page 254)	Nomad's Kebabs [LO] Jicama and Pomegranate Slaw [LO]	Easy Digestion Tea Kudzu Calming Pudding
Day 11				
Warm lemon water Sugar Balancer Tea Farmer's Wife's Breakfast [DB]	Easy French Pate [LO] Flaxseed Crackers [LO]	Jicama and Pomegranate Slaw [LO]	Butter Cod with Gremolata (page 240) Side salad of mixed bitter greens with lemon, EVOO, and sea salt	Kudzu Calming Pudding [LO] Nourishing Lattes, pick one
Day 12				
Warm lemon water Immune-Boosting Chicken Broth [LO] Farmer's Wife's Breakfast [LO]	Nourishing Lattes, pick one Flaxseed Crackers [LO]	Quick Salads—Four Ways, pick one	Butter Cod with Gremolata Side salad of mixed bitter greens with lemon, EVOO, and sea salt [NR]	Immune-Boosting Chicken Broth [LO] Raspberry Melties [LO]

Morning ritual/ breakfast	Snack (optional)	Lunch	Dinner	Bedtime ritual (optional)
Day 13				
Warm lemon water Sugar Balancer Tea Breakfast Casserole Two: Pork Chops and Apples	Energizing Matcha Lime Smoothie [DB]	Nutritious Quick Bowls, pick one [DB]	Rosemary and Garlic Stuffed Lamb Roast (page 251) Sauerkraut Carrot Salad [DB] (page 264)	Immune-Boosting Chicken Broth [LO] Raspberry Melties [LO]
Day 14				
Warm lemon water Parsnip Dill Pancake with Arugula and Smoked Salmon	Deep Green Spirulina Smoothie (page 197)	Nutritious Quick Bowls, pick one [DB]	Rosemary and Garlic Stuffed Lamb Roast [LO] Sauerkraut Carrot Salad [LO]	Flaxseed Crackers [LO] Raspberry Melties [LO]

Chapter 4

Detoxing Your Liver for Hormonal Balance

A healthy liver is the third leg of your hormonal balance stool. The liver plays a large role in regulating our hormones, but it is often overlooked when it comes to women's hormonal struggles. This is especially true with estrogen dominance and thyroid health. When I was first diagnosed with estrogen dominance, after I experienced breast lumps and hair loss, no doctor mentioned my liver. Through reading vastly on this topic, I learned of the liver's instrumental role in excreting metabolized (or "used") hormones. When the liver is overburdened, it may not be able to detoxify as quickly and efficiently, causing a hormone imbalance. By supporting my liver, I fixed my estrogen dominance and started feeling better than ever.

It's hard to know from any specific set of symptoms whether you have a toxic liver.

Ambiguous symptoms such as fatigue, allergies, insomnia, poor skin, and yellow eye whites may be signs of liver distress. Sensitivity to perfumes and smells, an adverse reaction to hormone-replacement therapy, and elevated LDL (or "bad" cholesterol) or liver enzyme levels such as alanine transaminase (ALT) and aspartate transaminase (AST) are indicative of liver-related problems. Experiencing pain under your right rib cage can also point to liver problems. Some practitioners believe that round brown spots on the skin are a sign of a taxed liver.

THE LIVER AND HORMONE CONNECTION

Think of your liver as a sieve. Everything you breathe, ingest, or apply on the skin gets into your bloodstream and eventually passes through the liver. It's the largest organ of the body, and the only organ that can regenerate itself.

Your liver performs about two hundred vital functions, most of which are key for overall health and hormone balance. It metabolizes drugs and alcohol and assimilates and stores fat-soluble vitamins (A, D, E, and K) and minerals such as iron. The liver converts the inactive T4 thyroid hormone to the active T3 hormone and eliminates fat-soluble toxins such as pesticides, preservatives, food additives, heavy metals, pollutants, plastics, and other environmental chemicals. It produces bile, which is critical to fat digestion (good fats and cholesterol are the precursors for steroid hormones); the bile also helps evacuate steroid hormones such as estrogen metabolites, progesterone, and testosterone. A sluggish liver can be a big contributor to estrogen dominance because of a buildup of harmful estrogenic metabolites that are the leading causes of estrogenic cancers, among other symptoms.

Your liver needs to eliminate metabolized or "used up" hormones to make space for new ones. The liver's detoxification happens in two phases. Phase 1, known as "oxidation," breaks the toxins up into less harmful compounds. Key nutrients needed in phase 1 detoxification are cruciferous vegetables, adequate proteins, vitamin B, choline (found in eggs and avocado), magnesium, iron, milk thistle, glutathione, and flavonoids (such as catechins found in matcha green tea).

In phase 2, known as "conjugation," the toxins are combined with another compound that will safely evacuate them by six detoxification pathways. Vitamins B6 and B12, folate, and beets (root and leaves) support the methylation pathway that clears estrogen, dopamine, histamine, and heavy metals. Sulfur, found in cruciferous vegetables, onion, garlic, and eggs, supports the sulfation pathway that

The Liver Detox Guide has been a life-changer for me. After detoxing my liver, I noticed that I had no more hair loss, my TPO [thyroperoxidase] antibodies went down, and I experienced much more energy, better sleep, and the disappearance of constant facial rosacea. As I continued on this protocol, my PMS and mood swings were gone and my anxiety greatly decreased. I even lost a few pounds, which was very motivating to make this a life-long change. —DEANNA SHANK

Want to geek out a little about the role of each detoxification pathway?

Great! Get the full lowdown from my website at www.HormonesBalance.com/book and learn more about each detoxification pathway's role, its inhibitors, and its activators.

clears estrogens, progesterone, thyroid hormones, DHEA, melatonin, histamine, and dopamine.

The other detoxification pathways are supported by compounds such as glycine (found in bone broth), calcium, magnesium, vitamin B, d-limonene (found in citrus peel), vitamin C, selenium, milk thistle, and N-acetylcysteine (NAC; the precursor for glutathione, the master detoxifier) to clear a myriad of hormones, neurotransmitters, and toxins, including bacteria, parasites, heavy metals, and pesticides.

If either of the detoxification phases is not working well, you will experience hormonal imbalances.

 ### Don't Throw Away the Lemon Rind!

The skin of lemons, limes, and oranges contains the medicinal d-limonene that eliminates carcinogenic metabolites in the liver. Before juicing, I like to grate the skins of citrus fruit to make citrus zest and use it as a flavorful addition to salad dressings, soups, and smoothies.

Pick This Superweed

Dandelion might be a common weed, but like all bitter greens, it stimulates stomach acid and bile production. Add dandelion greens to your salads or sauté or juice them. Dandelion root is a liver tonic; see my favorite teas and lattes on pages 302–313.

How Your Gallbladder Affects Your Hormone Balance

The liver produces bile and the gallbladder stores and releases it when you eat fat-containing foods. The bile helps the liver to excrete hormones like excess estrogen and its harmful metabolites. This explains why women who have their gallbladders removed often suffer from symptoms of estrogen dominance a few months after the surgery. If you are contemplating having your gallbladder removed or if it has already been removed, read about additional solutions at www.HormonesBalance.com/book.

Detoxify Your Liver with Cruciferous Vegetables

Cruciferous vegetables belong to the *Brassica* genus of vegetables and are rich in potent liver-supporting, anticarcinogenic, and hormone-balancing compounds: diindolylmethane (DIM), sulforaphane, and selenium. Cruciferous vegetables include cabbage, broccoli (including my favorite, broccoli sprouts), cauliflower, kale, bok choy, arugula, mustard greens, collard greens, turnips, radishes, rutabaga, and watercress.

The In-Out Guide to Reducing Toxins in Your Life

Use this guide to help you reduce your exposure to toxins.

OUT	IN	Brands I use or recommend
Skincare products like body and facial creams and lotions from major brands	Coconut oil, almond oil, jojoba oil, sesame oil, rose hip oil	Annmarie Gianni, John Masters Organics, Hugo Naturals, The Spa Dr., Juice Beauty
Body wash from major brands	Natural soaps made from organic oils, fats, or glycerine	Dr. Bronner's, Hugo Naturals, soaps sold at farmers' markets
Cosmetics, makeup from major brands	Cosmetics made with nontoxic and organic ingredients	Juice Beauty, Mineral Fusion, Annmarie Gianni, Beautycounter, Alima Pure, W3LL PEOPLE
Perfumes from major brands	Perfumes made with essential oils	Annmarie Gianni
Shampoos from major brands	Shampoos made with nontoxic and organic ingredients	John Masters Organics, Hugo Naturals, Morrocco Method (mud-based), Acure
Sunscreen containing retinyl palmitate (vitamin A) or oxybenzone	Sunscreens containing mineral oils, zinc oxide, and titanium dioxide	All Good, Annmarie Gianni, Juice Beauty, Badger, DeVita
Laundry detergent from major brands	Detergents free of phthalates, optical whiteners, and bleach	Seventh Generation, GreenShield Organic, Biokleen, Ecover
House-cleaning products from major brands	Products free of parabens, phthalates, or "fragrances"	Seventh Generation, Attitude, AspenClean, Biokleen
Fabric softener	½ cup baking soda in wash water, or wool dryer balls	Woolzies, BaaLLS
Tap water or water filtered with cheap or fridge filters. Avoid water in plastic bottles in the long term.	Kitchen or house three-stage filters that remove bacteria, fluoride, and heavy metals. Reverse osmosis filters if water source is highly contaminated.	Berkey, Aquasana
Nonstick cookware	Enamel, cast iron, glass, stainless steel	Lodge, Le Creuset, All-Clad
Air fresheners	Essential oil ultrasonic diffuser	Marsboy
House dust	Dust-free home!	IQAir filtration system, vacuum with HEPA filter, wet dusting, dusting with microfiber cloths
Plastic bottles	Stainless steel or glass bottles	Klean Kanteen, Lifefactory
Plastic lids on coffee cups	Get your own porcelain mug with a silicon lid	EcoJarz mason jar lids in stainless steel or silicon
Plastic containers for food storage	Glass containers	Frigoverre, Pyrex, Ball mason jars

OUT	IN	Brands I use or recommend
Canned food	Food in glass, especially tomatoes	Eden Foods
New house products such as furniture, mattresses, or carpet padding	Ask what fire retardant it contains. Be mindful of and/or avoid items containing PBDEs, antimony, formaldehyde, boric acid, and other brominated chemicals.	N/A

TOXINS IN SKINCARE AND HOUSEHOLD PRODUCTS AFFECT YOUR LIVER

The chemicals found in daily-use products add stress to the already taxed liver. According to the Environmental Working Group (EWG), a nonprofit organization focused on environmental health issues, women use an average of twelve products and get exposed to 168 unique chemical compounds every single day. Here are a few of the "bad boys," used extensively in most skincare and household-cleaning products:

Bisphenol A (BPA) in plastic bottles

Parabens synthetic preservatives

Phthalates make products smell "nice"

Triclosan an antibacterial agent

Aluminum makes deodorants more effective

Sodium lauryl/laureth a foaming agent

Formaldehyde a bonding agent

Synthetic colors make products look good

Perfluorinated chemicals (PFCs) used in nonstick cookware

What are endocrine disruptors?

They are chemicals that may interfere with the body's endocrine system (the network of glands that includes the pineal gland, pituitary gland, pancreas, ovaries, testes, thyroid gland, parathyroid gland, and adrenal glands) and produce adverse hormonal, reproductive, neurological, and immune effects in the body.

How can you trust your skincare or cosmetic brand?

Shop at health stores you trust. Their buyers do due diligence so you don't have to.

Check the toxic load of your favorite brands at the Environmental Working Group's Skin Deep Cosmetics Database (www.EWG.org /Skindeep) of more than sixty-four thousand products. Seek out "EWG Verified" products that are free of nearly all harmful chemicals.

Review the ingredients list on product packaging or at a company's website.

An All-Purpose Cleaner That Really Works

1 cup white vinegar
2 cups water
10 drops of any of these essential oils: tea tree, rosemary, lavender, cloves, lemon, lime, cinnamon, or eucalyptus.

For more on how to avoid endocrine-disrupting chemicals and replace them in skincare and house-cleaning products with herbs, spices, essential oils, and other natural solutions, go to www.HerbsforBalance.com.

LIVER DETOX GUIDE

Use this guide to help you put the content of this chapter plus additional strategies into action by following these simple suggestions. To download a digital version of this guide, go to www .HormonesBalance.com/book. Print it out and hang it in your kitchen to help make this new routine easy to follow. I recommend you adopt this protocol for one to three months. Your body will tell you if it needs more.

ADD TO DIET (+)

Stomach acid. Aids liver function and enzyme production for maximum detoxification. Add 2 tablespoons lemon, lime, apple cider vinegar, or sauerkraut juice before breakfast or each meal, or take HCl pills, if stomach acid is low (refer to page 36).

Fiber. Aids the liver in moving toxins out. Add 2 to 3 tablespoons insoluble fiber per day, such as ground flaxseeds, chia seeds, or psyllium husk.

Bitter greens. Promote bile excretion to help move toxins out. Found in raw radishes and juiced and steamed dandelion leaves and mustard greens. Add 2 servings per day.

Cruciferous vegetables. They are rich in diindolylmethane (DIM), which helps detoxification pathways. Found in broccoli, kale, Brussels sprouts, arugula, cauliflower, collard greens, and bok choy.

Vitamin B–rich food. Supports all major detoxification pathways. The foods richest in vitamin B are chicken, beef, and lamb livers. Alternatively, purchase a vitamin B complex supplement from a quality source.

Citrus peel. Rich in limonene—an activator in methylation pathway detoxification. Use in dressings, baking, smoothies, and juicing.

Choline-rich food. Supports the methylation pathway. Found in eggs (if tolerated) and avocados.

Sulfur. Supports the sulfation detoxification pathway. Found in egg yolks, broccoli, onion, and garlic or as a supplement (methylsulfonyl-methane, MSM). Consider the Detox Complete Kit on HormoneBalanceNutritionals.com.

Vitamin C–rich food. Helps the glutathionylation detoxification pathway. Highest amounts are found in camu camu or goji berries. Add ½ teaspoon camu camu powder to smoothies or porridge every day.

Selenium. Helps break toxins down. Found in Brazil nuts, sardines, anchovies, herring, chicken breast, turkey meat, mustard of all types, curry powder, milk thistle, and turmeric. I supplement with 200 micrograms per day.

Sea vegetables. Excellent chelator of heavy metals. Try kelp (kombu), nori, wakame, and arame in soups, stews, and salads. Not recommended for Hashimoto's patients with elevated antibodies.

Magnesium. Replenish by starting with 500 milligrams and go up to 1,500 milligrams, if needed. Preferred forms: glycerinate, citrate (can cause loose stool or diarrhea) or malate; avoid magnesium oxide. Maintain healthy levels of magnesium by regularly consuming kelp, cacao, pumpkin seeds, Brazil nuts, buckwheat, almonds, and cashews, if tolerated.

Milk thistle powder. Used in Western herbalism for centuries. Take 1 teaspoon per day in a smoothie or with water. Caution: Can be estrogenic for some.

REMOVE FROM DIET (−)

Food intolerances. Gluten, dairy, eggs, soy, corn, sugar, nightshades, yeast, citrus, nuts, and seeds are common culprits in creating digestive issues that inhibit liver function. Do the Elimination Diet (page 44) to identify your sensitivities.

Medications. Can inhibit detoxification pathways. Includes, but not limited to, antibiotics, antacids, birth control pills, NSAIDs (aspirin, acetaminophen, ibuprofen), and steroids such as corticosteroids.

Fluoride. Inhibits detoxification. Found in tap water (in the United States and Australia, but not in most European countries). Use a fluoride-removing water filter.

Other. Avoid fried food, coffee, and alcohol, as they take a lot of liver resources to clear out.

ADD TO LIFESTYLE (+)

Castor oil packs. These help relax detoxification pathways. Apply castor oil on the liver area and cover with a towel presoaked in castor oil for 30 minutes to an hour, then cover with a hot water bottle. Start with four times per week, then reduce to once per week.

Magnesium oil. Magnesium is a great relaxer and a facilitator of many metabolic processes. Apply topically on the liver area at bedtime. Can be done daily. Mix with coconut, sesame, or almond oil if it stings your skin.

Epson salt baths. Epsom salt is magnesium sulfate. It opens up detoxification pathways. Use weekly, according to package instructions.

Sauna. Try steam and infrared saunas two times per week.

Lymphatic massage. Try lymphatic massage by a professional, or search online for how to administer it to yourself.

In bed by 10 p.m. Liver detoxification happens between 1 and 3 a.m., during deep sleep.

REMOVE FROM LIFESTYLE (–)

Chemicals in skincare and cleaning products. These create an additional load on the liver. See the list of toxins and clean product options in this chapter.

Smoking. Smoking cigarettes and marijuana adds a toxic load to the liver.

Late-night snacking. This causes an additional load on the liver and its detoxification work, which happens late at night.

Liver Detox 14-Day Sample Meal Plan for Two

For the Liver Detox Meal Plan, follow the Elimination Diet 14-Day Meal Plan for Two (page 52) and add the above recommendations to your daily routine.

BEFORE PROCEEDING TO PHASE II

Be sure to have balanced the three legs of your Hormonal Foundation: your digestion, your sugar levels, and your liver. If the Elimination Diet was not enough to restore your gut, proceed to Chapter 5 and go deeper with more therapeutic protocols. Otherwise, hop to Chapter 6 to learn about various hormone- and condition-specific guides and meal plans.

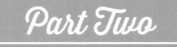

Part Two

Phase II: Your Hormonal Refinement

Completing Phase I might have resolved most of your symptoms, many related to hormonal imbalances. If that is not the case, you may need to go deeper by implementing the guides in this section.

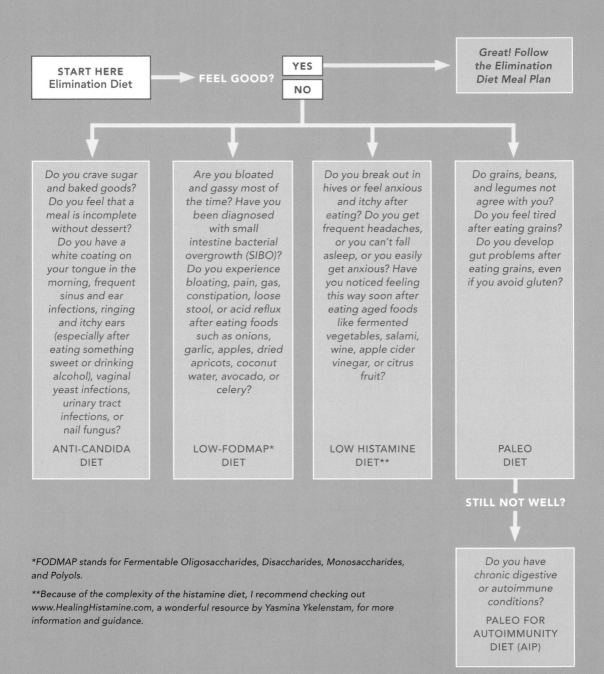

START HERE Elimination Diet → **FEEL GOOD?**

YES → Great! Follow the Elimination Diet Meal Plan

NO ↓

Do you crave sugar and baked goods? Do you feel that a meal is incomplete without dessert? Do you have a white coating on your tongue in the morning, frequent sinus and ear infections, ringing and itchy ears (especially after eating something sweet or drinking alcohol), vaginal yeast infections, urinary tract infections, or nail fungus?

ANTI-CANDIDA DIET

Are you bloated and gassy most of the time? Have you been diagnosed with small intestine bacterial overgrowth (SIBO)? Do you experience bloating, pain, gas, constipation, loose stool, or acid reflux after eating foods such as onions, garlic, apples, dried apricots, coconut water, avocado, or celery?

LOW-FODMAP* DIET

Do you break out in hives or feel anxious and itchy after eating? Do you get frequent headaches, or you can't fall asleep, or you easily get anxious? Have you noticed feeling this way soon after eating aged foods like fermented vegetables, salami, wine, apple cider vinegar, or citrus fruit?

LOW HISTAMINE DIET**

Do you crave grains, beans, and legumes not agree with you? Do you feel tired after eating grains? Do you develop gut problems after eating grains, even if you avoid gluten?

PALEO DIET

STILL NOT WELL? ↓

Do you have chronic digestive or autoimmune conditions?
PALEO FOR AUTOIMMUNITY DIET (AIP)

*FODMAP stands for Fermentable Oligosaccharides, Disaccharides, Monosaccharides, and Polyols.

**Because of the complexity of the histamine diet, I recommend checking out www.HealingHistamine.com, a wonderful resource by Yasmina Ykelenstam, for more information and guidance.

Chapter 5

How to Pick a Therapeutic Diet

GOING BEYOND THE ELIMINATION DIET

You've completed the Elimination Diet, identified your food intolerances, and eliminated those foods from your diet. And you feel *better*, but not as well as you'd like to. If this happens to you, one of the medicinal diets in this chapter may help further resolve your symptoms. It is not uncommon to have to go deeper into another diet to heal your digestion and reduce inflammation. Your hormones will thank you for that.

Use the chart on the opposite page (and your Food Mood Poop Journal) to help you find the diet that's right for you.

ANTI-CANDIDA DIET GUIDE AND MEAL PLAN

Candida is a fungus (a form of yeast) that is part of the gut flora—a group of microorganisms that can live in your mouth, intestine, and reproductive organs and on your skin. When not enough beneficial bacteria are present in a given body tissue to keep Candida under control, Candida weakens the intestinal wall and begins to release toxins throughout the body. As the toxins spread, they damage our body tissues and organs, wreaking havoc in the immune system.

Candida is infamously hard to diagnose, and many stool and blood tests miss it. I have found that listening to your symptoms and performing the quick and easy Candida Saliva Test (page 39) are the best diagnostic tools.

For best results, I recommend a four-week anti-Candida diet free of all grains (not just gluten) and fermented foods. Stay away from kombucha, coconut water kefir, and kvass throughout the Candida diet because they contain sugar. You can reintroduce grains in week 5, followed by fermented foods (such as sauerkraut or dill pickles) in week 6, but observe how your body reacts to

Anti-Candida Food List

A diet of processed foods high in sugars and simple carbohydrates encourages Candida overgrowth because yeast thrives on sugars. Avoid these foods:

Sugars and sweeteners

Artificial sweeteners
Chocolate
  (unless sugar free)
Coconut nectar
Honey
Molasses
Rice syrup
Sugar

Alcohol

Beer
Cider
Liquors
Spirits
Wine

Grains and gluten

Gluten grains such as wheat, rye, spelt, or barley found in breads, pastas, cakes, cookies, and burritos.

Best to avoid all other nongluten grains such as rice, amaranth, millet, corn, buckwheat, and quinoa for the first four weeks.

Fruit

Fruit in all forms: fresh, dried, canned, and juiced. Half of a green apple or a handful of berries is acceptable.

Vegetables

Beets
Carrots
Peas
Potatoes
Sweet potatoes
Yams

Meats

Cured meats
Processed meats
Smoked or vacuum-packed meats

Fish and seafood

All fish except for wild salmon and sardines
All shellfish

Dairy

Butter
Buttermilk
Cheese
Cream
Milk
Whey

Beverages

Coffee
Diet and regular soda
Energy drinks
Fruit juices
Tea—black and green

Nuts and seeds

All nuts, if sensitive to them
Cashews (unless scalded)
Peanuts
Pistachios (unless scalded)

Beans and legumes

Beans
Chickpeas
Lentils
Soy products, including soy milk, soy cheese, and tofu

Additives and preservatives

Citric acid
Anything you can't pronounce!

Fermented foods

Avoid for the first four weeks:
Dilled pickles
Sauerkraut
Yogurt, even nondairy
Kefir, even nondairy
Kimchi

Avoid completely:
Coconut water kefir
Fermented drinks made of fruit juice and grains
Kombucha
Kvass

Mushrooms

Button mushrooms
Champignon
Oyster mushrooms
Maitake
Porcinis
Shiitake

Vinegars

Vinegars such as white, rice, wine vinegar
Apple cider vinegar for the first four weeks

Fats and oils

Canola oil
Corn oil
Soy oil
Oils in processed foods
Peanut oil

these foods. Some people see their Candida symptoms return.

If your Candida does not clear up after following my anti-Candida diet and herbal protocol, you may have undetected food intolerances, oxalate sensitivity, heavy metal toxicity, parasites, or a compromised immune system. Work with a skilled practitioner who can order the right lab tests to uncover the underlying causes of the yeast overgrowth.

Everything that is not on this table is great to eat. Focus on the foods you can eat rather than the few temporary foods you will be removing. A typical anti-Candida diet consists of lots of protein and plenty of green leafy vegetables. Follow the Anti-Candida Meal Plan below.

You can download anti-Candida supplements and prescriptions from www.HormonesBalance.com/book.

Anti-Candida 14-Day Sample Meal Plan for Two

For warm lemon water: Add 2 tablespoons freshly squeezed lemon to 8 to 16 ounces warm water. Lime juice may also be used.

Pau D'Arco tea: Steep 1½ tablespoons Pau D'Arco bark in 3 cups hot water for 15 minutes; sip throughout the day.

Bone broth: Sip 1 to 2 cups per day with a dash of coconut milk, freshly grated ginger, lemon juice, and sea salt.

Abbreviations
[NR] No recipe
[LO] Leftovers
[MA] Made ahead; full recipe or parts of
[DB] Double the recipe
EVOO Extra virgin olive oil

WEEK 1

Morning ritual/ breakfast	Snack (optional)	Lunch	Dinner	Bedtime ritual (optional)
Day 1				
Warm lemon water Pau D'Arco Tea Farmer's Wife's Breakfast [DB] (page 182)	Nourishing Lattes, pick one (page 309)	Nutritious Quick Bowls, pick one [DB] (page 232)	Icelandic Fish Stew (page 214)	Immune-Boosting Chicken Broth [MA] (page 158); freeze half for next week Raspberry Melties [DB] (page 338)
Day 2				
Warm lemon water Pau D'Arco Tea Farmer's Wife's Breakfast [LO]	Energizing Matcha Lime Smoothie [DB] (page 191)	Nutritious Quick Bowls, pick one [DB]	Icelandic Fish Stew [LO]	Easy Digestion Tea (page 305) Kudzu Calming Pudding (page 348)

Morning ritual/ breakfast	Snack (optional)	Lunch	Dinner	Bedtime ritual (optional)
Day 3				
Warm lemon water Pau D'Arco Tea Breakfast Casserole One: Salmon and Broccoli (page 189)	Salmon and Avocado in Nori Sheets [DB] (page 298)	Icelandic Fish Stew [LO] Raspberry Melties [LO]	Fennel and Coriander Crusted Liver (page 246) Creamy Celeriac and Cauliflower Mash (page 267)	Easy Digestion Tea Kudzu Calming Pudding [LO]
Day 4				
Warm lemon water Pau D'Arco Tea Bacon, Oysters, and Collard Greens Stir Fry (page 204)	Salmon and Avocado in Nori Sheets [LO] Immune-Boosting Chicken Broth [LO]	Fennel and Coriander Crusted Liver [LO] Creamy Celeriac and Cauliflower Mash [LO]	Lamb with Collard Greens and Radishes (page 236) Side salad of mixed bitter greens with lemon, EVOO, and sea salt [NR]	Easy Digestion Tea Raspberry Melties [LO]
Day 5				
Warm lemon water Pau D'Arco Tea Coconut Kefir Chia Pudding (page 185)	Better Than Coffee Latte (page 312) Flaxseed Crackers [MA] (page 327)	Lamb with Collard Greens and Radishes [LO] Creamy Celeriac and Cauliflower Mash [LO]	Quick Detoxifying Soup (page 218)	Nourishing Lattes, pick one Raspberry Melties [LO]
Day 6				
Warm lemon water Pau D'Arco Tea Breakfast Casserole Two: Pork Chops and Apples (page 195)	Creamy Lime Pudding (page 342)	Quick Detoxifying Soup [LO] Flaxseed Crackers [LO]	Steam 'n Toss Veggies and Proteins on the Run (page 260)	Immune-Boosting Chicken Broth [LO] Zucchini Olive Muffin (page 205)
Day 7				
Warm lemon water Pau D'Arco Tea Parsnip Dill Pancake with Arugula and Smoked Salmon (page 199)	Decadent Chocolate Cherry Smoothie (page 207)	Quick Detoxifying Soup Flaxseed Crackers [LO]	Easy Chicken Curry Stew (page 212) Side salad of mixed bitter greens with lemon, EVOO, and sea salt [NR]	Nourishing Lattes, pick one Creamy Lime Pudding [LO]

WEEK 2

Morning ritual/ breakfast	Snack (optional)	Lunch	Dinner	Bedtime ritual (optional)
Day 8				
Warm lemon water Pau D'Arco Tea Breakfast Casserole One: Salmon and Broccoli	Creamy Lime Pudding [LO]	Nutritious Quick Bowls, pick one [DB] Flaxseed Crackers [LO]	Easy Chicken Curry Stew [LO] Side salad of mixed bitter greens with lemon, EVOO, and sea salt [NR]	Immune-Boosting Chicken Broth [LO] Raspberry Melties [LO]
Day 9				
Warm lemon water Pau D'Arco Tea Teff and Cherry Porridge (page 198)	Easy French Pate [MA] (page 290) Flaxseed Crackers [LO] Strawberry Ginger Ale [MA] (ferment takes 1 to 3 days) (page 318)	Steam 'n Toss Veggies and Proteins on the Run	Nomad's Kebabs (page 239) Jicama and Pomegranate Slaw (page 268)	Nourishing Lattes, pick one Raspberry Melties [LO]
Day 10				
Warm lemon water Pau D'Arco Tea Teff and Cherry Porridge [LO]	Easy French Pate [LO] Flaxseed Crackers [LO]	Quick Salads—Four Ways, pick one (page 254)	Nomad's Kebabs [LO] Jicama and Pomegranate Slaw [LO]	Easy Digestion Tea Kudzu Calming Pudding
Day 11				
Warm lemon water Pau D'Arco Tea Farmer's Wife's Breakfast [DB]	Easy French Pate [LO] Flaxseed Crackers [LO]	Jicama and Pomegranate Slaw [LO]	Butter Cod with Gremolata (page 240) Side salad of mixed bitter greens with lemon, EVOO, and sea salt [NR]	Kudzu Calming Pudding [LO] Nourishing Lattes, pick one
Day 12				
Warm lemon water Pau D'Arco Tea Farmer's Wife's Breakfast [LO]	Nourishing Lattes, pick one Flaxseed Crackers [LO]	Quick Salads— Four Ways, pick one	Butter Cod with Gremolata Quick Salads— Four Ways, pick one [LO]	Immune-Boosting Chicken Broth [LO] Raspberry Melties [LO]

Morning ritual/ breakfast	Snack (optional)	Lunch	Dinner	Bedtime ritual (optional)
Day 13				
Warm lemon water Pau D'Arco Tea Breakfast Casserole Two: Pork Chops and Apples	Energizing Matcha Lime Smoothie [DB]	Nutritious Quick Bowls, pick one [DB]	Rosemary and Garlic Stuffed Lamb Roast (page 251) Side salad of mixed bitter greens with lemon, EVOO, and sea salt [NR]	Immune-Boosting Chicken Broth [LO] Raspberry Melties [LO]
Day 14				
Warm lemon water Pau D'Arco Tea Breakfast Casserole One: Salmon and Broccoli	Deep Green Spirulina Smoothie (page 197)	Nutritious Quick Bowls, pick one [DB]	Rosemary and Garlic Stuffed Lamb Roast [LO] Side salad of mixed bitter greens with lemon, EVOO, and sea salt [NR]	Flaxseed Crackers [LO] Raspberry Melties [LO]

LOW-FODMAP DIET GUIDE AND MEAL PLAN

FODMAPs (Fermentable Oligosaccharides, Disaccharides, Monosaccharides, and Polyols) are carbohydrates (or forms of sugars) that are found in many foods. Not all carbohydrates are considered FODMAPs. A low-FODMAP diet limits foods high in fructose, oligos, lactose, fructose, and polyols. This diet was first used in Europe during the 1950s for people with IBS. It was then forgotten for several decades and only recently brought back into usage by Monash University in Melbourne, Australia. Today, it is used by anyone with chronic digestive dysbiosis, including SIBO and Crohn's disease, and those experiencing digestive upset when eating high-FODMAP foods.

Try the low-FODMAP diet after having done the Elimination Diet. You might have discovered, by keeping the Food Mood Poop Journal, that certain foods such as onions, garlic, or apples give you gas and make you bloat.

Will you be able to eat high-FODMAP foods again? Most likely, yes, if you repair your gut by restoring the digestive bacterial flora that helps to break down these sugars. I also used to be very sensitive to foods high in oligosaccharides such as onions, but I can eat them now.

There are two redeeming qualities about the low-FODMAP diet. One, you can have many of the high-FODMAP foods in small amounts. For example, even though almonds are high in oligos, a handful of nuts (about ten nuts) is still considered low in FODMAPs.

(Download Monash University's "Low FOD-MAP Diet" smartphone app to get the details.) And two, you might not be reacting to all the sugars I mention. For example, you might find that fructose (found in apples and cherries) triggers you but polyols (found in avocados, apricots, and blueberries) don't.

Many people with SIBO start on the low-FODMAP diet. I recommend modifying it and reducing all flours (even the ones low in FOD-MAPs) and fermented foods because most people do not tolerate them well. Diet alone will probably not be enough to heal SIBO, and it will probably be necessary for most people to start on rounds of herbal antibiotics. If you struggle with SIBO, get to know the work of Dr. Allison Siebecker and her website at www.siboinfo.com, which features plenty of SIBO resources, including options for testing and a listing of practitioners.

Low-FODMAP Food List

For a complete food list that is updated and expanded, please download Monash University's Low FODMAP Diet smartphone app (which also funds the university's research).

Low FODMAP (okay to consume)	High FODMAP (remove from diet)	Low FODMAP (okay to consume)	High FODMAP (remove from diet)
Meat and fish		**Dairy**	
Beef	Processed meats made with high-fructose corn syrup	*Not recommended, even though it is low FODMAP, because many people have a problem with dairy:*	*High-lactose dairy:*
Chicken			Buttermilk
Cold cuts like ham or turkey breast			Milk
Eggs		Lactose-free cheeses (camembert, cheddar, Colby, feta, cottage cheese, goat cheese, mozzarella, pecorino)	Creamy/cheesy sauces
Fish			Cream cheese
Lamb			Custard
Pork			Ice cream
Salami		Sheep or goat yogurt	Kefir
Seafood		Whipped cream	Milk (cow's, goat's, sheep's, condensed, evaporated)
Turkey		Lactose-free milk and yogurt	Soft cheeses (cottage, ricotta, etc.)
Venison			Sour cream
			Cow yogurt

Low FODMAP (okay to consume)	High FODMAP (remove from diet)
Nuts, seeds, legumes, and tubers	
Brazil nuts	Cashews
Hemp seeds	Soybeans, soy milk
Macadamia nuts	Beans
Pecans	Bulgur
Pumpkin seeds	Lentils
Tigernuts (according to the manufacturer)	Miso
Almonds (max. 10)	Pistachios
Hazelnuts (max. 10)	
Milks made from these nuts, seeds, and tubers	

Low FODMAP (okay to consume)	High FODMAP (remove from diet)
Grains	
Oats	Amaranth
Quinoa	Barley
Gluten-free foods made with the allowed grains	Bran
Buckwheat	Couscous
Corn	Gnocchi
Oatmeal (max. ½ cup)	Granola
Popcorn	Muesli
Rice (basmati, brown, white)	Rye
Tortilla chips	Semolina
	Spelt
	Wheat (breads, cakes, muffins, cereals, pasta)

Low FODMAP (okay to consume)	High FODMAP (remove from diet)
Vegetables	
Arugula	Artichoke
Bamboo shoots	Asparagus
Bean sprouts	Beans (black, broad, kidney, lima, soya)
Bell peppers	
Bok choy	Beets
Broccoli	Cassava
Butternut squash (max. ¼ cup)	Cauliflower
Cabbage (common and red)	Cabbage (savoy)
	Garlic
Carrots	Leeks (white parts)
Celery (max. 1½-inch stalk)	Mushrooms (portobello, shiitake, button, porcini)
Celeriac	Onions
Chickpeas (max. ¼ cup)	Peas (snow, sugar snap)
Chilies	Scallions, shallots (white parts)
Chives	
Collard greens	
Corn (max. ½ cob)	
Cucumber	
Eggplant	
Fennel bulb	
Green beans	
Ginger	
Kale	
Lettuce (butter, iceberg, radicchio)	
Leeks (green parts only)	
Mushrooms (oyster, champignons)	
Parsnip	
Potato	
Pumpkin	
Radish	
Scallions (green parts)	
Spinach	
Squash	
Sweet potato (max. ½ cup)	
Tomatoes (cherry, common, Roma)	
Turnip	
Zucchini	

Low FODMAP (okay to consume)	High FODMAP (remove from diet)

Fermented vegetables*

Low FODMAP (okay to consume)	High FODMAP (remove from diet)
Pickled cucumbers	*More than 1 tablespoon of:*
	Sauerkraut
	Kimchi

Fruit

Low FODMAP (okay to consume)	High FODMAP (remove from diet)
Bananas	Apples
Blueberries	Apricots
Cantaloupe	Avocados
Cranberries	Blackberries
Clementines	Cherries
Coconut, fresh (max. ½ cup)	Dates
	Figs
Grapes	Grapefruit
Melons	Goji berries
Kiwis	Mangos
Lemons	Peaches
Limes	Pears
Oranges	Plums
Pineapple	Pomegranates
Raspberries	Raisins
Rhubarb	Watermelon
Strawberries	

Condiments

Low FODMAP (okay to consume)	High FODMAP (remove from diet)
Balsamic vinegar (max. 1 tablespoon)	Hummus
Barbeque sauce	Tahini paste
Chutney (max. 1 tablespoon)	Ketchup with high-fructose corn syrup
Garlic-infused olive oil	
Strawberry jam	
Mayonnaise	
Mustard	
Soy sauce	
Tomato sauce	

Fats and oils

Low FODMAP (okay to consume)	High FODMAP (remove from diet)
Butter	
Garlic-infused olive oil	
Ghee	
Mayonnaise	
Avocado, coconut, olive, and sesame oils	

Sugars and confectionaries

Low FODMAP (okay to consume)	High FODMAP (remove from diet)
Cacao powder	Agave
Dark chocolate	Carob
Stevia	Honey
Sugar (raw, palm, brown, white)	Milk chocolate
Maple syrup	Date sugar
Golden syrup	
Coconut nectar (max. ½ tablespoon)	

Beverages

Low FODMAP (okay to consume)	High FODMAP (remove from diet)
Coffee	Coconut water
Tea	Dandelion infusion
Kvass	Fennel tea
Cranberry juice	

Prebiotics

Low FODMAP (okay to consume)	High FODMAP (remove from diet)
Cold potatoes	Fructooligosaccharides (FOS)
Cold rice	Inulin
	Oligofructose

Even though green cabbage is low in FODMAPs, more than 1 tablespoon fermented cabbage is high in polyols.

Low-FODMAP 14-Day Sample Meal Plan for Two

For warm lemon water: Add 2 tablespoons freshly squeezed lemon juice to 8 to 16 ounces warm water. Lime juice or apple cider vinegar may also be used.

Bone broth: Sip 1 to 2 cups per day with a dash of coconut milk, freshly grated ginger, lemon juice, and sea salt.

Abbreviations
[NR] No recipe
[LO] Leftovers
[MA] Made ahead; full recipe or parts of
[DB] Double the recipe
EVOO Extra virgin olive oil

WEEK 1

Morning ritual/ breakfast	Snack (optional)	Lunch	Dinner	Bedtime ritual (optional)
Day 1				
Warm lemon water Healing Bone Broth [MA] (page 162) Farmer's Wife's Breakfast [DB] (page 182)	Easy French Pate [MA] (page 290) Flaxseed Crackers [MA] (page 327)	Quick Salads—Four Ways, pick one (page 254); add Life-Giving Sprouts [MA] [DB] (page 163)	Creamy Rosemary Chicken [DB] (page 249) Creamy Celeriac and Cauliflower Mash (page 267) Steamed or sautéed greens or broccolini with EVOO and sea salt [NR]	Everyday Nourishing Tea (page 306) Raspberry Melties [DB] (page 338)
Day 2				
Warm lemon water Healing Bone Broth [LO] Farmer's Wife's Breakfast [LO]	Easy French Pate [LO] Flaxseed Crackers [LO]	Nutritious Quick Bowls, pick one [DB] (page 232); add Life-Giving Sprouts [LO]	Creamy Rosemary Chicken [LO] Creamy Celeriac and Cauliflower Mash [LO] Steamed or sautéed greens or broccolini with EVOO and sea salt [LO]	Liver Cleanser Tea (page 307) Raspberry Melties [LO]
Day 3				
Warm lemon water Breakfast Casserole One: Salmon and Broccoli (page 189); add Life-Giving Sprouts [LO]	Easy French Pate [LO] Flaxseed Crackers [LO]	Quick Salads—Four Ways, pick one (page 254) Healing Bone Broth [LO]	Fennel and Coriander Crusted Liver (page 246) Creamy Celeriac and Cauliflower Mash [LO]	Nourishing Lattes, pick one (page 309) Raspberry Melties [LO]

Morning ritual/ breakfast	Snack (optional)	Lunch	Dinner	Bedtime ritual (optional)
Day 4				
Daily Balancer Tea (page 306) Teff and Cherry Porridge (page 198)		Fennel and Coriander Crusted Liver [LO] Sautéed greens with EVOO, lemon, and sea salt [NR]	Quick Detoxifying Soup (page 218)	Healing Bone Broth [LO] Raspberry Melties [LO]
Day 5				
Warm lemon water Teff and Cherry Porridge [LO]	Energizing Matcha Lime Smoothie [DB] (page 191)	Quick Detoxifying Soup [LO] Raspberry Melties [LO]	Quick Salads—Four Ways, pick one Healing Bone Broth [LO]	Nourishing Lattes, pick one
Day 6				
Warm lemon water Farmer's Wife's Breakfast [DB]	Deep Green Spirulina Smoothie (page 197)	Nutritious Quick Bowls, pick one [DB] Healing Bone Broth [LO]	Icelandic Fish Stew (page 214) Side salad of mixed bitter greens with lemon, EVOO, and sea salt [NR]	Sugar Balancer Tea (page 308) Raspberry Melties [LO]
Day 7				
Warm lemon water Healing Bone Broth [LO] Farmer's Wife's Breakfast [LO]	Warming Chai Latte (page 310)	Icelandic Fish Stew [LO] Flaxseed Crackers [LO]	Japanese Seaweed and Cucumber Salad (page 273)	Liver Cleanser Tea Raspberry Melties [LO]

WEEK 2

Morning ritual/ breakfast	Snack (optional)	Lunch	Dinner	Bedtime ritual (optional)
Day 8				
Warm lemon water Icelandic Fish Stew [LO]	Decadent Chocolate Cherry Smoothie (page 207)	Japanese Seaweed and Cucumber Salad [LO]	Bacon, Oysters, and Collard Greens Stir Fry [DB] (page 204)	Immune-Boosting Chicken Broth (page 158)

Morning ritual/ breakfast	Snack (optional)	Lunch	Dinner	Bedtime ritual (optional)
Day 9				
Warm lemon water Breakfast Casserole Two: Pork Chops and Apples (page 195)	Matcha Frappe (page 299)	Bacon, Oysters, and Collard Greens Stir Fry [LO]	Easy Chicken Curry Stew (page 212); add Life-Giving Sprouts [LO]	Liver Cleanser Tea Raspberry Melties [LO]
Day 10				
Warm lemon water Coconut Kefir Chia Pudding (page 185)	Energizing Matcha Lime Smoothie	Quick Salads—Four Ways, pick one	Walnut Crusted Salmon [DB] (page 244) Fries Baked in Duck Fat (page 271)	Immune-Boosting Chicken Broth [LO]
Day 11				
Warm lemon water Adrenal Love Tea (page 305) Easy Chicken Curry Stew	Warming Chai Latte	Walnut Crusted Salmon [LO] Fries Baked in Duck Fat [LO]; add Life-Giving Sprouts [LO]	Seriously Mushroom Soup [LO]	Immune Booster Tea (page 303) Raspberry Melties [LO]
Day 12				
Warm lemon water Teff and Cherry Porridge	Immune-Boosting Chicken Broth [LO] Raspberry Melties [LO]	Steam 'n Toss Veggies and Proteins on the Run (page 260)	Nomad's Kebabs (page 239) Detoxing Beet and Carrot Salad (page 252); add Life-Giving Sprouts [LO]	Nourishing Lattes, pick one
Day 13				
Warm lemon water Adrenal Love Tea Teff and Cherry Porridge [LO]	Seed Bread with Figs [MA] (page 332)	Nomad's Kebabs [LO] Fresh greens with Life-Giving Sprouts [LO], EVOO, lemon, and sea salt [NR]	Nutritious Quick Bowls, pick one [DB] Immune-Boosting Chicken Broth [LO]	Immune Booster Tea Raspberry Melties [LO]
Day 14				
Warm lemon water Breakfast Casserole One: Salmon and Broccoli	Seed Bread with Figs [LO]	Sweet Potato and Sage Pancakes [LO] Fresh greens with Life-Giving Sprouts [LO], EVOO, lemon, and sea salt [NR]	Steam 'n Toss Veggies and Proteins on the Run	Immune-Boosting Chicken Broth [LO]

PALEO DIET GUIDE AND MEAL PLAN

The Paleo diet requires you to remove all grains, legumes, and beans. Remember that sometimes a hybrid approach is needed; for example, you might need to eliminate nuts or nightshades like tomatoes in order to feel good. Use your Food Mood Poop Journal during the first four weeks of the Paleo diet to hone in on the foods that cause symptoms.

If you wish to dive deeper into the Paleo diet and lifestyle, I recommend Diane Sanfilippo's Balanced Bites website (www.balancedbites.com) and her cookbook *Practical Paleo: A Customized Approach to Health and a Whole-Foods Lifestyle* (2nd ed., 2016).

Paleo Food List

	ADD (+)	REMOVE (−)
Meat and fish	Grass-fed, pastured animals Wild-caught fish	"Conventionally raised" animals Processed meats containing nitrates, additives, and preservatives
Dairy	None	All dairy
Nuts, seeds, legumes, and tubers	All nuts except peanuts All seeds Tigernuts Cassava	All beans All lentils Peanuts
Grains	None	All grains
Vegetables	All vegetables except potatoes Fermented vegetables Seaweed	Potatoes
Fruits	All fruit	Processed fruit Fruit juices with added sugar
Fats and oils	Refer to Fats and Oils (page 139)	Refer to Fats and Oils (page 139)
Nondairy beverages and yogurts	Bone and vegetable broths Coconut milk and yogurt Coconut water Tigernut milk Nut milks and yogurts Seed milks	Processed beverages and yogurts containing preservatives and additives

Paleo Diet 14-Day Sample Meal Plan for Two

For warm lemon water: Add 2 tablespoons freshly squeezed lemon juice to 8 to 16 ounces warm water. Lime juice or apple cider vinegar may also be used.

Bone broth: Sip 1 to 2 cups per day with a dash of coconut milk, freshly grated ginger, lemon juice, and sea salt.

Abbreviations
[NR] No recipe
[LO] Leftovers
[MA] Made ahead; full recipe or parts of
[DB] Double the recipe
EVOO Extra virgin olive oil

WEEK 1

Morning ritual/ breakfast	Snack (optional)	Lunch	Dinner	Bedtime ritual (optional)
Day 1				
Warm lemon water Healing Bone Broth [MA] (page 162) Farmer's Wife's Breakfast [DB] (page 182)	Salmon and Avocado in Nori Sheets [DB] (page 298)	Quick Salads—Four Ways, pick one (page 254)	Creamy Rosemary Chicken [DB] (page 249) Creamy Celeriac and Cauliflower Mash (page 267) Steamed or sautéed greens or broccolini with EVOO and sea salt [NR]	Everyday Nourishing Tea (page 306) Raspberry Melties [DB] (page 338)
Day 2				
Warm lemon water Healing Bone Broth [LO] Farmer's Wife's Breakfast [LO]	Salmon and Avocado in Nori Sheets [LO]	Nutritious Quick Bowls, pick Paleo [DB] (page 232)	Creamy Rosemary Chicken [LO] Creamy Celeriac and Cauliflower Mash [LO] Steamed or sautéed greens or broccolini with EVOO and sea salt [LO]	Liver Cleanser Tea (page 307) Raspberry Melties [LO]
Day 3				
Warm lemon water Ginger Beet Kvass [MA] (page 317) Breakfast Casserole One: Salmon and Broccoli (page 189)	Decadent Chocolate Cherry Smoothie (page 207)	Quick Salads—Four Ways, pick one Healing Bone Broth [LO]	Fennel and Coriander Crusted Liver (page 246) Creamy Celeriac and Cauliflower Mash [LO]	Nourishing Lattes, pick one (page 309) Raspberry Melties [LO]

Morning ritual/ breakfast	Snack (optional)	Lunch	Dinner	Bedtime ritual (optional)
Day 4				
Daily Balancer Tea (page 306) Deep Green Spirulina Smoothie (page 197)	Ginger Beet Kvass [LO]	Fennel and Coriander Crusted Liver [LO] Sautéed greens with EVOO, lemon, and sea salt [NR]	Seriously Mushroom Soup (page 216)	Healing Bone Broth [LO] Raspberry Melties [LO]
Day 5				
Warm lemon water Energizing Matcha Lime Smoothie [DB] (page 191)	Ginger Beet Kvass [LO]	Seriously Mushroom Soup [LO] Raspberry Melties [LO]	Quick Salads—Four Ways, pick one Healing Bone Broth [LO]	Nourishing Lattes, pick one
Day 6				
Warm lemon water Ginger Beet Kvass [LO] Farmer's Wife's Breakfast [DB]	Carrot and Beet Smoothie (page 203)	Nutritious Quick Bowls, pick Paleo [DB] Healing Bone Broth [LO]	Porcini Mushroom Beef Stew (page 224) Side salad of mixed bitter greens with lemon, EVOO, and sea salt [NR]	Sugar Balancer Tea (page 308) Raspberry Melties [LO]
Day 7				
Warm lemon water Healing Bone Broth [LO] Farmer's Wife's Breakfast [LO]	Better Than Coffee Latte (page 321)	Porcini Mushroom Beef Stew [LO] Ginger Beet Kvass [LO]	Japanese Seaweed and Cucumber Salad (page 273)	Liver Cleanser Tea Raspberry Melties [LO]

WEEK 2

Morning ritual/ breakfast	Snack (optional)	Lunch	Dinner	Bedtime ritual (optional)
Day 8				
Warm lemon water Porcini Mushroom Beef Stew [LO]	Decadent Chocolate Cherry Smoothie	Japanese Seaweed and Cucumber Salad [LO]	Bacon, Oysters, and Collard Greens Stir Fry [DB] (page 204)	Immune-Boosting Chicken Broth (page 158)

Morning ritual/ breakfast	Snack (optional)	Lunch	Dinner	Bedtime ritual (optional)
Day 9				
Warm lemon water Breakfast Casserole Two: Pork Chops and Apples (page 195) Fresh greens, lemon, EVOO, and sea salt [NR]	Matcha Frappe (page 299)	Bacon, Oysters, and Collard Greens Stir Fry [LO]	Seriously Mushroom Soup	Liver Cleanser Tea Raspberry Melties [LO]
Day 10				
Warm lemon water Seriously Mushroom Soup [LO]	Easy French Pate [MA] (page 290) with vegetable sticks [NR] or Flaxseed Crackers [MA] (page 327)	Quick Salads—Four Ways, pick one	Walnut Crusted Salmon [DB] (page 244) Detoxing Beet and Carrot Salad (page 252)	Immune-Boosting Chicken Broth [LO]
Day 11				
Warm lemon water Adrenal Love Tea (page 305) Energizing Matcha Lime Smoothie [DB]	Easy French Pate [LO] with vegetable sticks [NR] or Flaxseed Crackers [LO]	Walnut Crusted Salmon [LO] Detoxing Beet and Carrot Salad [LO]; add Life-Giving Sprouts [MA] [DB] (page 163)	Seriously Mushroom Soup [LO]	Immune Booster Tea (page 303) Raspberry Melties [LO]
Day 12				
Warm lemon water Deep Green Spirulina Smoothie (page 197)	Immune-Boosting Chicken Broth [LO] Raspberry Melties [LO]	Steam 'n Toss Veggies and Proteins on the Run (page 260)	Nomad's Kebabs (page 239) Detoxing Beet and Carrot Salad; add Life-Giving Sprouts [LO]	Nourishing Lattes, pick one
Day 13				
Warm lemon water Adrenal Love Tea Parsnip Dill Pancake with Arugula and Smoked Salmon [DB] (page 199)	Rosemary Pear Muffin (page 335)	Nomad's Kebabs [LO] Detoxing Beet and Carrot Salad [LO]; add Life-Giving Sprouts [LO]	Nutritious Quick Bowls, pick Paleo [DB] Immune-Boosting Chicken Broth [LO]	Immune Booster Tea Raspberry Melties [LO]

Morning ritual/ breakfast	Snack (optional)	Lunch	Dinner	Bedtime ritual (optional)
Day 14				
Warm lemon water Coconut Kefir Chia Pudding (page 185)	Rosemary Pear Muffin [LO]	Parsnip Dill Pancake with Arugula and Smoked Salmon [LO] Fresh greens with Life-Giving Sprouts [LO], EVOO, lemon, and sea salt [NR] Ginger Beet Kvass [LO]	Steam 'n Toss Veggies and Proteins on the Run	Immune-Boosting Chicken Broth [LO]

PALEO FOR AUTOIMMUNITY DIET GUIDE AND MEAL PLAN

The Paleo Autoimmune Protocol (AIP) is a diet that helps heal the immune system and gut by reducing inflammation in the intestines. A strict AIP diet isn't meant to last forever but is used as a temporary protocol to heal the intestines. The AIP diet is based on the Paleo way of eating that further restricts foods known to trigger inflammation, such as nightshades, eggs, nuts, and seeds.

If you want to dive deeper into the AIP diet and lifestyle, I recommend the website, blog, books, and cookbooks of Dr. Sarah Ballantyne (aka The Paleo Mom).

AIP Food List

	ADD (+)	REMOVE (−)
Meat and fish	Grass-fed, pastured animals	"Conventionally raised" animals
	Special focus on nutrient-dense foods such as bone broth, liver, and heart.	Processed meats containing nitrates, additives, and preservatives
	Wild-caught fish	Processed meats containing nightshades and non–AIP-compliant spices
Vegetables	All vegetables except nightshades	Nightshades: tomatoes, potatoes, peppers, eggplants, chilies, and goji berries
	Fermented vegetables	
	Seaweed	
Dairy	None	All dairy

	ADD (+)	REMOVE (−)
Eggs	None	All eggs
Grains	None	All grains
Sugars and sweeteners	Refer to Sugars and Sweeteners (page 138)	
Nuts, seeds, legumes, and tubers	Tigernuts Cassava	All nuts All seeds Beans Lentils Peanuts
Fruits	All fruit	Processed fruit Fruit juices with added sugar Goji berries
Fats and oils	Refer to Fats and Oils (page 139)	
Nondairy beverages and yogurts	Bone and vegetable broths Coconut milk and yogurt Coconut water Tigernut milk Nut milks and yogurts Seed milks	Processed beverages and yogurts containing preservatives and additives
Herbs and spices*	Basil Bay leaves Chamomile Chives Cilantro Dill Lavender Lemongrass Marjoram Mint Parsley Peppermint Rosemary Sage Spearmint Tarragon Thyme	Anise Caraway Curries Coriander Cumin Fennel seed Fenugreek Mustard Nutmeg Peppercorns

*In my experience, even though seed-based spices are not allowed with the AIP, some people can tolerate seed spices, especially when used in small amounts.

	ADD (+)	REMOVE (−)
Alcohol	No alcohol	
Condiments	Apple cider vinegar	Vinegar-based condiments
	Anchovies	Anything containing the above spices
	Arrowroot flour to prevent clumping	

Paleo for Autoimmunity Diet 14-Day Sample Meal Plan for Two

For warm lemon water: Add 2 tablespoons freshly squeezed lemon juice to 8 to 16 ounces warm water. Lime juice or apple cider vinegar may also be used.

Bone broth: Sip 1 to 2 cups per day with a dash of coconut milk, freshly grated ginger, lemon juice, and sea salt.

Abbreviations
[NR] No recipe
[LO] Leftovers
[MA] Made ahead; full recipe or parts of
[DB] Double the recipe
EVOO Extra virgin olive oil

WEEK 1

Morning ritual/ Breakfast	Snack (optional)	Lunch	Dinner	Bedtime ritual (optional)
Day 1				
Warm lemon water	Salmon and Avocado in Nori Sheets [DB] (page 298)	Quick Salads—Four Ways, pick one (page 254)	Creamy Rosemary Chicken [DB] (page 249)	Everyday Nourishing Tea (page 306)
Healing Bone Broth [MA] (page 162)			Creamy Celeriac and Cauliflower Mash (page 267)	Raspberry Melties [DB] (page 338)
Farmer's Wife's Breakfast [DB] (page 182)			Steamed or sautéed greens or broccolini with EVOO and sea salt [NR]	
Day 2				
Warm lemon water	Salmon and Avocado in Nori Sheets [LO]	Nutritious Quick Bowls, pick Paleo [DB] (page 232)	Creamy Rosemary Chicken [LO]	Liver Cleanser Tea (page 307)
Healing Bone Broth [LO]			Creamy Celeriac and Cauliflower Mash [LO]	Raspberry Melties [LO]
Farmer's Wife's Breakfast [LO]			Steamed or sautéed greens or broccolini with EVOO and sea salt [LO]	

Morning ritual/ Breakfast	Snack (optional)	Lunch	Dinner	Bedtime ritual (optional)
Day 3				
Warm lemon water Breakfast Casserole One: Salmon and Broccoli (page 189)	Ginger Beet Kvass [MA] (page 317)	Quick Salads—Four Ways, pick one Healing Bone Broth [LO]	Grain-Free Pizzas—Two Ways, pick one (page 228)	Nourishing Lattes, pick one (page 309) Raspberry Melties [LO]
Day 4				
Daily Balancer Tea (page 306) Bacon, Oysters, and Collard Greens Stir Fry (page 204)	Ginger Beet Kvass [LO]	Pan-fried wild salmon in ghee with sea salt [NR] Sautéed greens with EVOO, lemon, and sea salt [NR]	Quick Detoxifying Soup (page 218)	Healing Bone Broth [LO] Raspberry Melties [LO]
Day 5				
Warm lemon water Breakfast Casserole Two: Pork Chops and Apples (page 195)	Ginger Beet Kvass [LO]	Quick Detoxifying Soup [LO] Raspberry Melties [LO]	Quick Salads—Four Ways, pick one Healing Bone Broth [LO]	Nourishing Lattes, pick one
Day 6				
Warm lemon water Farmer's Wife's Breakfast [DB]	Ginger Beet Kvass [LO]	Nutritious Quick Bowls, pick Paleo [DB] Healing Bone Broth [LO]	Porcini Mushroom Beef Stew (page 224) Side salad of mixed bitter greens with lemon, EVOO, and sea salt [NR]	Sugar Balancer Tea (page 308) Raspberry Melties [LO]
Day 7				
Warm lemon water Healing Bone Broth [LO] Farmer's Wife's Breakfast [LO]	Nut and Seed Milks—pick tigernut milk, add a dash of cinnamon (page 300)	Porcini Mushroom Beef Stew [LO] Ginger Beet Kvass [LO]	Japanese Seaweed and Cucumber Salad (page 273)	Liver Cleanser Tea Raspberry Melties [LO]

WEEK 2

Morning ritual/ breakfast	Snack (optional)	Lunch	Dinner	Bedtime ritual (optional)
Day 8				
Warm lemon water Porcini Mushroom Beef Stew [LO]	Better Than Coffee Latte (page 321)	Japanese Seaweed and Cucumber Salad [LO]	Bacon, Oysters, and Collard Greens Stir Fry [DB]	Immune-Boosting Chicken Broth (page 158)
Day 9				
Warm lemon water Breakfast Casserole Two: Pork Chops and Apples Fresh greens, lemon, EVOO, and sea salt [NR]	Matcha Frappe (page 299)	Bacon, Oysters, and Collard Greens Stir Fry [LO]	Seriously Mushroom Soup (page 216)	Liver Cleanser Tea Raspberry Melties [LO]
Day 10				
Warm lemon water Seriously Mushroom Soup [LO]	Easy French Pate [MA] (page 290) with vegetable sticks [NR]	Quick Salads—Four Ways, pick one	Butter Cod with Gremolata (page 240) Fresh greens, lemon, EVOO, and sea salt [NR]	Immune-Boosting Chicken Broth [LO]
Day 11				
Warm lemon water Adrenal Love Tea Perfect French Crepes (page 208)	Easy French Pate [LO] with vegetable sticks [NR]	Butter Cod with Gremolata [LO] Fresh greens, lemon, EVOO, and sea salt [NR]; add Life-Giving Sprouts [MA] [DB] (page 163)	Seriously Mushroom Soup [LO]	Immune Booster Tea (page 303) Raspberry Melties [LO]
Day 12				
Warm lemon water Pan-fried wild salmon in ghee with sea salt [NR] Sautéed greens with EVOO, lemon, and sea salt [NR]	Immune-Boosting Chicken Broth [LO] Raspberry Melties [LO]	Steam 'n Toss Veggies and Proteins on the Run (page 260)	Nomad's Kebabs (page 239) Detoxing Beet and Carrot Salad (page 252); add Life-Giving Sprouts [LO]	Nourishing Lattes, pick one

Morning ritual/ Breakfast	Snack (optional)	Lunch	Dinner	Bedtime ritual (optional)
Day 13				
Warm lemon water Adrenal Love Tea Parsnip Dill Pancake with Arugula and Smoked Salmon [DB] (page 199)	Nut and Seed Milks—pick tigernut milk, add a dash of cinnamon	Nomad's Kebabs [LO] Detoxing Beet and Carrot Salad [LO]; add Life-Giving Sprouts [LO]	Nutritious Quick Bowls, pick Paleo [DB] Immune-Boosting Chicken Broth [LO]	Immune Booster Tea Raspberry Melties [LO]
Day 14				
Warm lemon water Breakfast Casserole One: Salmon and Broccoli	Matcha Frappe	Parsnip Dill Pancake with Arugula and Smoked Salmon [LO] Fresh greens with Life-Giving Sprouts [LO], EVOO, lemon, and sea salt [NR] Ginger Beet Kvass [LO]	Steam 'n Toss Veggies and Proteins on the Run	Immune-Boosting Chicken Broth [LO]

Chapter 6
Hormone- and Condition-Specific Guides and Meal Plans

Once you have established a strong Foundation for hormonal balance (remember that three-legged stool?) by healing your gut, balancing your sugar levels, and detoxifying your liver, you are ready to address your specific hormone imbalance or imbalances.

REVERSING ESTROGEN DOMINANCE

The key strategies for reversing estrogen dominance are to optimize your digestive health and support your liver and add foods and supplements that increase the "good estrogen" and help metabolize the harmful estrogen metabolites.

ADD (+)

Liver support. Continue following the Liver Detox Guide in Chapter 4.

Cruciferous vegetables. They are rich in diindolylmethane (DIM), which helps to block estradiol (E2). Found in cabbage, broccoli, kale, arugula, Brussels sprouts, radishes, cauliflower, and bok choy. Aim for 1 to 2 cups per day.

Bitter greens. They help produce bile to "flush out" metabolized estrogens. Found in radishes, dandelion, and artichokes. Minimum ½ cup per day.

Flaxseed. Even though it contains phytoestrogen, flax plays a dual role: increasing "good" estrogens but also mitigating the effects of harmful estrogen metabolites. Aim for 1 to 2 tablespoons freshly ground flaxseed per day.

Sprouts. Sprouts of cruciferous veggies have a highly estrogen-balancing quality. Aim for 2 to 3 tablespoons per day or ½ cup per day if you have breast lumps or cancer.

Turmeric. Counters the proliferative effect of estrogen on cancer cells. It's a powerful anti-inflammatory, too. Aim for 1 teaspoon per day.

Maca. An adaptogen that can rebalance estrogens and promote progesterone. Try 1 tablespoon per day. Caution: Maca does not work for everyone, so stop if estrogen dominance symptoms worsen. Pick Lepidium peruvianum Chacon (which shows the best clinical results) and the gelatinized (not raw) form.

Pomegranates. Known for their phytoestrogenic quality. Incorporate the seeds as a snack or add to smoothies and salads; ½ cup per week when in season, or drink freshly squeezed juice.

Seed Rotation Method. Days 1–14 of menstrual cycle: Support estrogen production by adding 1 tablespoon ground flaxseeds and 1 tablespoon ground pumpkin seeds per day.

Days 15–28: Promote progesterone production by adding 1 tablespoon ground sunflower seeds and 1 tablespoon ground sesame seeds.

Women in perimenopause or menopause can start seed rotation on any day.

Seeds should be raw and freshly ground and can be consumed with water, on salads, or in soups. (See the chart, right.)

Water filter. Invest in an all-house or under-the-counter water filter that removes fluoride, heavy metals, drugs, and hormones. I like Berkey and Aquasana brands. Brita and refrigerator filters are not good enough.

Supplements. To block and metabolize antagonistic estrogens, consider the EstraMetabolizer Kit on HormoneBalanceNutritionals.com.

Magnesium. Replenish by starting with 500 milligrams and go up to 1,500 milligrams, if needed. Preferred forms: glycerinate, citrate (can cause loose stool or diarrhea), or malate; avoid magnesium oxide. Maintain healthy

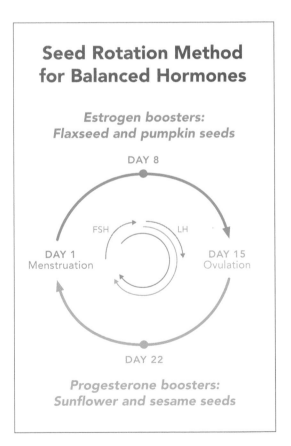

Seed Rotation Method for Balanced Hormones

Estrogen boosters:
Flaxseed and pumpkin seeds

DAY 8

FSH   LH

DAY 1
Menstruation

DAY 15
Ovulation

DAY 22

Progesterone boosters:
Sunflower and sesame seeds

levels of magnesium by regularly consuming kelp, cacao, pumpkin seeds, Brazil nuts, buckwheat, almonds, and cashews, if tolerated.

Chrysin or passionflower extract. Inhibits aromatization (the conversion of testosterone to estrogens). For dosing, follow instructions on the packaging. I like the brand Herb Pharm.

Clary sage essential oil. In Germany, clary sage oil is used to help ease menopausal discomfort and menstrual pain and regulate menstrual cycles. Combine four drops clary sage with 1 teaspoon carrier oil, such as jojoba, and rub on the abdomen or ovary area, bottom of the feet, behind the ear, or on the wrists.

REMOVE (–)

Conventionally grown vegetables. Chemicals used in fertilizers and pesticides are high in xenoestrogens (synthetic estrogens). Switch to organic food.

Conventionally raised animals. Eliminate estrogen-like hormones and antibiotics, which are given to conventionally raised animals, and switch to grass-fed and free-range meat.

Fish selection. Eliminate estrogen-like compounds found in fish feed and polluted waters. Pick fish using the tools found at Monterey Bay Aquarium Seafood Watch (www.seafoodwatch.org).

Soy. Avoid all soy products such as soy milk, tofu, fake meats, and soy derivatives (fillers, stabilizers, etc.). The exception is fermented organic soy in the form of tempeh and non-GMO soy lecithins, if tolerated.

Caffeine. Caffeine impairs estrogen detoxification. Reduce or eliminate coffee and black tea; substitute with roasted chicory root (for taste) or herbal noncaffeinated teas.

Alcohol. Alcohol can be estrogenic; limit to a maximum of three drinks per week.

Toxicity in skincare and cleaning products. Eliminate xenoestrogens found in BPAs, parabens, sodium lauryl/laureth sulfate (SLS), phthalates, and triclosan often used in skincare and household-cleaning products. Check out natural alternatives on page 73.

Birth control pills. Get off birth control pills; they contain synthetic estrogens and inhibit ovulation and thyroid function. Investigate other contraceptive options.

Stress. Stress and elevated cortisol levels block progesterone receptors, which exacerbates estrogen dominance. Reduce stress by bringing things into your life that make you happy and release oxytocin, like cuddling a child or a pet, getting a massage, taking long walks, enjoying a girlfriends' lunch, or having an orgasm!

Plastics. Avoid xenoestrogens by not drinking water from plastic water bottles and sipping coffee covered by plastic coffee lids. Don't microwave food in plastic containers.

Reversing Estrogen Dominance 14-Day Sample Meal Plan for Two

For warm lemon water: Add 2 tablespoons freshly squeezed lemon juice to 8 to 16 ounces warm water. Lime juice or apple cider vinegar may also be used.

Bone broth: Sip 1 to 2 cups per day with a dash of coconut milk, freshly grated ginger, lemon juice, and sea salt.

Abbreviations
[NR] No recipe
[LO] Leftovers
[MA] Made ahead; full recipe or parts of
[DB] Double the recipe
EVOO Extra virgin olive oil

WEEKS 1 AND 2

The follicular phase, day 1 (of your period) to day 14 of your cycle, needs an *estrogen* boost. Women in peri-menopause and menopause can start any time.

Morning ritual/ breakfast	Snack (optional)	Lunch	Dinner	Bedtime ritual (optional)
Days 1 and 8				
Warm lemon water Daily Balancer Tea (page 306) Farmer's Wife's Breakfast [DB] (page 182)	Flaxseed Crackers [MA] (page 327)	Quick Salads—Four Ways, pick one (page 254); add Life-Giving Sprouts [MA] (page 163)	Seriously Mushroom Soup (page 216) Jicama and Pomegranate Slaw (page 268)	Healing Bone Broth [MA] (page 162) Flaxseed and Pumpkin Seed Butter (page 281)
Days 2 and 9				
Warm lemon water Farmer's Wife's Breakfast [LO] Healing Bone Broth [LO]	Flaxseed Crackers [LO]	Seriously Mushroom Soup [LO] Jicama and Pomegranate Slaw [LO]	Nomad's Kebabs (page 239) Bitter greens with lemon, EVOO, and sea salt [NR]	Regular Cycle Tea (page 305) Flaxseed and Pumpkin Seed Butter [LO]
Days 3 and 10				
Warm lemon water Daily Balancer Tea Seriously Mushroom Soup [LO]	Flaxseed Crackers [LO]	Nomad's Kebabs [LO] Jicama and Pomegranate Slaw [LO]	Hearty Beet Stew (Borscht) (page 210)	Daily Balancer Tea Flaxseed and Pumpkin Seed Butter [LO]

Morning ritual/ breakfast	Snack (optional)	Lunch	Dinner	Bedtime ritual (optional)
Days 4 and 11				
Warm lemon water Sweet Potato and Sage Pancakes (page 179) Flaxseed and Pumpkin Seed Butter [LO]	Flaxseed Crackers [LO]	Hearty Beet Stew (Borscht) [LO]	Nutritious Quick Bowls [DB] (page 232)	Regular Cycle Tea Kudzu Calming Pudding (page 348)
Days 5 and 12				
Warm lemon water Regular Cycle Tea Sweet Potato and Sage Pancakes [LO]	Flaxseed Crackers [LO]	Hearty Beet Stew (Borscht) [LO]	Nutritious Quick Bowls, pick one [DB]	Daily Balancer Tea Flaxseed and Pumpkin Seed Butter [LO]
Days 6 and 13				
Warm lemon water Regular Cycle Tea Parsnip Dill Pancake with Arugula and Smoked Salmon (page 199)	Flaxseed Crackers [LO]	Quick Salads—Four Ways, pick one (page 254)	Walnut Crusted Salmon [DB] (page 244) Creamy Celeriac and Cauliflower Mash (page 267)	Daily Balancer Tea Flaxseed and Pumpkin Seed Butter [LO]
Days 7 and 14				
Warm lemon water Breakfast Casserole Two: Pork Chops and Apples (page 195)	Flaxseed Crackers [LO]	Walnut Crusted Salmon [LO] Creamy Celeriac and Cauliflower Mash [LO]	Honey Glazed Tarragon Chicken (page 226) Creamy Celeriac and Cauliflower Mash [LO]	Daily Balancer Tea Kudzu Calming Pudding

WEEKS 3 AND 4

The luteal phase, days 15 to 28 of your cycle, needs a *progesterone* boost. Women in perimenopause and menopause can start any time.

Morning ritual/ breakfast	Snack (optional)	Lunch	Dinner	Bedtime ritual (optional)
Days 15 and 22				
Warm lemon water Parsnip Dill Pancake with Arugula and Smoked Salmon	Daily Balancer Tea Pomegranate Crackers [MA] (page 324)	Quick Salads—Four Ways, pick one	Honey Glazed Tarragon Chicken [LO] Detoxing Beet and Carrot Salad (page 252)	Immune-Boosting Chicken Broth [MA] (page 158) Sesame and Sunflower Seed Butter (page 282)
Days 16 and 23				
Warm lemon water Teff and Cherry Porridge (page 198)	Energizing Matcha Lime Smoothie [DB] (page 191) Pomegranate Crackers [LO]	Detoxing Beet and Carrot Salad [LO]	Quick Detoxifying Soup (page 218) Sesame and Sunflower Seed Butter [LO]	PMS Tamer Tea (page 312)
Days 17 and 24				
Warm lemon water Teff and Cherry Porridge [LO]	Carrot and Beet Smoothie (page 203)	Quick Detoxifying Soup [LO] Bitter greens with lemon, EVOO, and sea salt [NR]	Nomad's Kebabs (page 239) Jicama and Pomegranate Slaw (page 268)	Immune-Boosting Chicken Broth [LO] Sesame and Sunflower Seed Butter [LO]
Days 18 and 25				
Warm lemon water Quick Detoxifying Soup [LO]	Immune-Boosting Chicken Broth [LO] Pomegranate Crackers [LO]	Nomad's Kebabs [LO] Jicama and Pomegranate Slaw [LO]	Butter Cod with Gremolata (page 240) Steamed or sautéed greens, lemon, and sea salt [NR]	PMS Tamer Tea Sesame and Sunflower Seed Butter [LO]
Days 19 and 26				
Warm lemon water Immune-Boosting Chicken Broth [LO] Parsnip Dill Pancake with Arugula and Smoked Salmon	PMS Tamer Tea Pomegranate Crackers [LO]	Butter Cod with Gremolata [LO] Jicama and Pomegranate Slaw [LO]	Fennel and Coriander Crusted Liver (page 246) Zesty and Creamy Collard Greens (page 261)	Immune-Boosting Chicken Broth [LO] Sesame and Sunflower Seed Butter [LO]

Morning ritual/ breakfast	Snack (optional)	Lunch	Dinner	Bedtime ritual (optional)
Days 20 and 27				
Warm lemon water	PMS Tamer Tea	Fennel and Coriander Crusted Liver [LO]	Bacon, Oysters, and Collard Greens Stir Fry	Liver Cleanser Tea (page 307)
Immune-Boosting Chicken Broth [LO]	Pomegranate Crackers [LO]	Zesty and Creamy Collard Greens [LO]	Mixed greens with lemon, EVOO, and sea salt [NR]	Sesame and Sunflower Seed Butter [LO]
Breakfast Casserole Two: Pork Chops and Apples				
Days 21 and 28				
Warm lemon water	Better Than Coffee Latte (page 313)	Creamy Rosemary Chicken (page 249)	Nutritious Quick Bowls, pick one [DB]; add Life-Giving Sprouts [LO]	PMS Tamer Tea
Applesauce Porridge (page 187)				Sesame and Sunflower Seed Butter [LO]

BOOSTING PROGESTERONE

No foods contain progesterone; therefore, the key strategy is to first rebalance your estrogen levels. Then, reduce inflammation and add nutrients that support the corpus luteum, the endocrine structure that produces progesterone.

ADD (+)

Reverse estrogen dominance. First, rebalance your estrogen levels with the Reversing Estrogen Dominance guide (page 103) to see estradiol, the "bad" estrogen, go down and not antagonize progesterone.

Seed rotation. Incorporate the highly effective Seed Rotation Method described on page 104.

Beets and carrots. Eating beets and carrots five days before your period can lessen PMS symptoms. See Carrot and Beet Smoothie (page 203) and Detoxing Beet and Carrot Salad (page 252).

Selenium. Facilitates the formation and integrity of the corpus luteum. Add four Brazil nuts to your diet daily or supplement with 200 mcg per day.

Vitamin B6. This key vitamin builds the corpus luteum, which secretes progesterone. To replenish, take vitamin B6 supplements until you remember your dreams. Then, maintain with vitamin B6–rich foods such as turkey, wild-caught tuna, beef, and chicken.

Herbal tinctures. Add Phytoprogest (Wise Woman Herbals); follow the instructions on the product packaging.

Vitex/chasteberry. If the above recommendations fail, try 200 milligrams standardized vitex extract before breakfast and stop five days before your period. Clinical trials in Germany show that vitex supports progesterone production.

Natural progesterone cream. If the above fail, work with a doctor to topically supplement with a bioidentical progesterone cream. Yam and soy creams do not work.

REMOVE (−)

Stress and high cortisol levels. Chronic stress diverts pregnenolone, the precursor hormone of cortisol and progesterone, to the production of cortisol, depleting progesterone levels. This is called "pregnenolone steal." Eliminate any form of physical, emotional, and chemical stress. Refer to the Adrenal Healing Guide (page 116) for recommendations.

Birth control pills. They deplete vitamin B6, which is instrumental in building the corpus luteum.

Overexercising. Hardcore cardio workouts like long-distance running, cycling, or Cross-Fit can create internal stress that can lead to pregnenolone steal.

Please use the Reversing Estrogen Dominance 14-Day Sample Meal Plan for Two (page 106), especially during weeks 3 and 4.

RESTORING THYROID HEALTH AND TREATING HASHIMOTO'S

The key strategy to regaining thyroid health is to first calm down the immune system, which is actively attacking the thyroid gland. Remove inflammatory foods and other factors such as stress and toxicity and add healing foods and nutrients. Autoimmunity can be complex; some people see results from removing just gluten; others (like me) require several years and many changes to see results in restoring thyroid health.

For more in-depth medical information about Hashimoto's disease, check out Dr. Izabella Wentz's blog (https://thyroidpharmacist .com) and books.

ADD (+)

Gut healing. Continue to follow the Gut-Healing Guide (page 41). Hashimoto's is an autoimmune condition, so gut healing is paramount.

Liver support. Continue to follow the Liver Detox Guide (page 75). The elimination of metabolized thyroid hormones and the conversion of T4 to T3 thyroid hormone depend on the health of the liver.

Adrenal support. Adopt the recommendations in the Adrenal Healing Guide (page 116). The adrenals modulate the immune system; tired adrenals mean a struggling immune system.

Cruciferous vegetables. They are rich in diindolylmethane (DIM), which supports liver detoxification and the conversion of T4 to T3 thyroid hormone. Eat them cooked, not raw. Aim for two servings per day.

Selenium. A master antioxidant, it helps to bring TPO antibody levels down. Add two to four brazil nuts to your diet daily or supplement with 200 mcg per day.

Zinc. Zinc is essential in immune function, detoxification, gut healing, and thyroid function and helps to convert the thyroid hormone T4 to T3. It's highest in oysters and present in beef, liver, pork, lobster, and chicken. If supplementing, pick zinc picolinate, 50 milligrams per day.

Flaxseed. Helps to keep the bowels moving, a common problem for people with Hashimoto's. Add 2 tablespoons per day. Avoid if causing digestive discomfort.

Turmeric. This is anti-inflammatory and helps to reduce TPO antibody levels. Add 1 teaspoon fresh turmeric per day or in a supplement form (follow manufacturer's dosage instructions).

Vitamin D. Low levels are found in most people with Hashimoto's. It's best to obtain vitamin D from regular sun exposure, but fish oil is also a good source. If supplemented, use 2,000 to 10,000 IU per day depending on your current vitamin D levels.

REMOVE (–)

Sugar fluctuation and cravings. Continue to follow the Sugar-Balancing Guide (page 64). Fluctuating sugar levels will inhibit thyroid function. Sugar cravings could be a sign of Candida inhibiting the conversion of T4 to T3 thyroid hormone.

Food intolerances. Continue with the Elimination Diet (page 44) to identify food intolerances that damage the gut lining and provoke the immune system. This is key to your recovery.

Toxicity. Eliminate toxins in food, skincare products, and cleaning products to support the immune system. Refer to the Liver Detox Guide (page 75) and Reversing Estrogen Dominance (page 103) for details.

Soy. Avoid all soy products and soy derivatives (fillers, stabilizers, etc.). The exception is organic miso, tempeh, and non-GMO soy lecithins, if tolerated.

Stress. Stress suppresses the immune system and inhibits the conversion of T4 to T3 thyroid hormone. Stress can be digestive, emotional, physical, or chemical. Find ways to keep stress to a minimum.

Fluoride. Eliminate fluoride from your drinking water by getting a good-quality filter. I like Berkey and Aquasana brands. Brita and refrigerator filters are not good enough.

Birth control pills. Get off birth control pills; they increase thyroxine-binding globulin, making less thyroid hormone available for your body.

BALANCE

Test for deficiencies. Many people with Hashimoto's are low on vitamins A, B1, B6, and B12 as well as magnesium, ferritin, zinc, and selenium. It is recommended to test for these deficiencies and then create a diet and supplementation plan depending on the test results.

Iodine. We need iodine for good brain and breast health, but supplementing with iodine can elevate TPO antibodies and make you feel worse. I recommend reducing your TPO antibody levels to less than 100 IU/mL before adding iodine-rich foods to your diet.

Restoring Thyroid Health and Treating Hashimoto's 14-Day Sample Meal Plan for Two

For warm lemon water: Add 2 tablespoons freshly squeezed lemon juice to 8 to 16 ounces warm water. Lime juice or apple cider vinegar may also be used.

Add 1 to 2 tablespoons collagen powder to smoothies, teas, soups, and stews at least once per day.

Bone broth: Sip 1 to 2 cups per day with a dash of coconut milk, freshly grated ginger, lemon juice, and sea salt.

Abbreviations
[NR] No recipe
[LO] Leftovers
[MA] Made ahead; full recipe or parts of
[DB] Double the recipe
EVOO Extra virgin olive oil

WEEK 1

Morning ritual/ breakfast	Snack (optional)	Lunch	Dinner	Bedtime ritual (optional)
Day 1				
Warm lemon water Healing Bone Broth [MA] (page 162) Farmer's Wife's Breakfast [DB] (page 182)	Salmon and Avocado in Nori Sheets [DB] (replace nori with steamed collard greens) (page 298)	Quick Salads—Four Ways, pick one (page 254)	Creamy Rosemary Chicken [DB] (page 249) Creamy Celeriac and Cauliflower Mash (page 267) Steamed or sautéed greens or broccolini with EVOO and sea salt [NR]	Immune Booster Tea (page 303) Four Brazil nuts

Morning ritual/ breakfast	Snack (optional)	Lunch	Dinner	Bedtime ritual (optional)
Day 2				
Warm lemon water Healing Bone Broth [LO] Farmer's Wife's Breakfast [LO]	Salmon and Avocado in Nori Sheets (replace nori with steamed collard greens) [LO] Four Brazil nuts	Nutritious Quick Bowls, pick one [DB] (page 232)	Creamy Rosemary Chicken [LO] Creamy Celeriac and Cauliflower Mash [LO] Steamed or sautéed greens or broccolini with EVOO and sea salt [LO]	Liver Cleanser Tea (page 307) Raspberry Melties [DB] (page 338)
Day 3				
Warm lemon water Ginger Beet Kvass [MA] (page 317) Breakfast Casserole One: Salmon and Broccoli (page 189)	Decadent Chocolate Cherry Smoothie (page 207)	Quick Salads—Four Ways, pick one Healing Bone Broth [LO]	Fennel and Coriander Crusted Liver (page 246) Creamy Celeriac and Cauliflower Mash [LO] Raspberry Melties [LO]	Nourishing Lattes, pick one (page 309) Four Brazil nuts
Day 4				
Daily Balancer Tea (page 306) Teff and Cherry Porridge (page 198)	Ginger Beet Kvass [LO] Four Brazil nuts	Fennel and Coriander Crusted Liver [LO] Sautéed greens with EVOO, lemon, and sea salt [NR]	Squash, Apple, and Turmeric Soup (page 222)	Healing Bone Broth [LO] Raspberry Melties [LO]
Day 5				
Warm lemon water Ginger Beet Kvass [LO] Teff and Cherry Porridge [LO]	Energizing Matcha Lime Smoothie [DB] (page 191)	Squash, Apple, and Turmeric Soup [LO] Raspberry Melties [LO]	Quick Salads—Four Ways, pick one Healing Bone Broth [LO]	Nourishing Lattes, pick one Four Brazil nuts
Day 6				
Warm lemon water Ginger Beet Kvass [LO] Farmer's Wife's Breakfast [DB]	Carrot and Beet Smoothie (page 203) Four Brazil nuts	Nutritious Quick Bowls, pick one [DB] Healing Bone Broth [LO]	Porcini Mushroom Beef Stew (page 224) Side salad of mixed bitter greens with lemon, EVOO, and sea salt [NR]	Sugar Balancer Tea (page 308) Raspberry Melties [LO]

Morning ritual/ breakfast	Snack (optional)	Lunch	Dinner	Bedtime ritual (optional)
Day 7				
Warm lemon water Healing Bone Broth [LO] Farmer's Wife's Breakfast [LO]	Better Than Coffee Latte (page 313) Four Brazil nuts	Porcini Mushroom Beef Stew [LO] Ginger Beet Kvass [LO]	Quick Salads—Four Ways, pick one	Liver Cleanser Tea Raspberry Melties [LO]

WEEK 2

Morning ritual/ breakfast	Snack (optional)	Lunch	Dinner	Bedtime ritual (optional)
Day 8				
Warm lemon water Porcini Mushroom Beef Stew [LO]	Decadent Chocolate Cherry Smoothie	Quick Salads—Four Ways, pick one	Bacon, Oysters, and Collard Greens Stir Fry [DB] (page 204)	Immune-Boosting Chicken Broth (page 158) Four Brazil nuts
Day 9				
Warm lemon water Breakfast Casserole Two: Pork Chops and Apples (page 195) Fresh greens, lemon, EVOO, and sea salt [NR]	Matcha Frappe (page 299) Four Brazil nuts	Bacon, Oysters, and Collard Greens Stir Fry [LO]	Seriously Mushroom Soup (page 216)	Liver Cleanser Tea Raspberry Melties [LO]
Day 10				
Warm lemon water Seriously Mushroom Soup [LO]	Easy French Pate [MA] (page 290) with vegetable sticks [NR] or Flaxseed Crackers [MA] (page 327) Four Brazil nuts	Quick Salads—Four Ways, pick one	Walnut Crusted Salmon [DB] (page 244) Detoxing Beet and Carrot Salad (page 252)	Immune-Boosting Chicken Broth [LO]

Morning ritual/ breakfast	Snack (optional)	Lunch	Dinner	Bedtime ritual (optional)
Day 11				
Warm lemon water Adrenal Love Tea (page 305) Teff and Cherry Porridge	Easy French Pate [LO] with vegetable sticks [NR] or Flaxseed Crackers [LO] Four Brazil nuts	Walnut Crusted Salmon [LO] Detoxing Beet and Carrot Salad [LO]; add Life-Giving Sprouts [MA] [DB] (page 163)	Seriously Mushroom Soup [LO]	Immune Booster Tea Raspberry Melties [LO]
Day 12				
Warm lemon water Teff and Cherry Porridge (LO)	Immune-Boosting Chicken Broth [LO] Raspberry Melties [LO]	Steam 'n Toss Veggies and Proteins on the Run (page 260)	Nomad's Kebabs (page 239) Detoxing Beet and Carrot Salad; add Life-Giving Sprouts [LO]	Nourishing Lattes, pick one Four Brazil Nuts
Day 13				
Warm lemon water Adrenal Love Tea Sweet Potato and Sage Pancakes (page 179)	Rosemary Pear Muffin (page 335) Matcha Frappe	Nomad's Kebabs [LO] Detoxing Beet and Carrot Salad [LO]; add Life-Giving Sprouts [LO]	Nutritious Quick Bowls, pick one [DB] Immune-Boosting Chicken Broth [LO] Four Brazil nuts	Immune Booster Tea Raspberry Melties [LO]
Day 14				
Warm lemon water Coconut Kefir Chia Pudding (page 185)	Rosemary Pear Muffin [LO] Four Brazil nuts	Sweet Potato and Sage Pancakes [LO] Fresh greens with Life-Giving Sprouts [LO], EVOO, lemon, and sea salt [NR] Ginger Beet Kvass [LO]	Steam 'n Toss Veggies and Proteins on the Run	Immune-Boosting Chicken Broth [LO]

ADRENAL HEALING

Nutrition plays one part in adrenal recovery, but good sleep and stress reduction are critical. The typical healing period is six months to one year. Adrenal fatigue affects every aspect of maintaining hormonal balance.

ADD (+)

PFF breakfast. Eat a breakfast rich in proteins, fat, and fiber (PFF) within one hour of rising. This will ensure stable sugar levels and help adrenal recovery.

Fat. Fat is the precursor for cortisol production by the adrenals and helps balance sugar levels. Learn how to pick the right fats with Fats and Oils (page 139). Add a minimum of 2 to 3 tablespoons per day.

Vitamin C. This is a critical vitamin in adrenal recovery. Highest levels of vitamin C are found in camu camu, a Peruvian berry. Add ½ teaspoon per day to smoothies or a glass of water.

Sea salt. Sodium loss can happen with adrenal dysfunction, so adding ½ teaspoon or more of sea salt per day is recommended. If you crave salt, add it generously to your diet unless you are dealing with hypertension.

Superfoods. Adrenals need superior nourishment. Add plenty of superfoods, such as bone and vegetable broths, and fermented and sprouted foods.

Sleep and pressing the pause button. Getting sufficient sleep and rest is critical in adrenal recovery. Food and supplements alone won't help if you are constantly on the run and not sleeping. Learn to slow down, do less during the day, say "no" more often to things and people, and find nourishing "me time" by getting a massage, spending time with your favorite person, getting hugs and cuddles, or having an orgasm.

Magnesium. Magnesium is a spark plug for the adrenals and is best absorbed before bed. To replenish, start with 500 milligrams and go up to 1,500 milligrams, if needed. The preferred forms are glycerinate, citrate (can cause loose stool or diarrhea), or malate; avoid magnesium oxide. Consider the topical gel called Quick Magnesium from Hormone BalanceNutritionals.com.

Vitamin B complex. B vitamins get quickly depleted during times of stress. Foods rich in vitamin Bs include liver, animal proteins, seaweed, mushrooms, sunflower seeds, and spinach.

Vitamin E. Vitamin E helps vitamin C to do its work, and it absorbs and neutralizes damaging free radical molecules inside the adrenal glands. Foods highest in vitamin E are sunflower seeds, almonds, and spinach. If supplementing, take 400 milligrams per day.

Supplements. Consider a blend of key vitamins, minerals, and herbs in the Adrenal Repair Kit on HormoneBalanceNutritionals.com.

REMOVE (−)

Stress. Stress originating from past or present physical exertion, emotional distress, unresolved trauma, digestive issues, or chemical exposure is the most common reason for adrenal dysfunction. Eliminating, reducing, and reframing stress are key to adrenal recovery.

Blood sugar fluctuation. The adrenals, among other things, are responsible for stabilizing blood sugar levels. Low or high sugar levels will worsen adrenal fatigue. Learn how to balance your sugar levels with the Sugar-Balancing Guide (page 64).

Coffee and caffeine. Coffee overstimulates the adrenals, even if mixed with fat. Switch to matcha green tea or caffeine-free herbal teas. Roasted chicory or dandelion root tea are good caffeine-free alternatives. Try the Better Than Coffee Latte (page 313).

Food intolerances. Gluten, dairy, eggs, soy, corn, sugar, nightshades, yeast, sometimes grains, and, of course, sugar can contribute to digestive distress and fluctuating sugar levels. After doing the Elimination Diet, you know what your sensitivities are; they are key to healing your adrenals.

Alcohol. Alcohol is sugar, and it stimulates the adrenals. If you must drink it, limit yourself to two to three drinks per week, always with or after food. Avoid drinking late at night as it may disturb your sleep and create additional spikes in blood sugar levels.

Excessive exercise. Be gentle on yourself and avoid excessive, especially cardiovascular, exercise such as running, biking, or Cross-Fit; it exhausts the adrenals even further. Yoga, tai chi, Pilates, swimming, hiking, or dancing are more soothing for the adrenals. You should feel rejuvenated after exercising, not tired (a sign that you did too much and the adrenals are not coping).

Sleep is key to adrenal recovery. Download *16 Hacks to Better Sleep* from www.HormonesBalance.com /book.

Adrenal Healing 14-Day Sample Meal Plan for Two

For warm lemon water: Add 2 tablespoons freshly squeezed lemon juice to 8 to 16 ounces warm water. Lime juice or apple cider vinegar may also be used.

Add 1 to 2 tablespoons collagen powder to smoothies, teas, soups, and stews at least once per day.

Bone broth: Sip 1 to 2 cups per day with a dash of coconut milk, freshly grated ginger, lemon juice, and sea salt.

Abbreviations
[NR] No recipe
[LO] Leftovers
[MA] Made ahead; full recipe or parts of
[DB] Double the recipe
EVOO Extra virgin olive oil

WEEK 1

Morning ritual/ breakfast	Snack (optional)	Lunch	Dinner	Bedtime ritual (optional)
Day 1				
Warm lemon water Breakfast Casserole One: Salmon and Broccoli (page 189)	Zucchini Olive Muffin [MA] (page 205) Deep Green Spirulina Smoothie (page 197)	Nutritious Quick Bowls, pick one [DB] (page 232)	Lamb with Collard Greens and Radishes (page 236)	Healing Bone Broth [MA] (page 162), freeze half for the following week
Day 2				
Warm lemon water Coconut Kefir Chia Pudding [DB] (page 185)	Hot Chocolate with Pink Roses (page 314)	Lamb with Collard Greens and Radishes [LO]	Quick Miso Soup [DB] (page 220); add Life-Giving Sprouts [MA] (page 163)	Zucchini Olive Muffin [LO]
Day 3				
Warm lemon water Coconut Kefir Chia Pudding [LO]	Decadent Chocolate Cherry Smoothie (page 207)	Quick Salads—Four Ways, pick one (page 254)	Quick Miso Soup [LO]; add Life-Giving Sprouts [LO]	Creamy Lime Pudding (page 342)
Day 4				
Warm lemon water Parsnip Dill Pancake with Arugula and Smoked Salmon (page 199)	Adrenal Love Tea (page 305) Creamy Lime Pudding [LO]	Steam 'n Toss Veggies and Proteins on the Run (page 260)	Rosemary and Garlic Stuffed Lamb Roast (page 251) Mixed greens, tossed with EVOO [NR] and Life-Giving Sprouts	Spiced Nut Butters, pick one (page 294)
Day 5				
Warm lemon water Farmer's Wife's Breakfast [DB] (page 182)	Spiced Nut Butters [LO]	Rosemary and Garlic Stuffed Lamb Roast [LO] Mixed greens, tossed with EVOO [NR] and Life-Giving Sprouts [LO]	Steam 'n Toss Veggies and Proteins on the Run	Healing Bone Broth [LO]

Morning ritual/ breakfast	Snack (optional)	Lunch	Dinner	Bedtime ritual (optional)
Day 6				
Warm lemon water Adrenal Love Tea Farmer's Wife's Breakfast [LO]	Hot Chocolate with Pink Roses	Quick Salads—Four Ways, pick one	Squash, Apple, and Turmeric Soup (page 222)	Zucchini Olive Muffin [LO]
Day 7				
Warm lemon water Parsnip Dill Pancake with Arugula and Smoked Salmon	Decadent Chocolate Cherry Smoothie	Squash, Apple, and Turmeric Soup [LO]	Nutritious Quick Bowls, pick one [DB]	Healing Bone Broth [LO]

WEEK 2

Morning ritual/ breakfast	Snack (optional)	Lunch	Dinner	Bedtime ritual (optional)
Day 8				
Warm lemon water Squash, Apple, and Turmeric Soup [LO] Raspberry and Green Tea Lime Melties (page 338)	Adrenal Love Tea Salmon and Avocado in Nori Sheets (page 298)	Japanese Seaweed and Cucumber Salad (page 273)	Butter Cod with Gremolata (page 240) Fries Baked in Duck Fat (page 271) Life-Giving Sprouts [MA]	Kudzu Calming Pudding (page 348)
Day 9				
Warm lemon water Teff and Cherry Porridge (page 198)	Adrenal Love Tea Salmon and Avocado in Nori Sheets [LO]	Butter Cod with Gremolata [LO] Fries Baked in Duck Fat [LO] Life-Giving Sprouts [LO]	Japanese Seaweed and Cucumber Salad [LO]	Kudzu Calming Pudding [LO]

Morning ritual/ breakfast	Snack (optional)	Lunch	Dinner	Bedtime ritual (optional)
Day 10				
Warm lemon water Teff and Cherry Porridge [LO] Hot Chocolate with Pink Roses	Zucchini Olive Muffin [LO] Better Than Coffee Latte (page 313)	Sticky Spare Ribs Casserole (page 242) Tuscan Shredded Fennel and Orange Salad (page 262)	Quick Salads—Four Ways, pick one	Spiced Nut Butters [LO]
Day 11				
Warm lemon water Breakfast Casserole Two: Pork Chops and Apples (page 195)	Deep Green Spirulina Smoothie	Sticky Spare Ribs Casserole [LO] Tuscan Shredded Fennel and Orange Salad [LO]	Steam 'n Toss Veggies and Proteins on the Run	Healing Bone Broth [LO]
Day 12				
Warm lemon water Coconut Kefir Chia Pudding	Raspberry and Green Tea Lime Melties	Nomad's Kebabs (page 239) Mixed greens, tossed with EVOO [NR] and Life-Giving Sprouts [LO]	Seriously Mushroom Soup (page 216)	Spiced Nut Butters [LO]
Day 13				
Warm lemon water Sweet Potato and Sage Pancakes (page 179)	Decadent Chocolate Cherry Smoothie	Seriously Mushroom Soup [LO]	Honey Glazed Tarragon Chicken (page 226) Creamy Celeriac and Cauliflower Mash (page 267)	Spiced Nut Butters [LO]
Day 14				
Warm lemon water Sweet Potato and Sage Pancakes [LO]	Deep Green Spirulina Smoothie	Honey Glazed Tarragon Chicken [LO] Creamy Celeriac and Cauliflower Mash [LO]	Grain-Free Pizza— Two Ways, pick one (page 228)	Healing Bone Broth [LO]

EASING THE TRANSITION INTO PERI/MENOPAUSE (LOW ESTROGEN)

An anti-inflammatory diet and lifestyle (such as reducing sugar, gluten, coffee, and alcohol and getting more sleep) help mitigate the most unpleasant perimenopause and menopause symptoms. Many women assume they no longer produce hormones when entering menopause, but that is not correct (you can't live without them). You will be producing fewer hormones, and supporting your body to relieve the symptoms will be as important as ever.

ADD (+)

PFF breakfast. Eat a breakfast rich in proteins, fat, and fiber (PFF) within one hour of rising. This will ensure stable sugar levels and feeling grounded. Many women report a reduction in hot flashes after changing to a PFF breakfast.

Calcium- and magnesium-rich food. Strengthening your bones is key; add bone broths (collagen helps bones), sardines with bones, green leafy vegetables, and sea vegetables such as kelp. If supplementing, take a calcium combo with magnesium and vitamins D3 and K2.

Superfoods. Add plenty of superfoods such as bone and vegetable broths, liver (try the Easy French Pate on page 290), sea vegetables, and fermented and sprouted foods. They will deliver daily doses of vitamins A, Bs, C, D3, E, and K2 as well as calcium, magnesium, zinc, and glutathione.

Flaxseeds. Along with their content of lignans, fiber, and omega 3 fatty acids, flaxseeds also help rebalance estrogens. Add 2 tablespoons freshly ground flaxseeds to your diet per day.

Fermented soy. A highly controversial food, it is recommended to eat soy in fermented form only—miso, tempeh, soy sauce, or natto—and avoid unfermented products like tofu, soy milk, and GMO lecithins. Avoid if you are sensitive to soy.

Liver support
Supporting the liver means keeping a "clean house" and making space for more hormone production. Continue following the Liver Detox Guide (page 75).

Broccoli sprouts. These are rich in sulforaphane, a potent antioxidant that helps with estrogen metabolism and is linked to reducing the risk of breast cancer. Also rich in glucosinolate, a sulfur-rich compound that supports liver detoxification and reduces menopause symptoms.

Acceptance and self-love. Menopause prepares us for many changes in the present and the future. Accepting how we look and feel, combined with a reflective sense of wisdom, can be liberating and healing. I recommend reading Christiane Northrup's books for support.

Herbal support. Herbs such as vitex/chasteberry, black cohosh, maca, licorice root, and dong quai are well documented to alleviate menopausal symptoms.

REMOVE (–)

Digestive distress. Gluten, dairy, eggs, soy, corn, sugar, nightshades, yeast, sometimes grains, and, of course, sugar can contribute to digestive distress and inflammation, which amplify menopausal symptoms. After doing the Elimination Diet, you will know what your sensitivities are; continue avoiding them.

Blood sugar fluctuation and cravings. Most highly symptomatic menopausal women experience a significant reduction of symptoms when their sugar levels are stable and cravings are contained. Adopt changes from the Sugar-Balancing Guide (page 64).

Coffee and alcohol. Coffee and alcohol inhibit the metabolism of "used" hormones and the production of new ones. Switch to matcha green tea or caffeine-free herbal teas. Roasted chicory or dandelion root tea offer the bitter taste without the caffeine. Avoid caffeine if you are sensitive to it. Reduce alcohol intake to two glasses of wine per week.

Unfermented soy. A highly controversial food, it is recommended to eat soy only in its fermented form—miso, tempeh, soy sauce, or natto—and avoid unfermented products like tofu, soy milk, and GMO lecithins.

Toxicity. Reduce the toxic load on your liver from nonorganic foods, processed foods, smoking, and xenoestrogens (synthetic estrogens) found in skincare and cleaning products. A healthy liver will alleviate the worst symptoms of menopause.

Stress. Many women despair over the changes menopause brings, stressing the adrenals even more. Embrace the wisdom that this phase of life offers.

Easing the Transition into Peri/Menopause (Low Estrogen) 14-Day Sample Meal Plan for Two

For warm lemon water: Add 2 tablespoons freshly squeezed lemon juice to 8 to 16 ounces warm water. Lime juice or apple cider vinegar may also be used.

Bone broth: Sip 1 to 2 cups per day with a dash of coconut milk, freshly grated ginger, lemon juice, and sea salt.

Abbreviations
[NR] No recipe
[LO] Leftovers
[MA] Made ahead; full recipe or parts of
[DB] Double the recipe
EVOO Extra virgin olive oil

WEEK 1

Morning ritual/ breakfast	Snack (optional)	Lunch	Dinner	Bedtime ritual (optional)
Day 1				
Warm lemon water Deep Green Spirulina Smoothie (page 197) Rosemary Pear Muffin (page 335)	Salmon and Avocado in Nori Sheets [DB] (page 298)	Quick Salads—Four Ways, pick one (page 254); add Life-Giving Sprouts [MA] [DB] (page 163)	Lamb with Collard Greens and Radishes (page 236) Side salad of mixed bitter greens with lemon, EVOO, and sea salt [NR]	Easy Menopause Latte (page 312) Flaxseed and Pumpkin Seed Butter (page 281)
Day 2				
Warm lemon water Daily Balancer (page 306) Lamb with Collard Greens and Radishes [LO]	Salmon and Avocado in Nori Sheets [LO] Better Than Coffee Latte (page 313)	Quick Bowls, pick one (page 232); add Life-Giving Sprouts [LO]	Grain-Free Pizza— Two Ways, pick one (page 228)	Rosemary Pear Muffin [LO] Healing Bone Broth [MA] (page 162), freeze half
Day 3				
Warm lemon water Daily Balancer Breakfast Casserole One: Salmon and Broccoli (page 189)	Japanese Seaweed and Cucumber Salad (page 273); add Life-Giving Sprouts [LO]	Quick Salads—Four Ways, pick one	Creamy Rosemary Chicken (page 249) Parsnip and Apple Coleslaw (page 258)	Liver Cleanser Tea (page 307) Flaxseed and Pumpkin Seed Butter [LO]
Day 4				
Warm lemon water Energizing Matcha Lime Smoothie [DB] (page 191) Rosemary Pear Muffin [LO]	Japanese Seaweed and Cucumber Salad Life-Giving Sprouts [LO]	Creamy Rosemary Chicken [LO] Parsnip and Apple Coleslaw [LO]	Seriously Mushroom Soup (page 216)	Easy Digestion Tea (page 305) Rosemary Pear Muffin [LO]
Day 5				
Warm lemon water Healing Bone Broth [LO] Breakfast Casserole Two: Pork Chops and Apples (page 195)	Deep Green Spirulina Smoothie	Seriously Mushroom Soup [LO] Parsnip and Apple Coleslaw; add Life-Giving Sprouts [MA] [DB]	Steam 'n Toss Veggies and Proteins on the Run (page 260)	Nourishing Lattes, pick one (page 309) Flaxseed and Pumpkin Seed Butter [LO]

Morning ritual/ breakfast	Snack (optional)	Lunch	Dinner	Bedtime ritual (optional)
Day 6				
Warm lemon water Teff and Cherry Porridge (page 198)	Decadent Chocolate Cherry Smoothie (page 207)	Seriously Mushroom Soup [LO]	Walnut Crusted Salmon [DB] (page 244) Side salad of mixed bitter greens with lemon, EVOO, and sea salt [NR]; add Life-Giving Sprouts [LO]	Liver Cleanser Tea Kudzu Calming Pudding (page 348)
Day 7				
Warm lemon water Teff and Cherry Porridge [LO]	Energizing Matcha Lime Smoothie [DB]	Walnut Crusted Salmon [LO] Side salad of mixed bitter greens with lemon, EVOO, and sea salt [NR]; add Life-Giving Sprouts [LO]	Quick Detoxifying Soup (page 218)	Nourishing Lattes, pick one Flaxseed and Pumpkin Seed Butter [LO]

WEEK 2

Morning ritual/ breakfast	Snack (optional)	Lunch	Dinner	Bedtime ritual (optional)
Day 8				
Warm lemon water Bacon, Oysters, and Collard Greens Stir Fry (page 204)	Energizing Matcha Lime Smoothie [DB]	Quick Detoxifying Soup [LO]; add Life-Giving Sprouts [LO]	Rosemary and Garlic Stuffed Lamb Roast (page 251) Zesty and Creamy Collard Greens (page 261)	Nourishing Lattes, pick one Ginger Orange Truffles (page 356)
Day 9				
Warm lemon water Daily Balancer Parsnip Dill Pancake with Arugula and Smoked Salmon (page 199)	Deep Green Spirulina Smoothie	Quick Detoxifying Soup [LO] Side salad of mixed bitter greens with lemon, EVOO, and sea salt [NR]; add Life-Giving Sprouts [MA] [DB]	Rosemary and Garlic Stuffed Lamb Roast [LO] Zesty and Creamy Collard Greens [LO]	Liver Cleanser Tea Flaxseed and Pumpkin Seed Butter [LO]

Morning ritual/ breakfast	Snack (optional)	Lunch	Dinner	Bedtime ritual (optional)
Day 10				
Warm lemon water Daily Balancer Coconut Kefir Chia Pudding [DB] (page 185)	Easy French Pate [MA] (page 290) Flaxseed Crackers (page 327)	Steam 'n Toss Veggies and Proteins on the Run; add Life-Giving Sprouts [LO]	Butter Cod with Gremolata (page 240) Creamy Celeriac and Cauliflower Mash (page 267)	Easy Digestion Tea Ginger Orange Truffles [LO]
Day 11				
Warm lemon water Coconut Kefir Chia Pudding [LO]	Easy French Pate [LO] Flaxseed Crackers [LO]	Butter Cod with Gremolata [LO] Creamy Celeriac and Cauliflower Mash [LO]	Bacon, Oysters, and Collard Greens Stir Fry (page 204) Jicama and Pomegranate Slaw (page 268)	Liver Cleanser Tea Flaxseed and Pumpkin Seed Butter [LO]
Day 12				
Warm lemon water Daily Balancer Breakfast Casserole One: Salmon and Broccoli	Salmon and Avocado in Nori Sheets [DB]	Jicama and Pomegranate Slaw [LO] Flaxseed Crackers [LO]	Honey Glazed Tarragon Chicken (page 226) Creamy Celeriac and Cauliflower Mash [LO] Jicama and Pomegranate Slaw [LO]	Easy Digestion Tea Ginger Orange Truffles [LO]
Day 13				
Warm lemon water Sweet Potato and Sage Pancakes (page 179)	Salmon and Avocado in Nori Sheets [LO] Flaxseed Crackers [LO]	Quick Salads—Four Ways, pick one; add Life-Giving Sprouts [MA]	Honey Glazed Tarragon Chicken [LO] Side salad of mixed bitter greens with lemon, EVOO, and sea salt [NR]	Nourishing Lattes, pick one Flaxseed and Pumpkin Seed Butter [LO] Mineral Vegetable Broth [MA] (page 160)
Day 14				
Warm lemon water Sweet Potato and Sage Pancakes [LO]	Energizing Matcha Lime Smoothie [DB] Flaxseed Crackers [LO]	Steam 'n Toss Veggies and Proteins on the Run	Quick Miso Soup (page 220); add Life-Giving Sprouts [LO]	Liver Cleanser Tea Ginger Orange Truffles [LO]

LOWERING HIGH TESTOSTERONE LEVELS AND TREATING PCOS

The key strategy for lowering high testosterone levels and treating PCOS is to stabilize your blood sugar levels and reduce inflammation, the two main causes of high testosterone in women. PCOS in women is most often caused by insulin resistance, high testosterone, and/ or birth control pills.

ADD (+)

Sugar-balancing protocol. Lower your intake of sugar (even from real food), processed carbohydrates (including cereals, flours, and protein powders), and alcohol. Continue following the Sugar-Balancing Guide (page 64), which you should have started before embarking on this guide.

PFF breakfast. Eat a breakfast rich in proteins, fat, and fiber (PFF) within one hour of rising. Avoid sugary, processed breakfasts such as cereals, rice puffs, and shakes and protein powders.

Fiber. Fiber helps reduce excess androgens by supporting the liver in excreting them. Add 2 to 3 tablespoons insoluble fiber per day, such as ground flaxseeds, chia seeds, or psyllium husk. Beans and green leafy vegetables are also great sources of fiber; add at least 2 cups per day to your diet.

Estrogen-lowering protocol. Testosterone is produced from estrogen; high estrogen can result in high testosterone. If your estrogen levels are elevated (which is often the case in women with PCOS), incorporate changes from the Reversing Estrogen Dominance guide (page 103). Estrogen dominance overstimulates the ovaries and can cause ovarian cysts and anovulation.

Protein-rich food and snacks. Sustaining sugar levels is key; look for PCOS-supporting meals and snacks in the Recipe Index by Protocol. Snacking on high-protein foods will stabilize your sugar levels.

Superfoods. Many women with PCOS are nutritionally depleted. Add plenty of superfoods like bone and vegetable broths, liver (pate), sea vegetables, and fermented and sprouted foods. They will deliver daily doses needed of vitamins A, Bs, C, D3, E, and K2 as well as calcium, magnesium, zinc, and glutathione.

Weight training. Increasing muscle mass will increase the surface area needed for insulin to enter and clear up excess glucose. Weight training and interval training produce great results for women with PCOS.

Herbal and supplement support. Herbs such as berberine, turmeric, and chromium picolinate are known to help increase the sensitivity of insulin receptors. Studies show that berberine is as effective as Metformin, without the harmful side effects. Consider the all-in-one PCOS Balance Kit on HormoneBalance Nutritionals.com.

REMOVE (−)

Blood sugar fluctuation and cravings. Reversing insulin resistance and stabilizing blood sugar levels are paramount in managing PCOS. Continue following the Sugar-Balancing Guide (page 64).

Dieting. Obsessive dieting, deprivation, counting calories, fad diets, diet pills, diet shakes, and weight-loss herbs are not a sustainable way of eating, losing weight, and embracing life. After following the Elimination Diet, you should have reduced inflammation and lost weight.

Coffee and alcohol. Coffee and alcohol increase blood sugar levels and amplify insulin resistance. If you must drink coffee or alcohol, do so with or after food. Add matcha tea for a slight kick, and try herbal teas for a new way of enjoying life.

Digestive distress. Gluten, dairy, eggs, soy, corn, sugar, nightshades, yeast, sometimes grains, and, of course, sugar can contribute to digestive distress and poor liver function, which cause inflammation, the underlying cause of PCOS. Continue the Elimination Diet to keep inflammation down.

Emotional well-being. Many women with PCOS experience low self-esteem, fear, pain, and guilt from the past and in the present, which can result in cortisol release. Cortisol increases blood sugar levels and amplifies the damaging effects of estrogen.

Excess weight. Belly fat produces estradiol, which contributes to the development of ovarian cysts. Losing weight through identifying your food sensitivities, supporting the liver, managing sugar levels, and exercising will help reduce estrogen overproduction.

Birth control pills. Pill-induced PCOS can be the cause of insulin resistance and can suppress ovulation.

Follow the Sugar-Balancing 14-Day Sample Meal Plan for Two on page 66.

RAISING LOW TESTOSTERONE LEVELS

No foods are full of testosterone. Nurturing your adrenals, balancing sugar levels, and lowering inflammation will create a conducive environment for your body to produce sufficient testosterone.

ADD (+)

Nurture your adrenals. Follow the Adrenal Healing Guide (page 116). Tired adrenals underproduce testosterone.

Balance sugar levels. If you are experiencing high sugar levels or cravings, implement the Sugar-Balancing Guide (page 64). High sugar levels cause low testosterone, making it less available for the body to utilize.

Zinc. Zinc inhibits the conversion of testosterone to estrogen. It's highest in oysters and present in beef, liver, pork, lobster, and chicken. If supplementing, pick zinc picolinate, 30 milligrams per day.

Chrysin. This prevents the conversion of testosterone to estrogen (through the inhibition of the aromatase enzyme). Use passionflower tincture; follow the manufacturer's instructions.

DHEA supplementation. If you have tried the above with poor results, speak to your doctor about supplementing with DHEA. Start with the lowest dose of 3 milligrams per day. Patients with estrogen receptor–positive cancers should avoid it.

REMOVE (–)

Stress. Be gentle on yourself and avoid excessive, especially cardiovascular, exercise such as running, biking, or CrossFit; it exhausts the adrenals even further. Yoga, tai chi, Pilates, swimming, hiking, or dancing are more soothing for the adrenals. You should feel rejuvenated after exercising, not tired (a sign that you did too much and the adrenals are not coping).

Inflammation from food. Continue the Elimination Diet; food intolerances cause inflammation and tax the adrenals.

Coffee and caffeine. Coffee overstimulates the adrenals, even if mixed with fat. Switch to matcha green tea or caffeine-free herbal teas. Roasted chicory or dandelion root tea are good caffeine-free alternatives; try the Better Than Coffee Latte (page 313).

Toxicity in skincare and cleaning products. Eliminate xenoestrogens found in BPAs, parabens, sodium lauryl/laureth sulfate (SLS), phthalates, and triclosan often used in skincare and household-cleaning products. Use the natural alternatives on page 73.

Raising Low Testosterone 14-Day Sample Meal Plan for Two

For warm lemon water: Add 2 tablespoons freshly squeezed lemon juice to 8 to 16 ounces warm water. Lime juice or apple cider vinegar may also be used.

Add ½ teaspoon camu camu per day (for vitamin C) to smoothies, salads, and bone broth.

Bone broth: Sip 1 to 2 cups per day with a dash of coconut milk, freshly grated ginger, lemon juice, and sea salt.

Abbreviations
[NR] No recipe
[LO] Leftovers
[MA] Made ahead; full recipe or parts of
[DB] Double the recipe
EVOO Extra virgin olive oil

WEEK 1

	Morning ritual/ breakfast	Snack (optional)	Lunch	Dinner	Bedtime ritual (optional)
Day 1	Warm lemon water Breakfast Casserole One: Salmon and Broccoli (page 189)	Zucchini Olive Muffin [MA] (page 205) Deep Green Spirulina Smoothie (page 197)	Nutritious Quick Bowls, pick one [DB] (page 232)	Lamb with Collard Greens and Radishes (page 236)	Healing Bone Broth [MA] (page 162), freeze half for the following week
Day 2	Warm lemon water Coconut Kefir Chia Pudding [DB] (page 185)	Hot Chocolate with Pink Roses (page 314)	Lamb with Collard Greens and Radishes [LO]	Quick Miso Soup [DB] (page 220) Life-Giving Sprouts [MA] (page 163)	Zucchini Olive Muffin [LO]
Day 3	Warm lemon water Coconut Kefir Chia Pudding [LO]	Decadent Chocolate Cherry Smoothie (page 207)	Quick Salads—Four Ways, pick one (page 254)	Quick Miso Soup [LO] Life-Giving Sprouts [LO]	Creamy Lime Pudding (page 342)
Day 4	Warm lemon water Parsnip Dill Pancake with Arugula and Smoked Salmon (page 199)	Adrenal Love Tea (page 305) Creamy Lime Pudding [LO]	Steam 'n Toss Veggies and Proteins on the Run (page 260)	Rosemary and Garlic Stuffed Lamb Roast (page 251) Mixed greens, tossed with EVOO [NR] with Life-Giving Sprouts [LO]	Spiced Nut Butters, pick one (page 294)
Day 5	Warm lemon water Farmer's Wife's Breakfast [DB] (page 182)	Spiced Nut Butters [LO]	Rosemary and Garlic Stuffed Lamb Roast [LO] Mixed greens, tossed with EVOO [NR] with Life-Giving Sprouts [LO]	Steam 'n Toss Veggies and Proteins on the Run	Healing Bone Broth [LO]

Morning ritual/ breakfast	Snack (optional)	Lunch	Dinner	Bedtime ritual (optional)
Day 6				
Warm lemon water Adrenal Love Tea Farmer's Wife's Breakfast [LO]	Hot Chocolate with Pink Roses	Quick Salads—Four Ways, pick one	Squash, Apple, and Turmeric Soup (page 222)	Zucchini Olive Muffin [LO]
Day 7				
Warm lemon water Bacon, Oysters, and Collard Greens Stir Fry (page 204)	Decadent Chocolate Cherry Smoothie	Squash, Apple, and Turmeric Soup [LO]	Nutritious Quick Bowls, pick one	Healing Bone Broth [LO]

WEEK 2

Morning ritual/ breakfast	Snack (optional)	Lunch	Dinner	Bedtime ritual (optional)
Day 8				
Warm lemon water Squash, Apple, and Turmeric Soup [LO] Raspberry and Green Tea Lime Melties (page 338)	Adrenal Love Tea Salmon and Avocado in Nori Sheets (page 298)	Japanese Seaweed and Cucumber Salad (page 273)	Butter Cod with Gremolata (page 240) Fries Baked in Duck Fat (page 271) Life-Giving Sprouts [MA]	Kudzu Calming Pudding (page 348)
Day 9				
Warm lemon water Teff and Cherry Porridge (page 198)	Adrenal Love Tea Salmon and Avocado in Nori Sheets [LO]	Butter Cod with Gremolata [LO] Fries Baked in Duck Fat [LO] Life-Giving Sprouts [LO]	Japanese Seaweed and Cucumber Salad [LO]	Kudzu Calming Pudding [LO]

Morning ritual/ breakfast	Snack (optional)	Lunch	Dinner	Bedtime ritual (optional)
Day 10				
Warm lemon water Teff and Cherry Porridge [LO] Hot Chocolate with Pink Roses	Zucchini Olive Muffin [LO] Better Than Coffee Latte (page 313)	Sticky Spare Ribs Casserole (page 242) Tuscan Shredded Fennel and Orange Salad (page 262)	Quick Salads—Four Ways, pick one	Spiced Nut Butters [LO]
Day 11				
Warm lemon water Breakfast Casserole Two: Pork Chops and Apples (page 195)	Deep Green Spirulina Smoothie (page 197)	Sticky Spare Ribs Casserole [LO] Tuscan Shredded Fennel and Orange Salad [LO]	Steam 'n Toss Veggies and Proteins on the Run	Healing Bone Broth [LO]
Day 12				
Warm lemon water Bacon, Oysters, and Collard Greens Stir Fry	Raspberry and Green Tea Lime Melties	Nomad's Kebabs (page 239) Mixed greens, tossed with EVOO [NR] with Life-Giving Sprouts [LO]	Seriously Mushroom Soup (page 216)	Spiced Nut Butters [LO]
Day 13				
Warm lemon water Sweet Potato and Sage Pancakes (page 179)	Decadent Chocolate Cherry Smoothie	Seriously Mushroom Soup [LO]	Honey Glazed Tarragon Chicken (page 226) Creamy Celeriac and Cauliflower Mash (page 267)	Spiced Nut Butters [LO]
Day 14				
Warm lemon water Sweet Potato and Sage Pancakes [LO]	Deep Green Spirulina Smoothie	Honey Glazed Tarragon Chicken [LO] Creamy Celeriac and Cauliflower Mash [LO]	Grain-Free Pizza—Two Ways, pick one (page 228)	Healing Bone Broth [LO]

Part Three

Techniques for Life

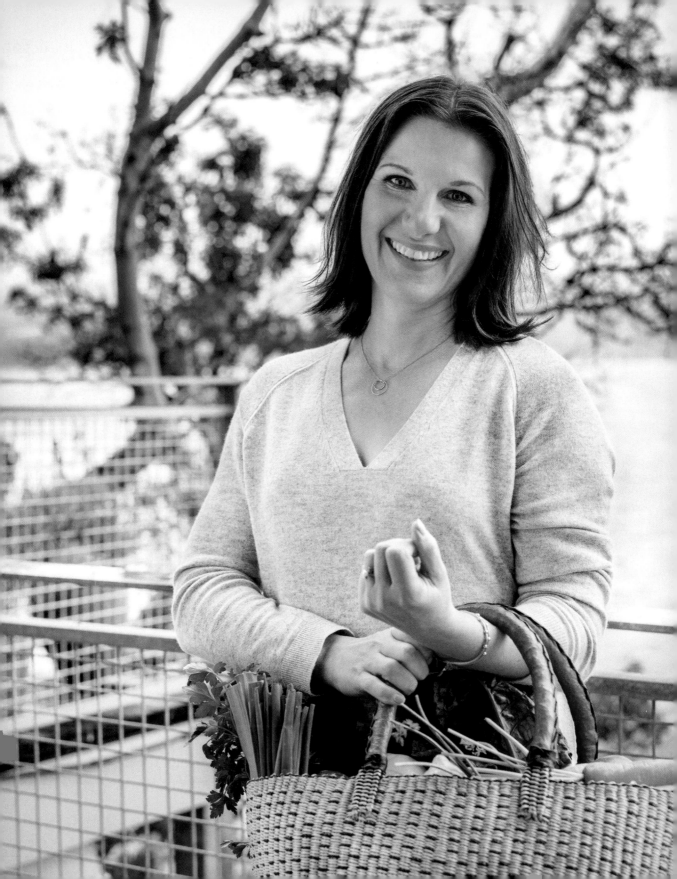

Chapter 7

Stocking Your Kitchen

IN-OUT ESSENTIALS

A well-stocked kitchen makes cooking and healing so much faster and easier. If the process of stocking your kitchen feels overwhelming, make one change every other week.

IN	OUT
FATS and OILS *See the complete lists in Fats and Oils (page 139).*	
Olive oil: unrefined, extra virgin, cold-pressed	Canola oil
Coconut oil: unrefined, organic	Safflower oil
Beef tallow from grass-fed cows	Sunflower oil
Ghee (clarified butter)	Margarine
Lard from pastured animals	Oil sprays
	Any refined oils, vegetable oils
GRAINS and LEGUMES	
Always whole grains; limit flours	Any packaged grains for "quick cooking" such as quick oats, quinoa flakes, or rice puffs
Brown rice*	
Amaranth*	Gluten (wheat, spelt, kamut, rye, couscous)
Millet*	Soy, unless fermented*
Quinoa*	All GMO grains
	Only if tolerated.

IN	OUT

VEGETABLES

IN	OUT
As much organic as possible	Nonorganic or conventional
Cruciferous vegetables	Canned or tinned
Seasonal and locally grown vegetables	Use cans only as "emergency" or "camping" food. Eden Foods has BPA-free cans.
Fermented vegetables	Glass bottles are better than cans (e.g., tomato paste)

CONDIMENTS

IN	OUT
Sea salt (Celtic salt from Utah, Himalayan salt)	Table salt, white salt, iodized salt
Homemade salad dressings (store in the refrigerator for a few weeks)	Bottled salad dressings and sauces unless refrigerated and compliant with this list

DAIRY

IN	OUT
Homemade nondairy yogurt (see Coconut Yogurt, page 164)	All commercial dairy products (milk, cheese, yogurt)
Homemade nondairy milk (see Nut and Seed Milks, page 300, and Coconut Cream, page 166)	

SUGAR

See the complete lists in Sugars and Sweeteners (page 138)

IN	OUT
Coconut nectar (my favorite)	High-fructose corn syrup
Maple syrup	White, processed sugar
Honey: raw, local, unheated	Aspartame
Stevia	Saccharin (Sweet'N Low)
	Sucralose (Splenda)
	Agave syrup

FISH

IN	OUT
Alaskan fish	All other farmed fish and seafood
Pacific Ocean fish	Atlantic Ocean fish and seafood
Farmed mussels	Any fish from China and Asia
Farmed oysters	Imported shrimp
Wild-caught pink shrimp from Oregon	Tuna (except troll- or pole-caught)
Wild-caught spot prawns from British Columbia	
Farmed rainbow trout, mackerel, and white fish	

IN	OUT

MEAT

IN	OUT
Organic, from pasture-raised, grass-fed animals only	"Conventional" meat from grain-fed, soy-fed animals
Homemade bone broth (see Healing Bone Broth, page 162, and Immune-Boosting Chicken Broth, page 158)	Avoid these preservatives: benzoates, nitrites, nitrates, sulfites, sorbates
Bone broths from small-batch makers	Stocks such as chicken or beef packaged in cartons
Organ meats like liver; only from pasture-raised animals	

SUPERFOODS

IN	OUT
Turmeric, fresh or powdered	Protein shakes and powders
Ground flaxseed	Excessive supplements
Oysters	Multilevel marketing (MLM) foods and supplements
Brazil nuts	
Liver	

SUGARS AND SWEETENERS

I've compiled this guide to sugars and sweeteners on the basis of three criteria: (1) the amount of fructose they contain (the less the better), (2) their glycemic load (how quickly a serving elevates your blood sugar levels), and (3) the degree of processing it takes to make the sugar. The "best to consume" sweeteners contain less than 40 percent fructose, and their glycemic index is less than 60 and glycemic load is less than 20 (which is a medium range).

Best to consume	Just okay	Best to avoid	Do not consume
Blackstrap molasses, molasses	Cane juice and sugar	Agave and agave nectar	Acesulfame potassium (Sweet One)
Coconut sugar (crystals and syrup)	Date sugar and syrup	Barley malt	Aspartame (Equal, NutraSweet)
Dates	Stevia (dry, green leaf, or extract*) (Stevia in the Raw, SweetLeaf)	Beet sugar	Saccharin (Sweet'N Low)
Honey (raw, unfiltered)	Monk fruit (mixed most often with erythritol)*	Brown rice syrup	Stevia (white, bleached, or highly processed, such as Truvia and Sun Crystals)
Maple syrup (Grade B)		Brown sugar	Sucralose (Splenda)
Yakon syrup		Carob syrup	
		Corn syrup	
		Dextran and dextrose	
		Ethyl maltol	
		Fructose	
		Fruit juice concentrate	
		Glucose	
		Golden sugar/syrup	
		Grape sugar	
		High-fructose corn syrup	
		Lactose	
		Malt syrup	
		Maltodextrin	
		Maltose	
		Manninol	
		Raw sugar	
		Sorbitol	
		Sorghum syrup	
		Sucrose	
		Turbinado	
		Table or white sugar	
		Xylitol	

Try not to use daily or for longer than three months.

FATS AND OILS

Invest in good-quality fats and oils as they are the backbone of your cooking and the source of HDL cholesterol, the "good" cholesterol and precursor to all of the sex hormones: pregnenolone, DHEA, testosterone, progesterone, cortisol, and estrogen.

Fats and oils	Smoking point, unrefined/refined	Best use
Highly stable oils and fats for high-temperature cooking		
Coconut oil*	350°F/450°F	*High-temperature cooking, like baking, sautéing, or frying*
Butter/ghee**	300°F/480°F	
Tallow/suet (beef fat)**	400°F	
Palm oil*	455°F	
Lard/bacon fat (pork fat)**	375°F	
Duck fat**	375°F	
Olive oil*	375°F	
Avocado oil*	520°F	
Cacao butter*	370°F	Used in making chocolate
Moderately stable; best used cold or in very-low-temperature cooking		
Macadamia nut oil*	410°F	*Moderate-heat cooking, like a quick sauté*
Sesame seed oil*	450°F	
Flaxseed oil	225°F	Cold use only (applies to flaxseed oil)
Other sources of good fats: avocados, olives, homemade dressings, fatty fish bone marrow, coconut milk, coconut butter, unsweetened dried coconut.		
Refined and unstable oils; should be avoided		
Safflower oil	225°F to 510°F	*Avoid these because of high omega 6 fatty acid content and/or the fact that they are chemically refined to prevent them from going rancid. These oils are most often sold as refined oils and are known to be highly inflammatory to the body.*
Canola oil	400°F	
Sunflower oil	225°F to 440°F	
Vegetable shortening	330°F	
Corn oil	445°F	
Soybean oil	495°F	
Walnut oil	400°F	
Grapeseed oil	420°F	
Other fats to avoid: spray oils, margarine, all vegetable oils and any hydrogenated oils.		

*Best organic and unrefined, purchased in dark bottles.
**Best from pasture-raised, grass-fed, organic sources.

BUYING AND PREPPING TIPS AND TRICKS

These are the foods, equipment, and brands I used in creating the recipes in this book, with some additional tips and tricks to help make cooking easier for you.

Foods

FATS

Ghee. To be truly dairy-free, the packaging needs to state "lactose-free" and "casein-free"; otherwise, it can't be used by people with a sensitivity to dairy. My favorite is Tin Star Foods, available online.

Brown butter. Despite its name, this is caramelized ghee (so it's dairy-free) and is used in top French restaurants. My favorite is Tin Star Foods, available online.

Coconut oil. Pick virgin, unrefined, cold-pressed, and organic.

Coconut butter. Also known as "coconut manna," this is blended coconut pulp and oil. Keep at room temperature and do not use with high heat. It makes a divine addition to smoothies and desserts or is wonderful just as a snack. My favorite brand is Artisana; available at many health stores and online.

Coconut milk. Buy full-fat milk, with as few preservatives and additives as possible. Most contain xanthan gum or guar gum; if you are sensitive, make your own (page 300). My favorite brands are Native Forest (BPA-free cans) and Thai Kitchen; available at most health stores and online.

Lard. Rendered pig fat is not to be feared; it contains 50 percent monounsaturated fats. Render your own or get ready-made, available at many health stores. My favorite brand is Fatworks; available at many health stores and online.

Duck fat. This is my absolute favorite; the rich flavor is the secret behind French cooking. My favorite brand is Fatworks; available at many health stores and online.

MEATS AND FISH

Meats. As much as you can, buy free-range and pasture-raised meats. The nutritional profile and healing properties excel compared with conventionally raised meats (not to mention the ethical and humane aspects!). Organic is better but not the best option. Most health stores offer pasture-raised meats, as do farmers' markets and local butchers. My favorite online butcher is Butcher Box (www.butcherbox.com).

Bone broths and stocks. The backbone of healthy cooking, homemade broths can't be compared to store-bought stocks that have no nutritional value and are packaged in cartons;

many add MSG (under various inconspicuous names) and preservatives. Make your own using my recipes and freeze for later use. Many health stores and farmers' markets sell frozen bone broths. My favorite online sellers are Bare Bones Broth and The Flavor Chef.

Collagen powder. This is a great quick addition to heal your gut if you have no time to make your own bone broths. My favorite brands are Bulletproof, Vital Proteins, and Great Lakes Gelatin; purchase them online.

Bacon. Buy uncured bacon that is free of nitrates and sugars.

Fish. Try your best to buy wild fish. Farmed fish is nutritionally inferior and can be outright harmful because of the added coloring and growth hormones and compounds used in the feed. Wild fish from the Pacific Ocean tends to be less contaminated than fish from the Atlantic. Avoid any fish and seafood from China and Thailand. My favorite is a wild Alaskan salmon. You can order online from Vital Choice Wild Seafood and Organics, a wonderful sustainable fishing company.

VEGETABLES, FRUITS, AND SEAWEED

Organic fruits and vegetables. Buy organic as much as you can for maximum nutrient density and to minimize hormone-disrupting chemicals. Use the Environmental Working Group's "Dirty Dozen" (https://www.ewg.org /foodnews/dirty_dozen_list.php) and "Clean Fifteen" (https://www.ewg.org/foodnews /clean_fifteen_list.php) lists for guidance. The Dirty Dozen contain the highest amounts of chemicals: strawberries, spinach, nectarines, apples, peaches, pears, cherries, grapes, celery, tomatoes, sweet bell pepper, and potatoes; try your best to buy these organic. The Clean Fifteen contain the lowest amounts of pesticides: sweet corn, avocados, pineapples, cabbage, onions, sweet peas (frozen), papayas, asparagus, mangos, eggplant, honeydew melon, kiwi, cantaloupe, cauliflower, and grapefruit.

Organic vegetables are becoming more mainstream, and most health stores offer them. They might be more expensive, but they will help you heal and prevent medical costs farther down the road. If cost or access to organic food is a challenge for you, check out local farmers' markets and community-supported agriculture (CSA) that offer veggie (and sometimes meat) boxes. LocalHarvest is a wonderful resource to help you find organic food sources near you (www.localharvest.org).

Citrus rind. When using skin peels from lemons, limes, and oranges, be sure to use organic fruit. They are rich in d-limonene, a potent liver detoxifier. Use a microplane grater or a zester.

Dried fruit. Get them unsulfured and with no added sugar.

Root vegetables. Do not peel them if they are organic; plenty of nutrients and beneficial soil bacteria are found in the skins (this is why you will see many of my recipes calling for unpeeled root vegetables).

Sauerkraut and other fermented foods. Buy the ones that are in the refrigerator in the store, in lacto-fermented form (it does not contain lactose or dairy!). Sauerkraut in vinegar contains no medicinal value and worsens Candida.

Fermentation starters. These include kefir starter (can be used for dairy and nondairy) and vegetable starter (use in brined medleys and krauts) to inoculate the ferments or yogurt starter. My favorite brands are Body Ecology and Cultures for Health; both can be purchased online.

Seaweed. You can get seaweed such as nori, kelp, wakame, arame, and hijiki from companies in California, Maine, Canada, or Australia. Avoid seaweed from China and Japan because of contamination. My favorite brands are Maine Coast Sea Vegetables, Emerald Cove, and Eden Foods.

GRAINS AND FLOURS

Cassava flour. This is not the same as tapioca flour. My favorite brand is Otto's Naturals. I've also tested the recipes with Anthony's Goods cassava flour. Buy them online.

Teff grain and flour—Teff is the smallest grain in the world and a nutritional powerhouse; it contains two times more protein than brown rice and helps maintain healthy blood sugar levels. Available from Bob's Red Mill.

Tigernut flour. Despite its name, this is a tuber, not a nut. It is hypoallergenic and can be tolerated by most people (unlike almond flour nowadays). It can replace almond flour in most recipes (although reduce the sugar amount, as it is sweeter than almond flour). It is rich in prebiotics and very high in fiber. My favorite brand is Organic Gemini; available at more health stores now and online.

SUGARS AND SWEETENERS

For the sugars and sweeteners I recommend, including the brands, see Sugars and Sweeteners (page 138).

CONDIMENTS

Salt. Use unprocessed sea salt (such as Celtic, from Utah) or pink Himalayan salt. Avoid iodized or white table salt as well as Kosher salt; they have been stripped of all trace minerals. For some variation and extra flavor, try smoked salts or my absolute favorite, truffle salt!

Rose water. This makes a wonderful addition to smoothies and desserts. Get it at your local Middle Eastern grocery or online.

Pomegranate molasses (or pomegranate syrup). Reduced pomegranate juice forms a tart, sweet, floral, thick syrup. Get it at a local Middle Eastern grocery or online.

Coconut aminos. This can be a 1:1 replacement for soy sauce (it's soy-free). Get it at a local health store or online.

AIP baking powder. Combine 1 tablespoon baking soda and 2 tablespoons cream of tartar. If making ahead, add 2 tablespoons arrowroot flour to prevent clumping.

HERBS, SPICES, TEA, AND WATER

Storing herbs and spices. Buy herbs and spices whole and grind them in small batches. Ground spices release therapeutic volatile oils and lose their potency in four weeks, so grind them when you need them. Store in air-tight containers. If you love spices and have as many of them as I do, invest in the AllSpice Wooden Spice Rack, which organizes sixty spice bottles in one vertical rack.

Cinnamon. If you use a lot of cinnamon in your cooking, get Ceylon cinnamon (true cinnamon, or *Cinnamomum verum*); it is a superior form with a low coumarin content compared with the commonly available Chinese cassia cinnamon. Coumarin can cause liver toxicity when consumed in large amounts or frequently. Buy Ceylon cinnamon at your local health store, herbal apothecary, or online.

Vanilla powder. I like to use this in nonbaked goods such as smoothies because it does not leave an alcoholic aftertaste. It can be replaced with vanilla extract. Get it at a local health store or online.

Matcha tea. This ceremonial Japanese tea is pricey, but you need only a teaspoon in most recipes. My favorite brands are DoMatcha and Teavana; buy at a local health store or online.

Rose petals. These are a soothing addition to any dessert or beverage; order them online.

Herbs for tea infusions, decoctions, and healing lattes. Buy the common herbs used in recipes at Mountain Rose Herbs.

Filtered water. Get the Berkey or Aquasana filters; Brita and fridge filters are not good enough.

Equipment

POTS AND PANS

In: Cast iron, cast iron coated with enamel, ceramic, glass, and heavy-bottomed stainless steel.

Out: Nonstick Teflon (the chemicals used to make the nonstick surfaces have been linked to health concerns), aluminum, and copper (gets leached into the food)

10-quart or larger stainless stockpot with lid

6-quart enamel cast iron pot, also known as a Dutch oven, with lid (Lodge brand)

12-inch ceramic nonstick skillet (GreenPan) or stainless steel

8-inch ceramic nonstick skillet (GreenPan) or stainless steel

5-quart stainless steel saucepan with lid

3-quart stainless steel saucepan with lid

1½-quart stainless steel saucepan with lid

BAKING DISHES

In: Stainless steel, silicon, glass

Out: Nonstick and aluminum (alternatively, use parchment paper or muffin paper cups so food does not touch the pans)

13 × 9-inch baking pan

11 × 7-inch baking pan

12-muffin stainless steel or silicon pan

12-mini-muffin stainless steel or silicon pan

9-inch or 9½-inch glass baking pie dish

9 × 5-inch bread baking pan

9 × 5¾ × 2-inch baking pan

ELECTRONIC EQUIPMENT

High-speed electric blender (Vitamix or Blendtec). Speed and motor power really matter. If you are on a budget, get a reconditioned unit from Vitamix's website or get one second-hand.

NutriBullet

14-cup food processor (Cuisinart). Quality really matters. A cheap food processor won't make silky smooth food such as nut butters, nut mayo, or pate.

Hand mixer

Coffee or spice grinder (have one for coffee and one for spices)

Immersion blender

KITCHEN GADGETS AND MORE

8-inch chef's knife. A good knife will cost you $200 to $300, but it will last for years and is totally worth it.

Paring knife

Knife sharpener. Use it daily or weekly to keep your knives sharp.

Four-sided grater

Microplane for grating citrus peel

Citrus squeezer. I can't live without this. No more hand squeezing and seed picking.

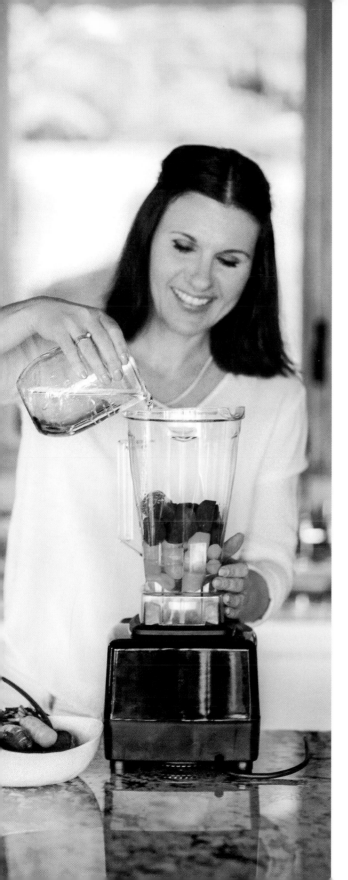

Wooden, stainless steel, or silicon spoons and spatulas

Large fine mesh strainer with handle

Small fine mesh strainer with handle

Glass storage containers. Avoid plastic, and never microwave food in plastic containers.

Glass measuring cup set

Oven thermometer

Parchment paper

Measuring cups and spoons

Large wooden cutting board for cutting fruit and vegetables

Medium plastic cutting board for cutting meat and fish

Chapter 8

Traditional Food Preparation Techniques

SOAKING AND SPROUTING

Soaking is the process of putting a whole seed or kernel in water for a period of time. After a seed or kernel has been soaked, it can be sprouted, or germinated. Sprouting transforms a dry, hard ball into a much richer source of vitamins and minerals and releases enzymes that break down proteins and carbohydrates. This process makes sprouts easier to digest, and they have a low glycemic index.

Many nuts, seeds, grains, and legumes can be sprouted. I recommend starting with broccoli seeds (Life-Giving Sprouts, page 163). Once you master these, there is no limit to what you can sprout. Get your kids involved. They are often much more willing to eat sprouts if they've grown them themselves!

To sprout nuts, use nuts that are raw (unpasteurized), unsalted, and whole. Commercially sold almonds in the United States are required to be sold pasteurized, so sprouting won't be possible (although you can buy small batches of unpasteurized almonds at some farmers' markets). Nuts sprout on the inside, so you will not see a sprout tail, as you do with seeds. You can eat the nuts as soon as they have soaked 6 to 8 hours. If you do not eat them within a couple of days, dehydrate them using a dehydrator or an oven set at a temperature lower than 150°F (I leave the oven door open to cool it since the lowest temperature most ovens offer is 170°F).

How long do sprouts take to grow? Most are ready to eat in just a few days. The longer the sprout time, the longer their tails will be.

Find the Soaking and Sprouting Guide for seeds and nuts at www.Hormones Balance.com/book.

Get started with sprouting by following the Life-Giving Sprouts recipe on page 163.

Add sprouts to salads, soups, stews (only at the end), and smoothies.

FERMENTING

Fermentation is the chemical breakdown of sugar into acid, alcohol, and gases by micro-organisms, such as yeast or bacteria. I'm delighted that fermented foods are making a comeback and gaining much love among American home cooks and posh chefs.

A fear of bacteria has made many people cautious about consuming fermented foods, but this fear is unjustified. I'm often asked if fermented foods are safe to consume during pregnancy and the answer is yes. People have been fermenting for generations, not only to improve the nutritional value of food but also to preserve it in the absence of refrigeration.

Every culinary culture features fermented foods—from Indian dosa (a rice and lentil crepe), Korean kimchi, Ethiopian injera (a teff crepe), Russian sauerkraut, German rye bread, and Peruvian chicha (corn beer) to Icelandic hákarl (fermented shark). Beer, wine, cheese, yogurt, and salami are all products of fermentation.

Benefits of Fermenting and Eating Fermented Foods

Helps metabolize fats. In Poland and Russia, lacto-fermented vegetables like dill pickles or sauerkraut always accompany a serving platter of sausages, ham, and cheese. Fermented vegetables stimulate stomach acid production that then helps release bile, which is essential in metabolizing the fats in rich foods. When metabolized, these fats are a source of cholesterol, the precursor to all of your sex hormones.

Restores the estrobolome. Fermented foods can help restore the estrobolome, a subset of gut bacteria that metabolize "bad" estrogens.

Probiotics. Fermented foods have millions of beneficial bacteria that can populate your gut and rebuild your digestive health.

Easily digestible. Fermented foods are more digestible. Many people can't stomach raw cabbage but feel revived eating sauerkraut. Soy milk can cause a lot of health issues, but in a fermented form like miso or tempeh, it's a healthful food (if you can tolerate soy).

Enhances nutritional value. Fermentation can also enhance the nutritional value of food. There are more bioavailable vitamin Bs in sauerkraut than in cabbage.

Which fermented foods should you eat and how much?

Each ferrnented food offers a different spectrum of beneficial bacteria. In their book *The Good Gut,* Justin and Erica Sonnenburg, of Stanford University, state that the diversity of the gut bacteria is more important than large amounts of just a few strains of bacteria. I recommend eating at least half a cup of fermented foods every day (but see the precautionary note below) and rotating them every week to get a variety of bacteria. Bacteria are transient and stay in the gut only from a few days to two weeks, so you need to replenish them regularly.

Do you need to take probiotics in pill form when eating fermented foods, or vice versa?

It depends on your current bacterial profile and what is missing from your gut. This is why some people feel no difference when taking one probiotic brand and experience huge health shifts when they switch to another. It's hard to know until you try a few brands. I recommend eating half a cup of fermented foods each day as well as supplementing with a high-quality probiotic.

Who should not consume fermented foods?

People with histamine intolerance, Candida yeast overgrowth, and sometimes IBS may not tolerate fermented foods at the beginning of their healing journey.

Fermenting at Home

You can ferment at home with a few basic ingredients. To get started, try my easy, delicious recipes for Coconut Yogurt (page 164), Preserved Lemon (page 170), Coconut Kefir Chia Pudding (page 185), Kohlrabi Kraut (page 275), Cultured Vegetable Medley—Four Ways (page 277), Grain-Free Sourdough Flatbread (page 329), Ginger Beet Kvass (page 317), Strawberry Ginger Ale (page 318), and Fizzy Orange, Carrot, and Beet Soda (page 320).

COOKING WITH ORGAN MEATS

The words "organ meats" probably make you roll your eyes and sigh "No way." But stay with me for a few minutes and read about this misunderstood group of superfoods.

Most people in North America dislike organ meats, such as liver, because their parents overcooked and underseasoned them. Yet in many cuisines, such as Spanish, French, Moroccan, and Chinese, organ meats are used to make some of the most celebrated delicacies. Europeans, Asians, Africans, and South Americans have a long history of honoring the whole animal from nose to tail, with nothing going to waste. In hunter-gatherer cultures, organ meats were considered precious and healthful and given to royalty and the sick.

This is no surprise; the nutritional density of organ meats is superior to other parts of an animal. For example, according to the U.S. Department of Agriculture National Nutrient Database, 100 grams cooked chicken livers contain 234 times more vitamin B12, 40 times more iron, and 10 times more zinc compared with 100 grams grilled chicken breast (which you will therefore not find in this cookbook!). Beef liver contains 16 times more vitamin D, 20 times more vitamin B12, 5,000 times more vitamin A, 2.5 times more iron, and 2.4 times more selenium than a pricey rib-eye steak.

To start exploring organ meats, try my Fennel and Coriander Crusted Liver (page 246) and Easy French Pate (page 290).

Always buy organ meats that come from healthy, pasture-raised animals.

 Since the liver filters toxins from the body, isn't it a "dirty" organ to eat? If I eat liver, won't I ingest those toxins?

No! The liver does filter toxins, but it does not store those toxins. They are excreted from the body as waste.

Chapter 9
Food Apothecary

Include these potent medicinal foods in your daily diet to rebalance your hormones.

20 HORMONE-BALANCING SUPERFOODS

Berries (strawberries, blueberries, blackberries, raspberries). Sugar balancing, anti-inflammatory, estrogen balancing, rich in antioxidants, rich in fiber

Brazil nuts. Mood boosting, thyroid supporting, cholesterol lowering, rich in selenium, support breast health

Broccoli sprouts. Support breast health, liver detoxing, detoxifying, anti-inflammatory, anticarcinogenic, immune boosting, rich in sulfurs

Butter and ghee. Gut healing, antifungal, anti-inflammatory, source of good fat for hormone production

Camu camu (a Peruvian berry). Liver detoxing, estrogen balancing, rich in vitamin C, immune boosting, adrenal supporting, anti-inflammatory

Citrus fruits. Liver detoxing (the peels), sugar balancing, alkalizing, rich in vitamin C, rich in antioxidants

Coconut oil. Sugar balancing, immune boosting, high in good fats, antifungal, antibacterial, energizing

Cruciferous vegetables. Liver detoxing, estrogen balancing, rich in antioxidants, anticarcinogenic, immune boosting, anti-inflammatory, rich in sulfurs, rich in fiber

Flaxseed. Gut healing, estrogen boosting, estrogen detoxifying, high in good fats, rich in zinc, rich in omega 3 fatty acids

Garlic. Gut healing, liver detoxing, antimicrobial, anti-inflammatory, alkalizing, rich in selenium

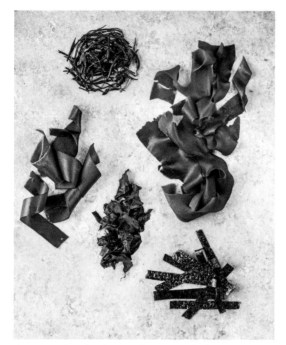

Seaweeds (clockwise from top left): hijiki, wakame, nori, dulse, kelp.

Gelatin. Gut healing, anti-inflammatory, rich in protein, immune boosting

Liver. Energizing, rich in protein, hormone balancing, nutrient dense, rich in iron, rich in niacin (vitamin B3), rich in vitamins B6 and B12

Onion. Liver detoxing, sugar balancing, rich in prebiotics, antibacterial, anti-inflammatory, anticarcinogenic, rich in sulfur

Pomegranates. Gut healing, anti-inflammatory, estrogen balancing, anticarcinogenic, rich in antioxidants, high in good fats

Pumpkin seeds. Estrogen balancing, support breast health, nutrient dense, immune boosting, rich in magnesium

Salmon. Thyroid balancing, antioxidant, anti-inflammatory, rich in omega 3 fatty acids, good source of protein

Sauerkraut. Gut healing, anti-inflammatory, rich in good bacteria, immune boosting

Seaweed. Sugar balancing, food for the brain and breasts, nutrient dense, detoxifying, high in fiber, rich in iodine and magnesium, rich in B vitamins

Sesame seeds. Estrogen balancing, rich in B vitamins, rich in minerals, progesterone boosting

Walnuts. Antioxidant, anti-inflammatory, rich in omega 3 fatty acids, rich in antioxidants

20 HORMONE POWER HERBS, SPICES, AND MUSHROOMS

Cacao. Anti-inflammatory, antioxidant, mood boosting, rich in magnesium

Cilantro. Sugar balancing, liver detoxing, antioxidant, estrogen balancing, progesterone boosting, antibacterial

Cinnamon. Anti-inflammatory, sugar balancing, insulin stabilizing

Cumin. Gut healing, antioxidant, antifungal, antispasmodic, diuretic, sugar balancing, immune boosting

Dandelion (root and leaf). Root: Liver detoxing, diuretic, sugar balancing; leaf: kidney cleansing, gut healing, sugar balancing, antibacterial, rich in fiber, diuretic

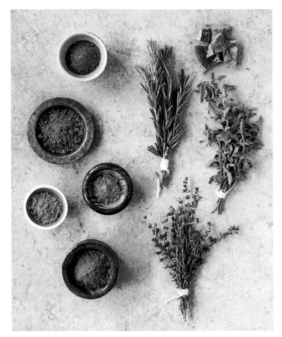

Clockwise from top left: Tulsi (holy basil), rosemary, reishi (brown and woody-looking), oregano, thyme, Ceylon cinnamon, turmeric, matcha (bright green), and cacao.

Dong quai (*Angelica sinensis*). Gut healing, liver detoxing, estrogen balancing, antispasmodic, antioxidant, anti-inflammatory, anticarcinogenic, supports breast health

Fennel. Gut healing, rich in vitamin C, antioxidant, anti-inflammatory, antibacterial, antifungal

Fenugreek. Gut healing, sugar balancing, estrogen balancing

Ginger. Gut healing, anti-inflammatory, antioxidant, anticarcinogenic

Maca. Sugar balancing, liver detoxing, estrogen balancing, progesterone boosting, energizing, anticarcinogenic

Matcha. Alkalizing, detoxifying, rich in antioxidants, anti-inflammatory, anticarcinogenic, calming and energizing at the same time

Medicinal mushrooms. Liver detoxing, sugar balancing, immune boosting, anticarcinogenic, rich in antioxidants, estrogen balancing

Oregano. Antifungal, antibacterial, antiviral, antioxidant, anti-inflammatory, nutrient dense, immune boosting

Parsley. Liver detoxing, nutrient dense, anticarcinogenic, immune boosting

Raspberry leaf. Sugar balancing, rich in antioxidants, astringent, antimicrobial, anticarcinogenic, uterus strengthening

Rosemary. Estrogen balancing, anticarcinogenic, anti-inflammatory, immune boosting

Slippery elm. Gut healing, estrogen balancing, anti-inflammatory

Thyme. Gut healing, sugar balancing, anti-inflammatory, anticarcinogenic, antibacterial, antispasmodic

Tulsi. Adrenal balancing, adaptogenic, anticarcinogenic, antioxidant

Turmeric. Anticarcinogenic, antioxidant, anti-inflammatory, immune boosting

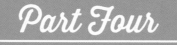

Recipes

Making Bone and Vegetable Broths

Bone broth is the latest health craze, but do not let the marketing buzz fool you into thinking it is just another fad. To differentiate between a fad and a sound practice, I ask, "Has this food been around for at least one hundred years?" In the case of bone broth, the answer is a resounding yes. In fact, bone broths are present in just about every culture, from Japanese pork bone broths simmering at the back of every mom-and-pop ramen shop, to chicken feet stocks bubbling away at a Peruvian market, and beef bone broths brewing at top-notch French restaurants. Broths stand alone and are the foundation for soups, stews, and sauces and a valuable addition to mashes and sautés.

Bone broths are touted as the new superfood for good reasons. Rich in the amino acid glutamine, bone broths are instrumental in helping to heal the gut, support growth of the villi, stimulate the immune system, and build muscles. Bone broths are also high in the amino acid proline, found in collagen, and have helped many women recover their healthy joints, lush hair, and plump skin. Another amino acid found in bone broths, glycine, is the precursor for glutathione, the master antioxidant and detoxifier. The fat tissue in bone marrow is a significant source of the hormone adiponectin, which helps maintain insulin sensitivity and break down fat and has been linked to a decreased risk of developing cardiovascular disease, diabetes, and obesity-associated cancers.

Bone broths contain very small amounts of calcium, even though the bones used in making broth are high in calcium. So why do so many women with osteopenia and osteoporosis report improvement of their bone density after they start drinking bone broth? It is because the collagen found in the bone broth helps to build collagen fibrils, which are the "scaffoldings" of the bones that allow the deposit of calcium and other minerals that build strong bones.

What bones should you use to make broth, and where can you buy them? Quality is key. Make bone broths only from bones of pastured animals and wild-caught fish, and use only organic vegetables. Use a variety of bones: marrow bones, ribs, knuckles, necks, feet, heads, carcasses, and wings. A great way to obtain the best bones and bits is to make friends with a farmer at a local farmers' market.

Why does your broth not gel? This is a frequent question and a common issue that happens for two reasons. First, there may not be enough soft-tissue bits such as knuckles, necks, or feet in your broth. These impart collagen, which is what makes the broth congeal when cooled. Second, you might have cooked the broth on high heat for too long, which can break down the collagen; the best bone broths are simmered. Slow is good.

 Many health stores now sell small-batch bone broths made by local food makers. Most are frozen. Do not fall for broths packaged in cartons. A lot of them are full of MSG (which goes under many inconspicuous names, including yeast extract), preservatives, and additives, and many are not even made from real bones.

Make-Your-Own Bone Broth

Make your own signature bone broth using these simple steps. Roasting the bones is optional, but it will produce a far richer-tasting broth.

Roasting the bones: To roast the bones, preheat the oven to 450°F. Line the roasting pan with the parchment paper, arrange the bones in the pan in a single layer, and roast for about 20 minutes, or until the bones are brown. Turn the bones to brown the other side, switch to the broiler setting, and roast for another 10 minutes to get an even browning.

Add the bones to the stockpot: Beef bones, knuckles, necks; lamb bones, knuckles, necks; pig bones, ribs, knuckles, or feet; chicken bones, feet, necks, or carcass; turkey bones and necks; fish heads, bones, and tails (from white fish such as cod).

Add the chopped vegetables: Onions with skins on, unpeeled garlic, leeks, carrots, parsnips, celery, celeriac (celery root), sweet potatoes, or zucchinis.

Add the vinegar: Use ½ cup vinegar to 6 quarts water.

Add your choices of seasonings: Whole peppercorns, bay leaf, thyme, fresh ginger, fresh turmeric, lemongrass, star anise, kelp seaweed, or parsley (add at the end).

Add 4 to 6 quarts filtered water.

Simmer: Lamb and beef: 24 to 36 hours; Chicken and turkey: 12 to 24 hours; Vegetables: 24 hours; Fish: 8 hours.

Strain and store.

MAKES 5 quarts

EQUIPMENT 10-quart stockpot or larger (you can also use a pressure cooker or slow cooker), parchment paper (if roasting), roasting pan or rimmed baking sheet (if roasting), fine-mesh sieve and a wide-mouthed funnel, and five 1-quart jars

Bones (3 to 5 pounds)

Chopped vegetables (2 to 3 pounds)

Apple cider vinegar (½ cup)

Herbs, spices, and seaweed to taste

PALEO

AIP Omit adding all seed spices such as peppercorns

ANTI-CANDIDA Omit root vegetables such as carrots, sweet potatoes, and parsnips

LOW FODMAP Omit vegetables such as celery (celeriac is fine), sweet potatoes, onions, and garlic. Only use the green parts of leeks.

Immune-Boosting Chicken Broth

Gut healing, cold fighting, reviving

We could all benefit from providing more support to our immune systems. I have fortified this stock, the proverbial "Jewish penicillin," with traditional Chinese medicinal herbs—astralagus root, reishi mushroom, and burdock root—known for their superb immune-boosting properties. The longer you simmer the stock, the more nutrients it will contain. Top restaurants know that the secret to the best chicken stock is to use chicken feet. On your next visit to a farmers' market, ask a farmer to save you some chicken feet, and I promise you that your stock will never be the same. Most ethnic supermarkets sell frozen chicken feet.

MAKES 4 quarts

PREP TIME 15 minutes

COOKING TIME 24 hours

EQUIPMENT See page 157 except four 1-quart mason jars

PALEO

AIP *Omit the peppercorns.*

ANTI-CANDIDA *Omit the carrots.*

LOW FODMAP *Replace the onion with the green part of one leek. Omit the garlic, burdock root, and astralagus; the latter has not been tested, so it's best to avoid.*

Place all of the ingredients except the parsley in a stockpot. Cover, bring to a boil, and then reduce to a simmer. Cook for 24 hours.

Add parsley 10 minutes before finishing.

Strain the broth through a fine-mesh sieve and transfer to the mason jars.

Allow the broth to cool to room temperature before refrigerating or freezing.

Keeps well in the refrigerator for up to 7 days and in the freezer for up to 6 months. If freezing, leave a 1-inch headspace.

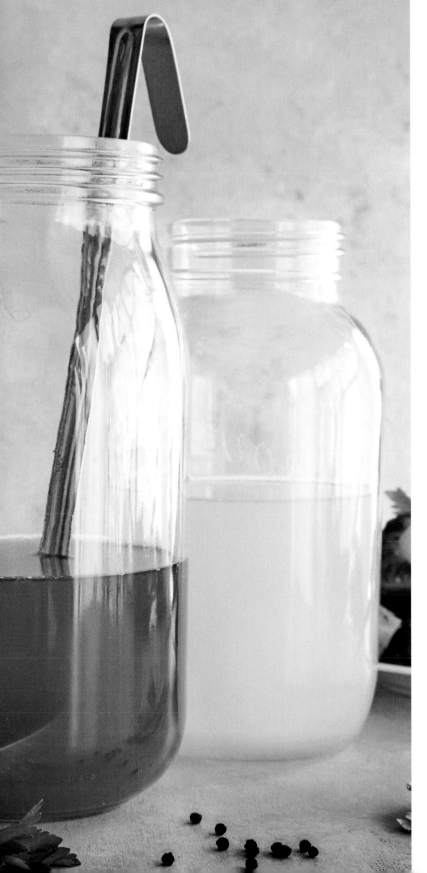

1 whole chicken or 2 to 3 pounds leftover roasted chicken carcass, bones, knuckles, wings, and neck

4 chicken feet (optional)

1 unpeeled onion, coarsely chopped

1 large unpeeled carrot, coarsely chopped

3 cloves unpeeled garlic, crushed

2 tablespoons apple cider vinegar

1½-inch fresh ginger root, sliced

1 teaspoon black peppercorns

8-inch kelp strip

3-inch dried astralagus roots

1 large dried reishi mushroom

1 tablespoon dried burdock root

4½ quarts cold filtered water

1 bunch of flat-leaf parsley

Mineral Vegetable Broth

Liver detoxing, nutrient dense, anticarcinogenic

MAKES 6 quarts

PREP TIME 15 minutes

COOKING TIME 4 hours

EQUIPMENT See page 157 except six 1-quart mason jars

4 large unpeeled carrots, coarsely chopped

2 unpeeled yellow onions, quartered

2 large unpeeled parsnips, coarsely chopped

1 leek, including the green parts, coarsely chopped

1 bunch celery, coarsely chopped

1 unpeeled sweet potato, coarsely chopped

1 fennel bulb, coarsely chopped

3 cloves peeled garlic, crushed

3-inch fresh ginger root, crushed

8-inch kelp strip

8 black peppercorns

8 whole allspice or juniper berries

1 teaspoon sea salt

1 bay leaf

6½ quarts cold filtered water

½ bunch of curly-leaf parsley

This recipe calls for the skin of the onions to be left on as it is high in flavanoids such as quercetin, which is great for circulation and slows down histamine release, the key cause of inflammatory reactions, including allergies and sensitivities. Kelp not only is a taste enhancer but also contains a full range of minerals such as calcium, magnesium, potassium, iron, iodine, and fucoidan, a documented anticarcinogenic agent.

Put all of the ingredients except the parsley in a stockpot, cover, and bring to a boil.

Reduce heat and simmer covered for 4 hours.

Add parsley 10 minutes before finishing.

Strain the broth through a fine-mesh sieve and transfer to the mason jars.

Allow the broth to cool to room temperature before refrigerating or freezing.

This broth will keep well in the refrigerator for up to 10 days and in the freezer for up to 6 months.

PALEO

AIP

ANTI-CANDIDA *Replace carrots and sweet potato with extra fennel bulb and celery or add one zucchini, coarsely chopped.*

LOW FODMAP *Omit the garlic, replace the onions with one green part of a leek and use only the green parts of the two additional leeks (that's a total of three leeks). Replace the celery with two fennel bulbs and the sweet potato with an unpeeled small pumpkin.*

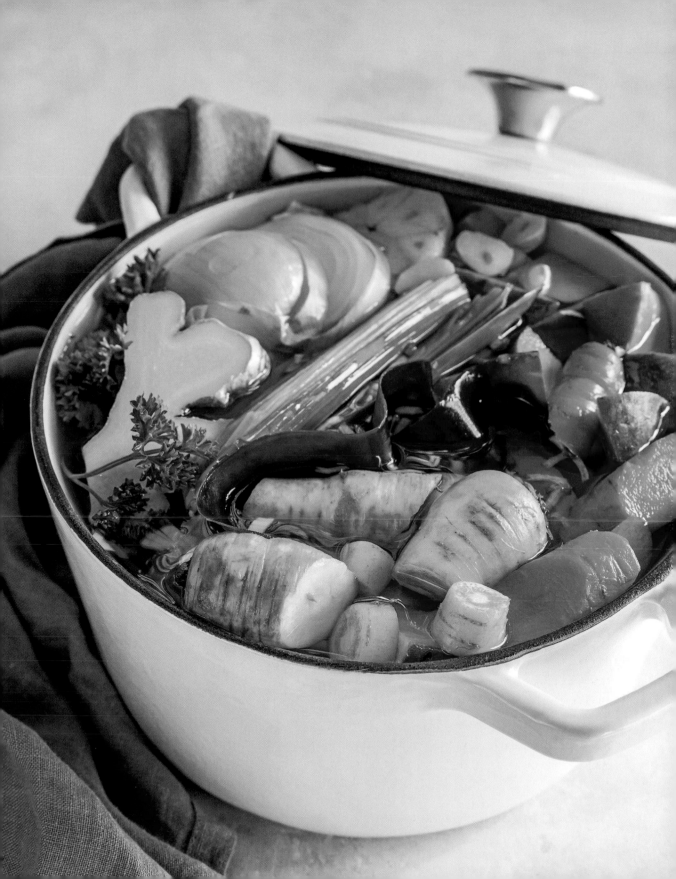

Healing Bone Broth

Gut healing, nutrient dense, boosts immunity

MAKES 6 quarts

PREP TIME 20 minutes

COOKING TIME 12 to 72 hours

EQUIPMENT See page 157 except six 1-quart mason jars

6 pounds beef marrow and/or knuckle bones

1 cow foot (optional)

2 medium unpeeled onions, coarsely chopped

2 unpeeled carrots, coarsely chopped

4 celery stalks, coarsely chopped

½ cup apple cider vinegar

2-inch fresh ginger, coarsely chopped

8-inch kelp strip

2 bay leaves

Several sprigs of thyme

1 teaspoon black peppercorns

6 quarts cold filtered water

1 bunch of parsley

PALEO

AIP *Omit the black peppercorns.*

ANTI-CANDIDA

LOW FODMAP *Omit onions or replace with the green parts of two leeks. Omit the celery or replace with ½ celeriac (celery root).*

Preheat the oven to 450°F.

Roast the bones (see page 157).

Transfer the bones to a stockpot. Save the fat that has run off the bones for later use, or discard. Add to the pot onions, carrots, celery, cider vinegar, ginger, kelp, bay leaves, thyme, and peppercorns. Add the water and cover. Bring to a boil and reduce to a simmer.

Check the broth after 1 hour and remove any scum that has risen to the top. Simmer for 12 to 72 hours. The slower and longer the simmer, the more nutritionally dense and flavorful the broth will be. If using a 10-quart stockpot, after about 12 hours, remove the melted fat with a large spoon.

Add parsley 10 minutes before finishing.

Remove all bones with tongs and discard. Strain the broth through a fine-mesh sieve and transfer to the mason jars.

Once the broth is cooled to room temperature, refrigerate or freeze.

Keeps well in the refrigerator for up to 7 days and in the freezer for up to 6 months. If freezing, leave a 1-inch headspace.

Life-Giving Sprouts

Liver detoxing, estrogen balancing, anticarcinogenic

Medical research has shown that broccoli sprouts can prevent and even shrink estrogenic breast cancers in women because of sulforaphane, a compound that kills cancer stem cells. Read more on the healing power of sprouts in Soaking and Sprouting (page 146).

Wash the mason jar with regular soap (do not use antibacterial soap), and sterilize it with boiling water.

Add the seeds to the jar and fill it with a few inches of filtered water. Soak the seeds for 6 to 12 hours.

Drain the seeds in the strainer, rinse well, and drain again.

Return the seeds to the mason jar. Cover the jar with cheesecloth and secure with an elastic band.

Place the jar at a 45-degree angle in a well-ventilated place, ideally between 68°F and 72°F.

Drain and rinse the sprouts every 12 hours. Strain well each time so little to no water is left in the jar.

When sprouts reach 1 to 1½ inches in length, place them in a large bowl of water. Gently swirl them so the seed shells separate and float to the top. Scoop up and discard the shells.

Place a paper towel in an airtight container, transfer the well-rinsed sprouts to the container, seal, and keep in the refrigerator.

Sprouts keep well in the refrigerator for up to a week.

MAKES 2 cups sprouts

PREP TIME 10 minutes

GROWING TIME 4 to 5 days

EQUIPMENT 1-quart mason jar, fine-mesh sieve, cheesecloth (100 percent cotton) or coffee filter, rubber band, large bowl

1 tablespoon sprouting broccoli seeds

1 tablespoon sprouting red clover seeds

Filtered water

PALEO

AIP Rinse well to remove all of the seed shells. If you are very sensitive to seed shells, do not eat sprouts until your digestion improves.

ANTI-CANDIDA

LOW FODMAP

Coconut Yogurt

Gut healing, estrogen balancing, rich in probiotics

Giving up dairy does not have to be hard when you can make this creamy dairy-free yogurt. I used arrowroot flour to thicken its otherwise runny consistency. In place of the vegan yogurt starter, you can also use ¼ capsule of any good-quality probiotic but you might have to lengthen the fermentation time. The yogurt is ready when it reaches a tart flavor.

MAKES Two 12-ounce jars

SERVES 4

PREP TIME 30 minutes

FERMENTATION TIME
6 to 12 hours

EQUIPMENT Whisk, thermometer, yogurt maker (preferred), slow cooker, two 12-ounce jars

Two 13½-ounce cans full-fat coconut milk

2 tablespoons arrowroot or tapioca flour

1 packet Cultures for Health Vegan Yogurt Starter

PALEO

AIP

ANTI-CANDIDA *Eat only after the first 4 weeks of the anti-Candida diet.*

LOW FODMAP *Eat no more than 1 tablespoon per day.*

Wash the jars well (do not use antibacterial soap).

Pour the coconut milk in a saucepan and whisk in the arrowroot flour. Heat to 140°F, stirring occasionally. Cool to 110°F.

Whisk in the yogurt starter and transfer to the glass jars.

Place the jars in the yogurt maker and ferment for 6 to 12 hours or until the yogurt becomes tart. If using a slow cooker, set it to "warm," wrap the jars in a hand towel, put the lid on the cooker, and monitor the temperature; it should be between 108°F and 110°F. This might require leaving the cooker lid ajar.

Transfer the yogurt to the refrigerator, where it will thicken further.

Keeps well in the refrigerator for up to 5 days.

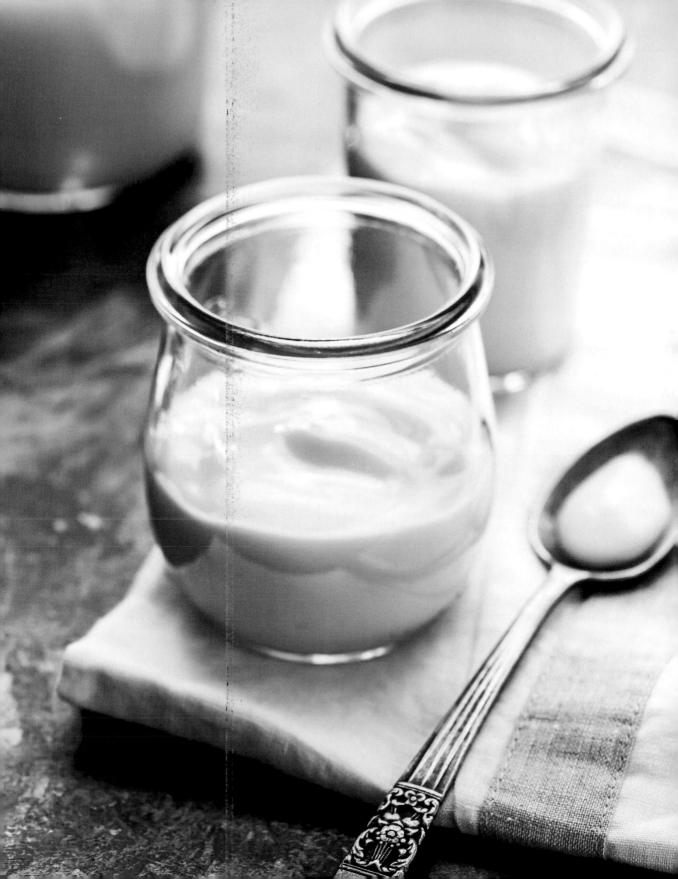

Whipped Coconut Cream

High in good fats, antibacterial ⏲ Less than 30 minutes

This rich, luxurious comfort food will end your dairy whipped cream cravings. The key to success is to keep the coconut fat and mixing bowl cold. A warm cream will turn into an unappealing curd. Use full-fat coconut milk and save the drained coconut water for smoothies. If you do not have a hand mixer, use a whisk but work quickly so the fat does not get warm. Keep a can of coconut milk in the fridge so when you feel like making the cream, it will be there, ready to go.

MAKES 1½ cups

CHILLING TIME 24 hours

PREP TIME 15 minutes

EQUIPMENT Electric hand mixer or whisk

1 13½-ounce can full-fat coconut milk, chilled in the refrigerator

1 tablespoon coconut syrup or Grade B maple syrup

1 teaspoon vanilla powder

Pinch of sea salt

PALEO

AIP

ANTI-CANDIDA Replace the syrup with three drops liquid stevia.

LOW FODMAP

Chill a medium glass bowl in the freezer for 10 minutes.

Meanwhile, remove the coconut milk from the refrigerator, open the can, and drain off the coconut water. Set it aside.

Scoop the coconut fat into the chilled bowl and whip for about 1 minute or until light and fluffy.

Whip in the coconut syrup, vanilla powder, and salt.

Use right away or refrigerate in a glass jar for up to 24 hours.

Homemade Applesauce

Rich in antioxidants, anticarcinogenic, rich in fiber ⏱ Less than 30 minutes

Applesauce is easy to make, a delicious snack, and a versatile ingredient to add to other recipes, such as Sweet Potato and Sage Pancakes (page 179) or Perfect French Crepes (page 208). This is a very basic recipe, but feel free to jazz it up by adding spices like cinnamon, cloves, cardamom, anise seed, or allspice. Royal Gala apples will make a sweeter sauce than tart Granny Smith apples.

Place the apples and the water in the pot, cover, and bring to a boil.

Reduce to medium heat and cook covered for 15 to 20 minutes or until the apples are very soft.

Cool for 5 minutes and puree to a desired consistency with the blender.

Transfer to the mason jars and refrigerate.

Keeps in the refrigerator for up to a week and in the freezer up to 3 months.

MAKES 6 cups

PREP TIME 8 minutes

COOKING TIME 20 minutes

EQUIPMENT 6-quart Dutch oven or heavy-bottomed pot with lid, immersion blender or electric blender, four 12-ounce mason jars

3 to 4 pounds unpeeled Royal Gala or Granny Smith apples, cored and coarsely chopped

½ cup water

PALEO

AIP

LOW FODMAP Replace the apples with pumpkin (but not butternut squash).

Creamy Egg-Free Mayo—Four Ways

Rich in magnesium, manganese, and copper 🕐 Less than 30 minutes

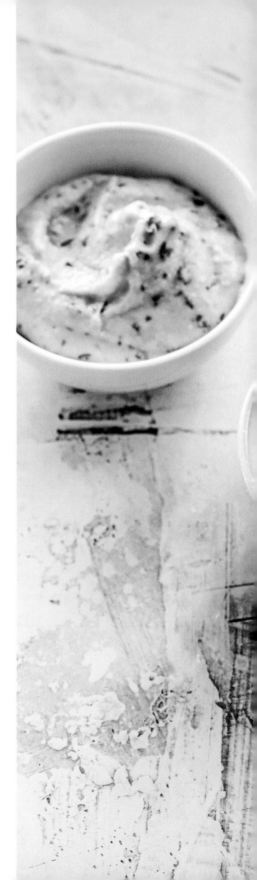

You will enjoy these delicious spreads and dips even if you do not tolerate eggs. Soaking the cashews makes them easier to digest. Watch out for store-bought egg-free mayo options, as many contain inflammatory canola oil, stabilizers, and additives.

In a medium bowl, cover the cashews with hot water and soak for 15 minutes.

Strain and transfer the cashews to the blender. Discard the water.

Add all of the remaining ingredients to the blender.

Puree on high until silky smooth, about 2 minutes. Stop and scrape the sides, if needed.

Transfer to the mason jars.

Keeps well in the refrigerator for up to 2 weeks or the freezer up to 3 months.

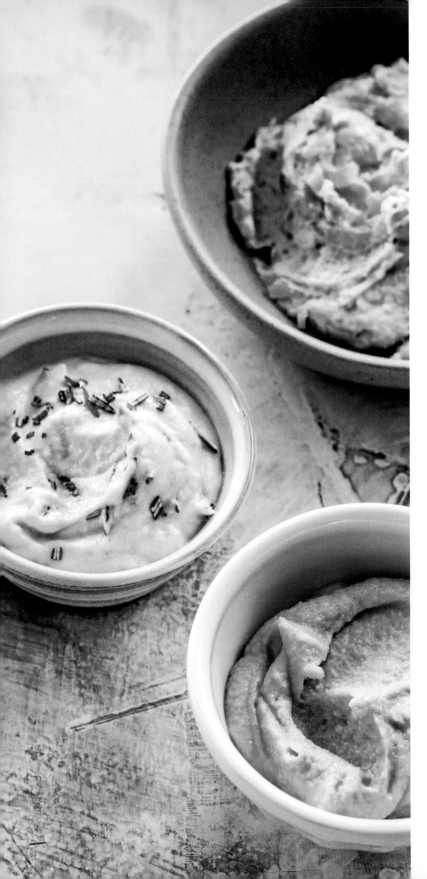

MAKES Two 6-ounce jars

SERVES About 16

PREP TIME 20 minutes

MAKING TIME 5 minutes

EQUIPMENT High-speed electric blender or food processor, two 6-ounce mason jars

CLASSIC MAYO

2 cups raw cashews

¼ cup filtered water

3 tablespoons Dijon mustard

2 tablespoons freshly squeezed lemon juice

1 teaspoon sea salt

½ cup extra virgin olive oil

PRESERVED LEMON MAYO

Classic Mayo (above), but reduce the salt to ½ teaspoon

¾ Preserved Lemon (page 170), seeds removed, coarsely chopped

HORSERADISH MAYO

Classic Mayo (above)

¼ cup freshly grated horseradish root

1 teaspoon dried rosemary

SEAWEED MAYO

Classic Mayo (above)

3 tablespoons dried wakame, soaked in lukewarm water for 5 minutes

4 to 6 anchovy fillets, coarsely chopped

PALEO
ANTI-CANDIDA

Preserved Lemon

Liver detoxing, alkalizing, rich in probiotics

I regularly use preserved lemon, adding it to salads, soups, dressings, and seasoning because of its exquisite umami flavor. The fermentation process transforms the lemon peel's bitterness into a unique taste that will amaze you. Preserved lemon is also high in probiotics and contains liver-detoxing essential oils in the peel. Use the rind and discard the pulp. It is a staple condiment in North Africa and is available at any Middle Eastern grocery.

MAKES 4 preserved lemons

PREP TIME 15 minutes

MAKING TIME 60 to 80 days

EQUIPMENT One 16-ounce mason jar

8 Meyer lemons

6 tablespoons sea salt

2 cinnamon sticks, broken into rough pieces (optional)

5 coriander seeds (optional)

2 cloves (optional)

PALEO

AIP Do not include the coriander seeds.

ANTI-CANDIDA

LOW FODMAP

Sanitize the mason jar by washing it with soap and hot water. Do not use antibacterial soap.

Wash the lemons with boiling water. Cut four of them lengthwise to quarter, but do not cut all the way so the lemon quarters remain connected at the base.

Place 1 tablespoon sea salt at the bottom of the jar. Stuff one quartered lemon into the bottom of the jar, with the base of the lemon down. Pack it in tightly and press down to release the juice. Top with 1 tablespoon salt and the spices. Repeat, topping the other three quartered lemons with salt. Cover all lemons with salt on top.

Juice the remaining four lemons and pour the juice into the jar. The lemons should be fully submerged. If they aren't completely covered, place a small glass container in the mason jar to press the lemons down under the liquid, or add more lemon juice. Do not use a metal or plastic container.

Tighten the lid of the jar and place it in a warm place away from direct sunlight.

Turn the jar upside down every few days.

Ferment for 60 days and check for readiness; the lemon rind should be very soft and no longer taste bitter. If it is not, ferment for up to another 20 days.

Transfer to the refrigerator.

Keeps well in the refrigerator for up to 2 years.

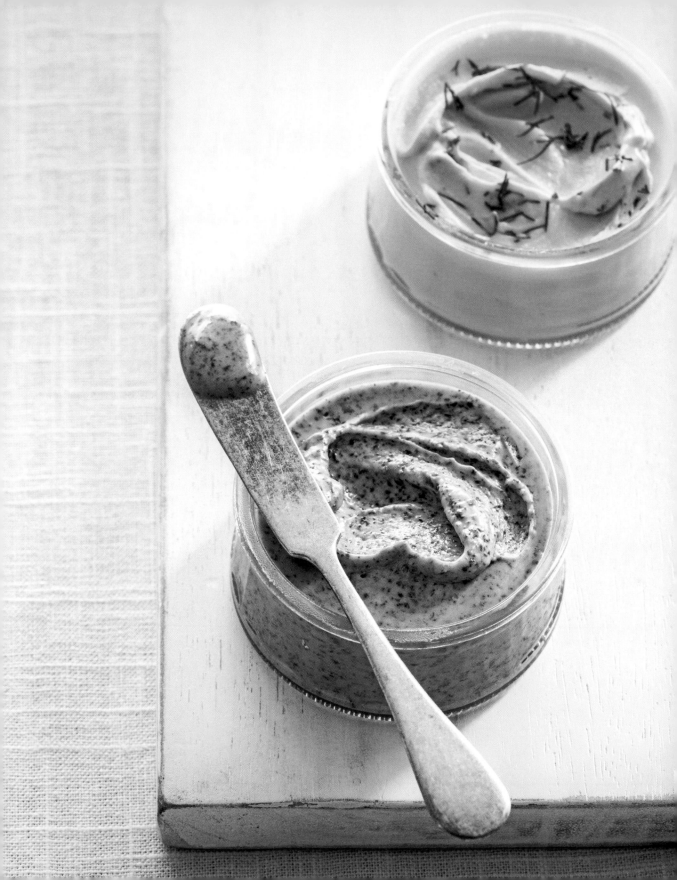

Whipped Herbal Butter—Two Ways

Nutrient dense, rich in antioxidants ⏱ Less than 30 minutes

Do you find yourself with leftover herbs in the fridge that go to waste because you don't use them quickly enough? Turning them into herbal butters not only preserves them but makes them a flavorful and rich addition to sandwiches, salads, steamed vegetables, roast meats, and grilled fish. Be sure to melt the ghee without heating it too much so it does not cook the herbs when added to the blender. Be creative and make your own butters. Two of my favorite butters are made with dill/cilantro/mint and rosemary/thyme/parsley. Whipping is an optional step. I often just pour the unwhipped blend into a mason jar and call it a day. Whipped butter has a fluffy, light texture, but it tastes exactly the same as unwhipped butter.

Place all of the ingredients in the blender and puree until silky smooth.

Transfer to the mason jar and refrigerate until the butter hardens, about 12 hours.

To make whipped butter, transfer the hardened butter to a medium bowl and whip it with a hand mixer until light and fluffy, about 2 minutes.

Return the whipped butter to the mason jar and refrigerate.

Keeps well in the refrigerator for up to 2 weeks.

MAKES One 12-ounce mason jar (each blend)

SERVINGS About 16 tablespoons

PREP TIME 15 minutes

EQUIPMENT High-speed electric blender or food processor, electric hand mixer

BASIL AND GARLIC BUTTER

1 cup firmly packed fresh basil

½ cup extra virgin olive oil

½ cup ghee, melted

1 clove garlic, crushed

½ teaspoon smoked sea salt or sea salt

DILL AND LEMON BUTTER

1 cup firmly packed fresh dill

½ cup extra virgin olive oil

½ cup ghee, melted

½ tablespoon freshly squeezed lemon juice

½ teaspoon smoked sea salt or sea salt

PALEO

AIP

ANTI-CANDIDA

LOW FODMAP Omit the garlic, or use garlic-infused olive oil.

Fabulous Spice Mixes

Gut healing, versatile 🕐 Less than 30 minutes

PREP TIME 15 minutes

ROASTING TIME 4 minutes
(only some recipes)

EQUIPMENT Spice (or coffee)
grinder, 10-inch skillet

Use these spice mixes to quickly turn a dish into something extraordinary.

All of the spice mixes should be kept for no longer than 6 months.

PALEO

AIP *Avoid any seed-based spices that include, for instance, fennel, peppercorn, cumin, or coriander seeds.*

ANTI-CANDIDA

LOW FODMAP *Replace onion and garlic with two pinches asafetida.*

Five-Spice Mix (Chinese Spice)

MAKES 4 tablespoons

2 tablespoons broken
pieces star anise

1 teaspoon black peppercorns

2 teaspoons cloves

2 teaspoons fennel seeds

1 tablespoon finely chopped
cinnamon stick

This is an excellent spice to use with roasted vegetables and rich meats like lamb, pork, or chicken thighs. Use it to season Breakfast Casserole Two: Pork Chops and Apples (page 195), Sticky Spare Ribs Casserole (page 242), and Fries Baked in Duck Fat (page 271).

In a skillet, toast over medium heat the star anise, peppercorns, cloves, and fennel seeds for 3 minutes or until they impart a wonderful fragrance. Cool, add the cinnamon, and grind to a powder. Transfer to an airtight container and label.

Ras el Hanout (Moroccan Spice)

Ras el Hanout in Arabic means "top of the shop," because it's the merchant's best spice mix. Use it in stews and soups and with root vegetable fries. Also use it to season Fries Baked in Duck Fat (page 271).

Place all of the ingredients except the saffron in a spice grinder and grind to a powder. Add the saffron, transfer to an airtight container, and label.

MAKES 4 tablespoons

2 teaspoons dried ginger

2 teaspoons coriander seeds

1½ teaspoons cumin seeds

1½ teaspoons cardamom seeds

1½ teaspoons black peppercorns

1¼ teaspoons nutmeg powder

1½ teaspoons allspice

1 teaspoon finely chopped cinnamon stick

¼ teaspoon dried turmeric powder

Generous pinch of saffron threads (optional)

Herbes de Provence

This spice blend from the south of France quickly transforms grilled fish, seafood, and meats into delicious dishes.

In a medium bowl, combine all of the ingredients. Transfer to an airtight container and label.

MAKES 4 tablespoons

1½ tablespoons dried thyme

1 tablespoon dried basil

1 tablespoon dried oregano

½ tablespoon crushed fennel seed

½ tablespoon crushed dried rosemary

½ tablespoon crushed dried lavender flowers

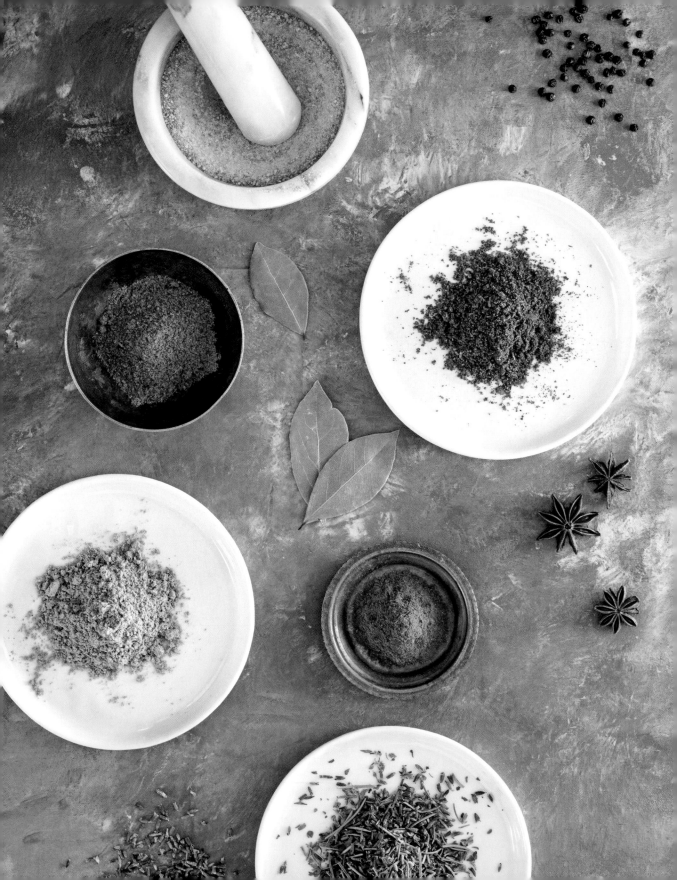

Garam Masala (Indian Spice)

Use this classic Indian spice mixture to make Fries Baked in Duck Fat (page 271), Easy Chicken Curry Stew (page 212), and Flaxseed Crackers (Estrogen Boosters) (page 327).

Over high heat, toast all of the ingredients in a skillet for about 3 minutes or until the cumin starts to pop. Cool and grind to a powder. Transfer to an airtight container and label.

MAKES 8 tablespoons

2-inch cinnamon stick, broken into pieces

2 bay leaves, broken into pieces

⅓ cup coriander seeds

¼ cup cumin seeds

1 tablespoon cardamom pods, crushed

1 tablespoon whole black peppercorns

2 teaspoons whole cloves

Savory Delight

Use this mix to flavor soups, stews, or when frying meat and fish.

Place all of the ingredients in a spice grinder and grind to a powder. Transfer to an airtight container and label.

MAKES ¼ cup

2 tablespoons whole fennel seeds

2 tablespoons whole coriander seeds

1 tablespoon whole cumin seeds

1 tablespoon whole anise seed

1 tablespoon granulated garlic

1 tablespoon granulated onion

Salt Brine for Cultured Vegetables

🕐 Less than 30 minutes

Use this salt brine to make the Cultured Vegetable Medley—Four Ways (page 277). Whenever I have leftover or excess carrots, parsnips, cauliflower, or kohlrabi, I turn them into quick ferments. This simple method transforms vegetables into probiotic-rich powerhouses. Be sure to use filtered water that is free of fluoride and chlorine.

Warm up the water in a saucepan over medium heat, add the salt, and stir until completely dissolved. Once cooled to room temperature, use in recipes as directed.

MAKES 2 quarts

PREP TIME 10 minutes

2 quarts filtered water
6 tablespoons sea salt

PALEO
AIP
ANTI-CANDIDA
LOW FODMAP

Sweet Potato and Sage Pancakes

Source of sustained energy, rich in phytonutrients and fiber

Do you crave a sweet breakfast but want to heal and thrive? This dish is for you. These pancakes are rich in fiber; vitamins A, C, and B6 (essential in progesterone production); and manganese; and the sweet potato, applesauce, and flaxseed will sustain you until lunch.

MAKES 6 pancakes

SERVES 2 to 3

PREP TIME 15 minutes

COOKING TIME 30 minutes

EQUIPMENT Whisk, rimmed baking sheet, parchment paper

3 tablespoons ground flaxseed

⅓ cup hot water

1 cup firmly packed shredded unpeeled sweet potato

¾ cup Homemade Applesauce (page 167)

2 tablespoons unrefined extra virgin olive oil

1 tablespoon freshly squeezed lemon juice

2 teaspoons dried sage

1 cup brown rice flour

¾ teaspoon baking soda

¼ teaspoon sea salt

ANTI-CANDIDA *Eat only after the first 4 weeks of the anti-Candida diet. After that, eat only one to two pancakes per week. Avoid syrup as a topping.*

LOW FODMAP *Replace sweet potato with pumpkin. If you have SIBO, limit to one pancake per day or omit.*

Preheat the oven to 400°F.

In a small bowl, whisk the flaxseed with water and set aside for 5 minutes.

In a medium bowl, mix sweet potato, applesauce, olive oil, lemon juice, sage, and the flaxseed slurry.

In another medium bowl, mix the flour, baking soda, and salt.

Add the wet ingredients to the dry ingredients and stir well to combine.

Line a baking sheet with parchment paper and grease it with ghee or olive oil.

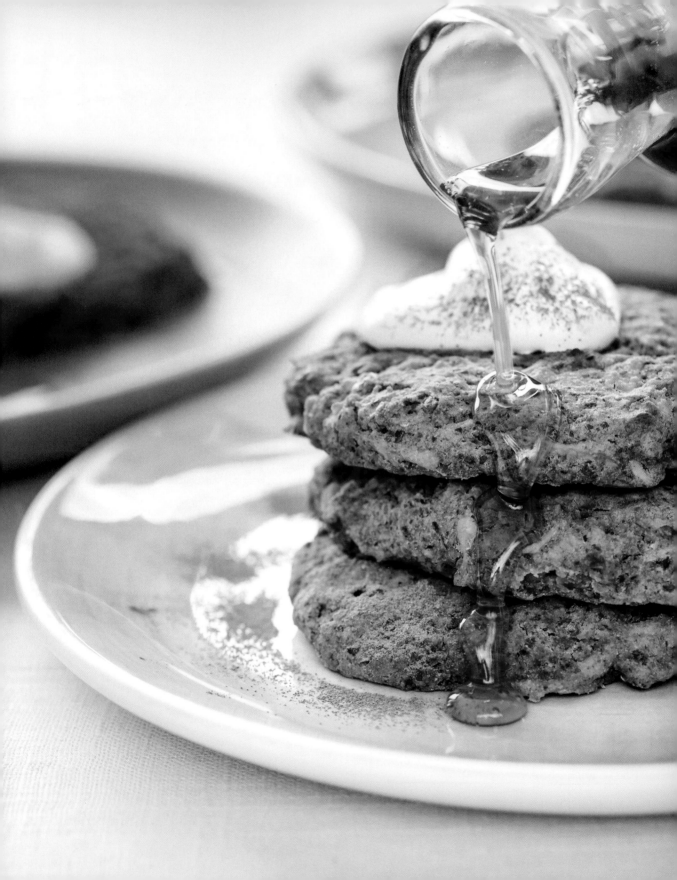

Scoop out slightly less than ½ cup batter and roll it in your palms to form a ball. Place it on the baking sheet and press down to form a ¼-inch-thick pancake. Repeat the process.

Bake for 20 minutes or until brown.

Serve topped with a dollop of Coconut Yogurt (page 164) or Whipped Coconut Cream (page 166), a drizzle of Grade B maple syrup, and a sprinkle of ground cinnamon.

Keep refrigerated in an airtight container for up to 3 days. Reheat in a skillet with a dash of ghee.

Farmer's Wife's Breakfast

Sugar balancing, liver detoxing, rich in proteins

When I lived in California, I visited the local farmers' market every Sunday. It was my little ritual to honor the start of the week. This recipe was inspired by the formidable woman who served many of these breakfasts at the market. Feel free to modify the patties by replacing half of the lamb with ground pork, bison, beef, chicken, or turkey. Experiment with different herbs, spices, or even fruits that resonate with you and help you to feel energetically balanced. Perhaps some cumin, nutmeg, and apricots or dried cherries?

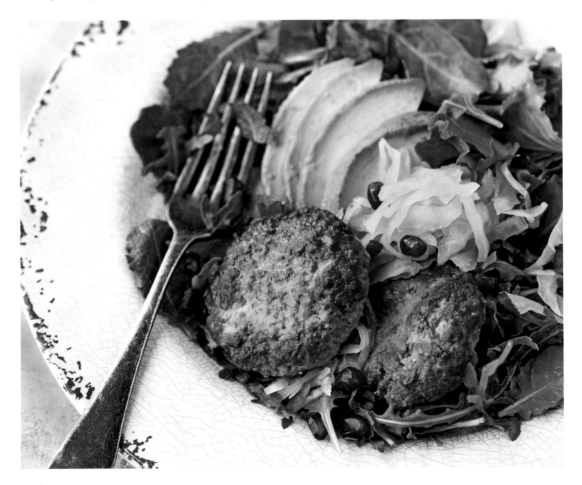

To make the patties, in a large bowl, knead together the lamb, fennel seed, apple cider vinegar, coconut aminos, and salt.

Using your hands, form the mixture into twelve patties.

In a skillet over medium-high heat, heat 1½ teaspoons ghee. Place six patties in the hot skillet and fry for 4 minutes or until brown. Flip and fry for 3 minutes. Set aside. Add the remaining ghee to the skillet and fry the remaining patties.

To make the salad, in a medium bowl, toss the greens with the olive oil, lemon, and salt until well coated.

To serve, place half the salad on each plate and top with two patties and half the avocado, sauerkraut, and pomegranate seeds. Store the remaining patties for the next day's breakfast.

Patties keeps well in the refrigerator for up to 5 days or in the freezer for up to 3 months.

PALEO

AIP *Replace the fennel seed with thyme or oregano.*

ANTI-CANDIDA *Avoid Kohlrabi Kraut or sauerkraut for the first 4 weeks of the anti-Candida diet.*

LOW FODMAP *Eat only ⅛ of the avocado per serving, or avoid. Eat no more than 1 tablespoon Kohlrabi Kraut or sauerkraut per day.*

MAKES 12 patties
(freeze the balance)

SERVES 2

PREP TIME 20 minutes

COOKING TIME 30 minutes

EQUIPMENT 11-inch skillet

LAMB PATTIES

1 pound ground lamb

2 tablespoons ground fennel seed

2 tablespoons apple cider vinegar

2 tablespoons coconut aminos

1 teaspoon smoked sea salt

1 tablespoon ghee, divided

SALAD

2 handfuls of greens such as arugula, mizuna, baby kale, or baby spinach

2 tablespoons extra virgin olive oil

1 tablespoon freshly squeezed lemon juice

Dash of sea salt

SIDES

1 ripe avocado, peeled, pitted, and sliced

1 cup Kohlrabi Kraut (page 275) or store-bought sauerkraut

½ cup fresh pomegranate seeds

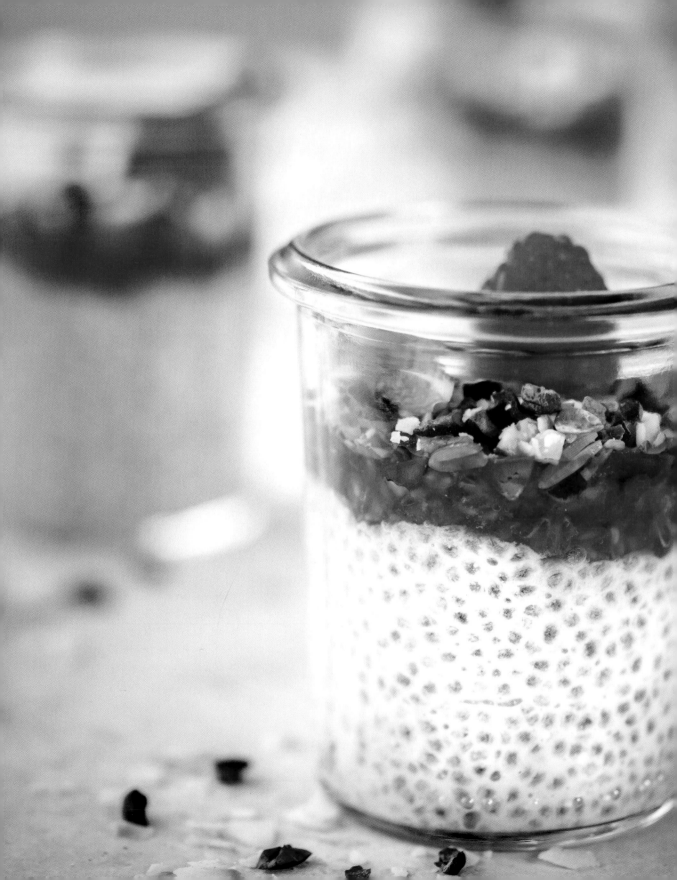

Coconut Kefir Chia Pudding

Gut healing, rich in probiotics, rich in fiber

Add more probiotics to your day by turning coconut milk into a tart and refreshing kefir. Coconut nectar facilitates the fermentation process, and though the nectar is high in sugar, most of the sugar will be eaten by the kefir grains. The fermentation speed will depend on the freshness of the kefir packet and the temperature of the room, which ideally should be between 68°F and 72°F. I keep my kefir going for 48 hours, as I like it tart. If you are new to fermentation, taste it after 12 hours in a warmer kitchen and 24 hours in a cooler one. Longer fermentation means a tarter taste, less sugar, and a higher count of probiotics.

Sterilize the glass jar by washing it with hot water and regular soap (do not use antibacterial soap).

In a medium saucepan over low heat, heat the coconut milk and water until it is warm to the touch. Whisk in the chia seeds, coconut nectar, kefir starter, maca, and vanilla powder.

Transfer to the glass jar, cover the jar with a paper towel, and secure it with a rubber band.

Check for tartness after 12 hours of fermentation. If it is not tart yet, keep it going for another 12 to 24 hours. The kefir should taste like sour cream.

To serve, garnish with any of the topping options.

Keeps well in the refrigerator for up to 5 days.

PALEO

ANTI-CANDIDA *Do not consume during the first 4 weeks of the anti-Candida diet. Reduce the coconut nectar to 1 tablespoon.*

LOW FODMAP *Maca has not been tested; it is best to omit it.*

SERVES 2

PREP TIME 10 minutes

FERMENTATION TIME 12 to 24 hours

EQUIPMENT Whisk, 1-quart glass jar, rubber band

One 13.66-ounce can full-fat coconut milk

1 cup mineral water (avoid tap water)

½ cup chia seeds

2 tablespoons coconut nectar

½ packet Body Ecology Kefir Starter

2 teaspoons maca (optional)

1 teaspoon vanilla powder

Topping options: Berries, nuts, seeds, cacao nibs, coconut flakes, or fresh mint

Seed Rotation Porridge—Two Ways

Estrogen balancing, progesterone boosting, rich in fiber ⏱ Less than 30 minutes

MAKES 2 servings

PREP TIME 10 minutes

WARMING TIME 5 minutes

PALEO

LOW FODMAP Replace cherries with blueberries and applesauce with pumpkin puree.

These simple recipes are a great way to incorporate the Seed Rotation Method (page 104) into your diet. Use Squash Porridge to rebalance your estrogen levels during the luteal phase and Applesauce Porridge to boost your progesterone levels during the follicular phase. Menopausal women can eat either one of the porridges throughout the month.

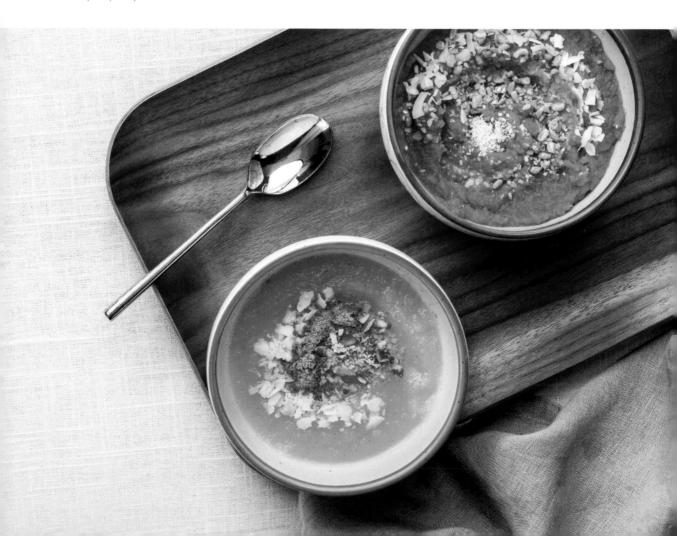

Squash Porridge (estrogen balancing)

PORRIDGE

1 15-ounce can butternut squash puree

¾ cup filtered water

½ cup unsweetened shredded coconut

3 tablespoons chia seeds

2 tablespoons ghee

1 tablespoon freshly squeezed lemon juice

2 teaspoons ground allspice

1 teaspoon vanilla extract

½ teaspoon turmeric powder

1 cup frozen tart cherries

Dash of fine sea salt

TOPPING

2 tablespoons freshly ground flaxseed

2 tablespoons freshly ground
raw pumpkin seeds

Applesauce Porridge (progesterone boosting)

PORRIDGE

2 cups unsweetened Homemade
Applesauce (page 167)

½ cup filtered water

½ cup unsweetened shredded coconut

2 tablespoons ghee

3 tablespoons chia seeds

1 tablespoon ground cinnamon

1 teaspoon vanilla extract

Dash of fine sea salt

TOPPING

2 tablespoons ground raw sesame seeds

2 tablespoons ground raw sunflower seeds

Place all of the porridge ingredients in a medium-size pan and heat through until the porridge thickens, about 5 minutes.

Ladle into serving bowls and sprinkle with the topping ingredients. Serve warm.

The porridges keep well in the refrigerator for up to 5 days.

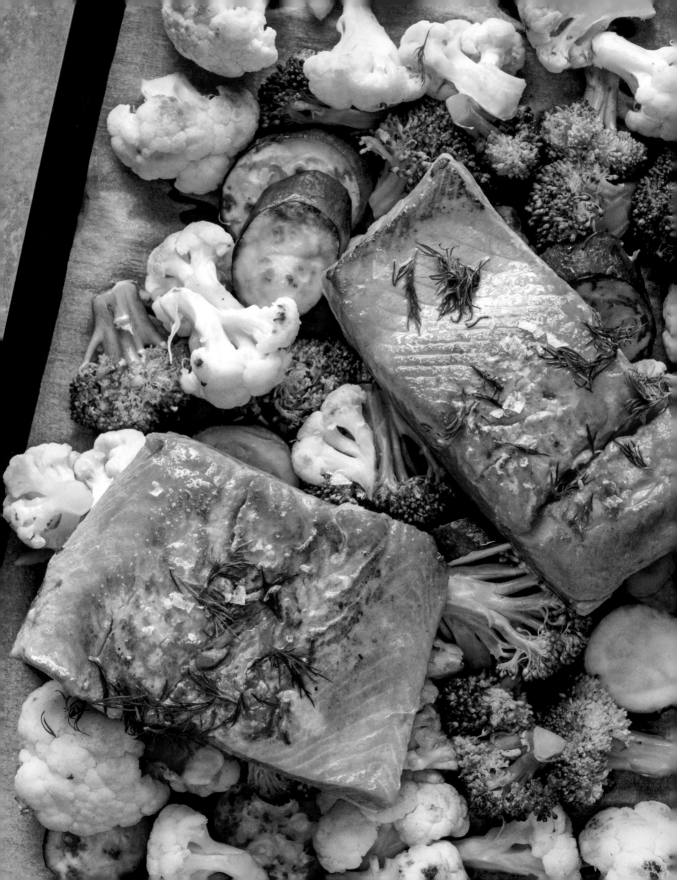

Breakfast Casserole One: Salmon and Broccoli

Estrogen balancing, sugar balancing, rich in proteins ⏱ Less than 30 minutes

I developed breakfast casserole recipes for busy women who don't have time to make an elaborate breakfast but want to avoid the high sugar content of most grab-and-go options. The method is simple: Put coarsely chopped vegetables and protein in a dish and bake while you get ready for your day. You can save time by chopping the vegetables and placing them in the baking dish the night before.

Preheat the oven to 400°F.

Grease the baking pan with olive oil. Place the cauliflower, broccoli, and zucchini in the pan. Sprinkle the vegetables with ½ teaspoon salt, drizzle with the olive oil, and toss until well coated.

Place the salmon on top of the vegetables. Spoon the ghee over each fillet and sprinkle with ½ teaspoon salt and the dill.

Bake uncovered for 15 to 20 minutes, or until the fish easily flakes away when tested with a fork.

Serve and eat right away.

Keeps well in the refrigerator for up to 3 days.

PALEO

AIP

ANTI-CANDIDA

LOW FODMAP *Replace the cauliflower with broccoli or zucchini.*

SERVES 2

PREP TIME 10 minutes

COOKING TIME
15 to 20 minutes

EQUIPMENT 13 × 9-inch
baking dish

2 tablespoons extra virgin olive oil, plus additional for greasing

1 small head cauliflower, stemmed and coarsely chopped

1 small head broccoli, stemmed and coarsely chopped

1 small zucchini, cut into ½-inch slices

1 teaspoon sea salt, divided

2 salmon fillets (about 1 pound)

1 tablespoon ghee

1 teaspoon dried dill or 2 teaspoons fresh dill

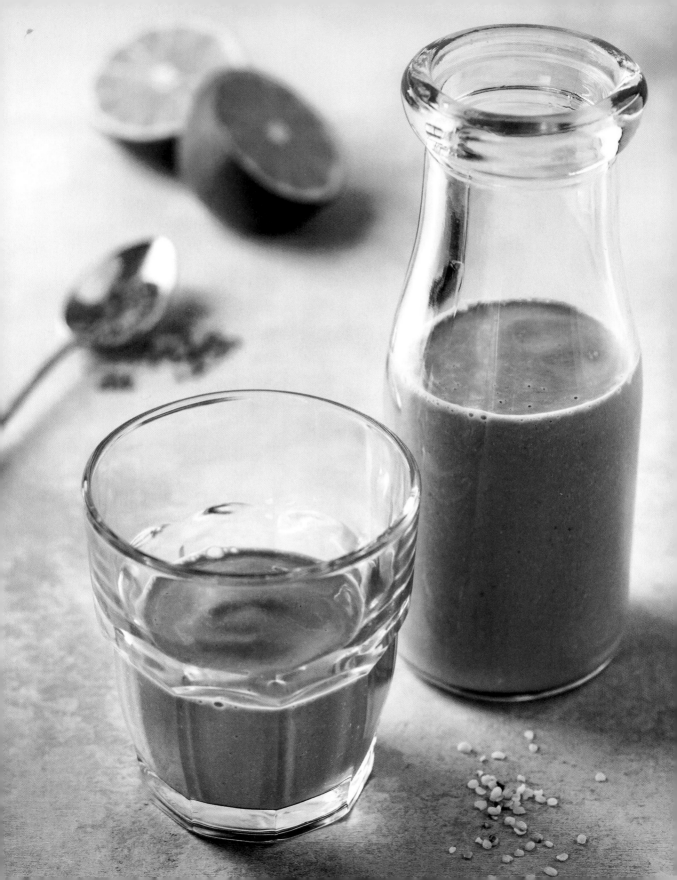

Energizing Matcha Lime Smoothie

Liver detoxing, sugar balancing, estrogen balancing ⏱ Less than 30 minutes

Is getting out of bed in the morning a struggle? Kick-start your day with this rich, creamy smoothie instead of coffee and avoid disruptive caffeine highs and lows. Matcha, a type of green tea from Japan, contains caffeine but causes a steady energy boost rather than a spike. Arugula, flaxseed, and maca (called "Peruvian ginseng" because of its natural stimulating qualities, which are similar to the benefits found in the commonly known ginseng-related herbs) support your estrogen levels. Cinnamon effectively stabilizes blood sugar levels.

Add all of the ingredients to a blender and puree until silky smooth.

PALEO

ANTI-CANDIDA *Replace the date with four drops liquid stevia.*

LOW FODMAP *Replace the avocado with 2 tablespoons coconut butter; replace the date with 1½ teaspoons maple syrup. Omit the maca.*

SERVES 1

PREP TIME 15 minutes

EQUIPMENT High-speed electric blender

1½ cups filtered water

1 cup loosely packed fresh arugula leaves or mixed greens, such as baby spinach, mizuna, or lettuce

½ ripe avocado, peeled, pitted, and sliced

1 Medjool date, pitted

4 Brazil nuts

3 tablespoons freshly squeezed lime juice

2 tablespoons ground flaxseed

1 tablespoon ghee

1 tablespoon maca

1½ tablespoons hemp seed

1 teaspoon freshly ground ginger root

1 teaspoon matcha green tea

¼ teaspoon ground cinnamon

Dash of sea salt

Grain-Free Sunday Brunch Pancakes with Mixed Berries

Sugar balancing, rich in vitamins A and C, rich in potassium

SERVES 2

PREP TIME 15 minutes

COOKING TIME 20 minutes

EQUIPMENT High-speed blender or a good food processor, 15-inch ceramic nonstick skillet with lid

PANCAKES

2 medium green plantains, about 1½ pounds

1 tablespoon freshly squeezed lime juice

¼ cup ghee, lard, or coconut oil, melted

Generous pinch of sea salt

2 teaspoons ghee or coconut oil, divided

BERRY TOPPING

1 cup mixed fresh berries

2 tablespoons coconut butter

1 teaspoon freshly squeezed lime juice

1 teaspoon vanilla extract

Pinch of sea salt

The pancake breakfast many of us grew up with was rich in processed flour and a generous pour of maple syrup, resulting in an immediate blood sugar spike, followed by a sharp drop several hours later. Replacing processed flour with green plantains, which are high in starch but not sugar, will stabilize your blood sugar levels and keep you energized throughout the day. Spongy and moist with a neutral flavor, these pancakes pair well with sweet or savory toppings (see the Variation). The savory topping is great if you are doing the anti-Candida diet or trying to avoid sweet breakfasts.

Peel and slice the plantains into ½-inch rounds.

Place the plantains, lime juice, ghee, and salt in a blender and blend until smooth. Add up to 2 tablespoons water if the batter is too thick and the blades don't easily turn. If you are not using a high-speed blender, you might need to stop the machine and scrape down the sides of the container with a spatula a few times to help the ingredients combine thoroughly.

Heat the skillet over medium heat. Add 1 teaspoon ghee.

When the ghee has melted, pour half of the batter into the skillet and spread evenly with a spatula. Cover loosely, with the lid ajar. Cook on low-medium heat for 10 minutes, or until the top of the pancake is dry; then flip it.

Cook for another 2 to 3 minutes, until brown. Repeat.

To make the berry topping, place berries, coconut butter, lime juice, vanilla extract, and sea salt in a small bowl and mash with a fork. Serve half on top of each pancake.

Variation: Bacon and Greens Topping

Divide ingredients in half and place on top of each pancake.

PALEO

AIP *Remove seeds from the broccoli sprouts.*

LOW FODMAP *Skip the avocado.*

1 ripe avocado, peeled, pitted, and sliced

4 bacon slices, fried or oven-roasted at 350°F for 20 minutes

Handful of arugula leaves

Handful of broccoli sprouts

1 teaspoon extra virgin olive oil

Pinch of sea salt

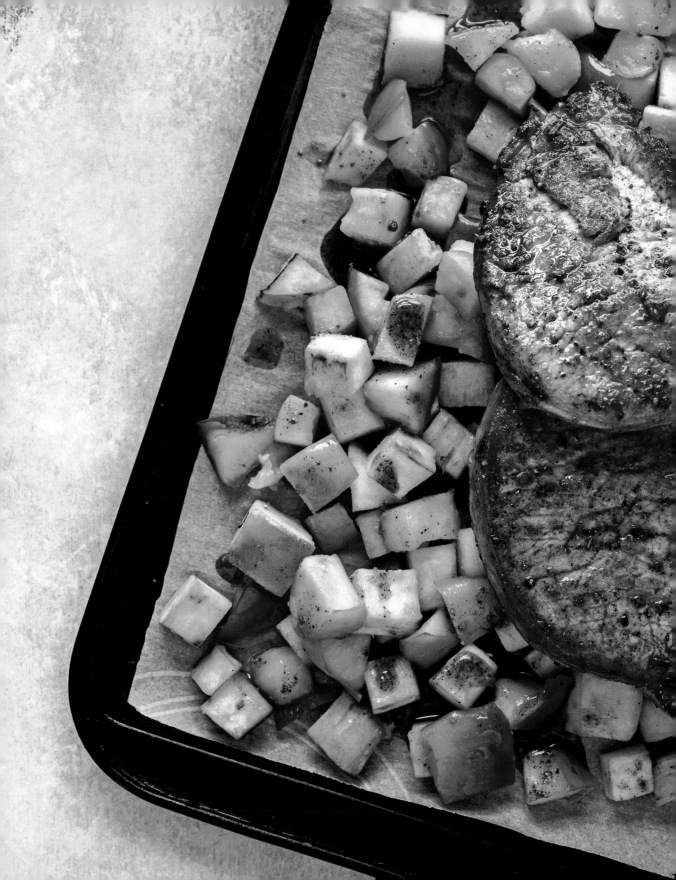

Breakfast Casserole Two: Pork Chops and Apples

Sugar balancing, estrogen balancing, rich in proteins ⏱ Less than 30 minutes

One of our online community members wisely said: "To change my nights, I had to change my mornings." Breakfasts like this one significantly helped her improve her sleep. Expect more benefits from adapting to a PFF breakfast; such as fewer sugar cravings, more energy and mental acuity.

Preheat the oven to 400°F.

Grease the baking dish with olive oil. Place the celeriac and apples in the pan, drizzle with the olive oil, and sprinkle with sea salt. Toss until well coated.

In a small bowl, make a slurry of the spice mix, smoked sea salt, and ghee.

Glaze the pork chops on both sides with the spice slurry and place on top of the vegetables.

Bake uncovered for 15 minutes. Turn the pork chops over and bake for another 15 minutes.

Serve right away.

Keeps well in the refrigerator for up to 5 days.

PALEO

AIP *Replace the Five-Spice Mix with ground cinnamon.*

ANTI-CANDIDA *Omit apples or replace by adding 2 cups parsnip and celeriac. Or, replace with squash such as acorn or delicata.*

LOW FODMAP *Omit apples or replace by adding 2 cups parsnip and celeriac.*

SERVES 2

PREP TIME 20 minutes

COOKING TIME 30 minutes

EQUIPMENT 13 × 9-inch baking dish

2 cups ⅓-inch cubes peeled celeriac or parsnip

2 small unpeeled apples, cored and coarsely chopped

1 tablespoon extra virgin olive oil

Pinch of sea salt

1 teaspoon Five-Spice Mix (page 174)

¼ teaspoon smoked sea salt or truffle sea salt

2 teaspoons ghee, melted

2 pork rib chops

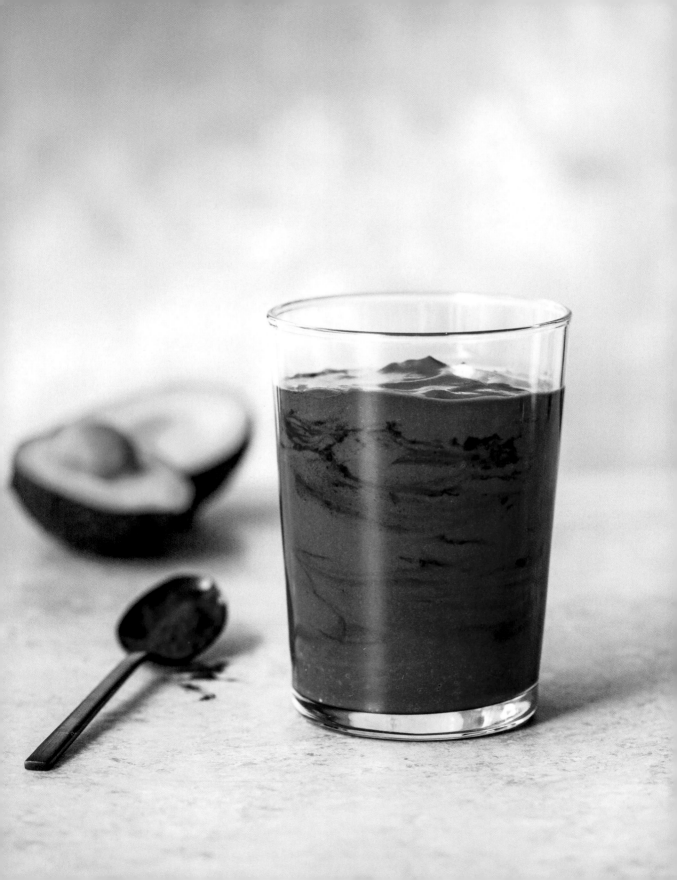

Deep Green Spirulina Smoothie

Estrogen balancing, rich in iodine, supports breast health ⏱ Less than 30 minutes

It might feel strange to use the sea-tasting spirulina in a smoothie, but you will be in for a pleasant surprise. Many women have told me that they feel energized and clear in their minds after having this smoothie and they end up craving it. I'm not surprised—rich in iodine, spirulina can boost your mental function, energy levels, and breast health, especially if you are low in iodine. In spite of its wonderful benefits, about 30 percent of the population is sensitive to spirulina. Hashimoto's patients should omit it due to a high iodine content.

Add all of the ingredients to a blender and puree until silky smooth.

PALEO

ANTI-CANDIDA *Replace the pear with a handful of berries.*

SERVES 2

PREP TIME 10 minutes

EQUIPMENT High-speed electric blender

2½ cups filtered water

1 ripe avocado, peeled, pitted, and sliced

1 ripe Bartlett pear, coarsely chopped

½ cup firmly packed broccoli sprouts

2 tablespoons spirulina powder

3 tablespoons freshly squeezed lemon juice

2 tablespoons freshly ground flaxseed

2 tablespoons pumpkin seeds

½ teaspoon camu camu

Dash of sea salt

Teff and Cherry Porridge

Low in sugar, rich in proteins ⏱ Less than 30 minutes

I do not recommend eating carbohydrates for breakfast as they can leave you feeling hungry way before lunch and cause your energy level to crash in the middle of the day. But for those times when you crave a hot cereal, try teff. An ancient grain originally from Ethiopia, teff contains 20 percent protein (which is the highest content among all grains) so it will sustain your energy throughout the day. It is also high in thiamine (vitamin B1), which helps with thyroid health and mental functions. When toasted, teff imparts a heavenly nutty flavor. This porridge is a staple in my home.

SERVES 4

PREP TIME 5 minutes

COOKING TIME 25 minutes

EQUIPMENT Deep 9-inch skillet or sauté pan with lid

PORRIDGE

1 cup teff grain (not flour)

3 cups water

¼ cup cacao butter, ghee, or coconut butter

1 teaspoon ground cloves

1 teaspoon vanilla powder

¼ teaspoon sea salt

1½ cups sweet or sour frozen cherries

TOPPINGS

½ cup toasted coconut flakes

¼ cup raw pecans, coarsely chopped

2 tablespoons Grade B maple syrup (optional)

In a skillet over high heat, toast the teff, stirring frequently, for 4 minutes or until it starts to pop.

Take the skillet off the heat and carefully and slowly add the water, cacao butter, cloves, vanilla powder, and salt. Return the skillet to the stove and bring to a boil. Reduce the heat to medium low, cover, and cook for 10 minutes, stirring occasionally.

Fold in the cherries and cook for another 2 minutes. Stir frequently so the porridge does not stick to the bottom of the pan.

Remove the porridge from the heat and let it cool for 5 minutes before serving.

Ladle into bowls and top with coconut flakes, pecans, and maple syrup. Serve right away.

Keeps well in the refrigerator for up to 5 days.

ANTI-CANDIDA *Avoid during the first 4 weeks of the anti-Candida diet. Replace cherries with fresh or frozen blueberries. Replace the maple syrup with three drops of stevia.*

LOW FODMAP *Replace cherries with fresh or frozen blueberries.*

Parsnip Dill Pancake with Arugula and Smoked Salmon

Sugar balancing, estrogen balancing, rich in omega 3 ◑ Less than 30 minutes

This is a decadent breakfast inspired by some of the most common ingredients available in arctic Iceland, where I've lived. Parsnips will sustain your energy, salmon will deliver omega 3 fatty acids, and the tossed arugula salad will help detoxify from antagonistic estrogen. Brown butter provides an additional nutty and caramelized flavor (see Buying and Prepping Tips and Tricks, page 140).

MAKES 4 pancakes

SERVES 2

PREP TIME 20 minutes

COOKING TIME 8 minutes

EQUIPMENT 11-inch skillet or bigger

In a medium bowl, knead all of the pancake ingredients except the ghee until a sticky batter is formed. If the pancake batter is too dry, add water 1 teaspoon at the time until it becomes sticky.

In a skillet over medium-high heat, melt the ghee.

Scoop out one-quarter of the batter, roll it in your hands, and press it down to form a ¼-inch-thick pancake. Repeat to make four pancakes.

Place each pancake in the skillet and press down again with your hand or a spatula. Fry for 5 minutes or until brown and easy to lift up. Flip and fry for another 2 to 3 minutes.

PANCAKES

1½ cups tightly packed shredded peeled parsnips

½ cup cold water

⅓ cup plus 1 tablespoon cassava flour

2 teaspoons arrowroot flour

¾ teaspoon sea salt

1 tablespoon ghee or brown butter

PALEO

AIP Replace mayo with a drizzle of olive oil.

ANTI-CANDIDA Replace the balsamic vinegar with apple cider vinegar and three drops of stevia.

LOW FODMAP Omit mayo or replace with any of the dollops in Chapter 15. Only use the green part of the scallions.

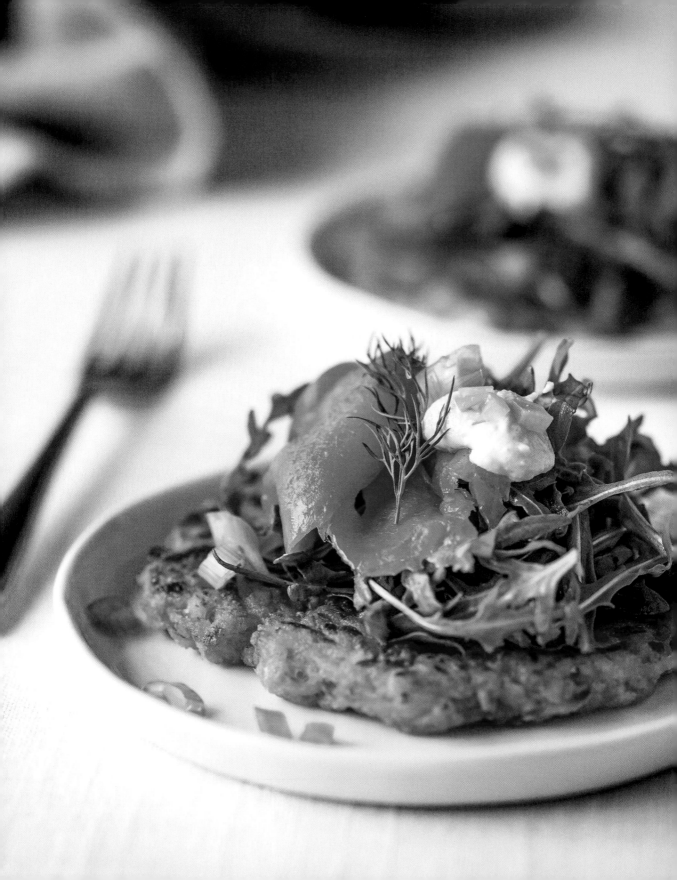

While the pancakes are frying, make the arugula salad. In a separate medium bowl, toss all of the salad ingredients.

Serve each pancake topped with salad, a slice of salmon, a dollop of Preserved Lemon Mayo, and a sprinkle of scallions and dill.

Serve and eat immediately.

ARUGULA SALAD TOPPING

1 cup lightly packed arugula leaves

1 tablespoon extra virgin olive oil

½ teaspoon balsamic vinegar

Pinch of fine sea salt

ADDITIONAL TOPPINGS

4 slices smoked salmon

2 tablespoons Preserved Lemon Mayo (page 169) (optional)

2 teaspoons finely chopped scallions

1 teaspoon dried dill or 2 teaspoons finely chopped fresh dill

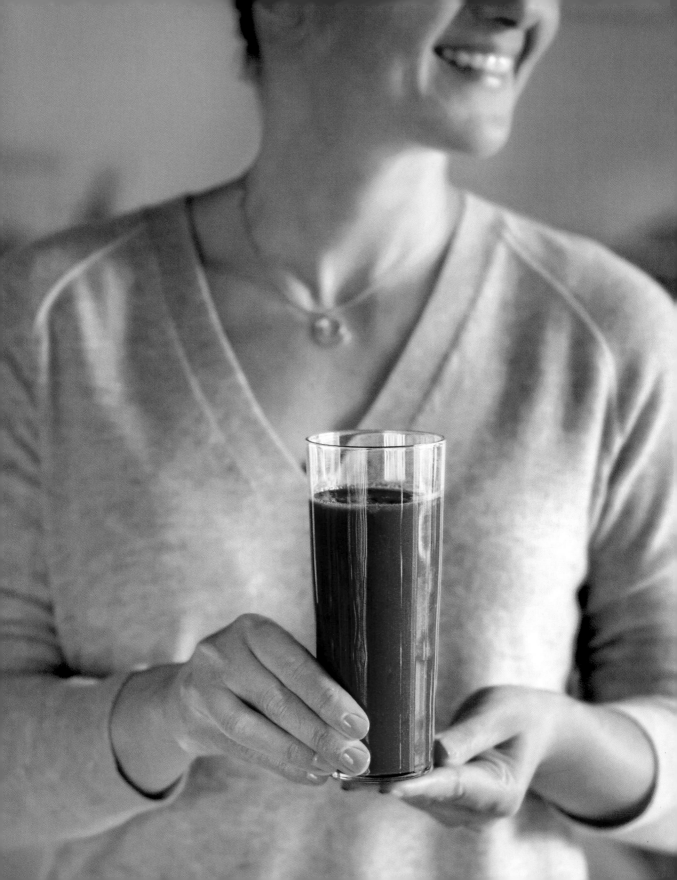

Carrot and Beet Smoothie

Estrogen balancing, progesterone boosting, rich in fiber, high in good fats ⏱ Less than 30 minutes

Try this smoothie if you are struggling with PMS; drink one glass per day during the 5 days before your period. Beets support the liver in estrogen detoxification, and carrots support progesterone production. If you can't tolerate almonds, replace them with other nuts such as raw walnuts, macadamia nuts, hazelnuts, or pecans. Adding hemp seed will boost the content of omega 3 fatty acids, which is anti-inflammatory and can help mitigate PMS symptoms.

Add all of the ingredients to a blender and puree until silky smooth.

Refrigerate in an airtight container for up to 3 days.

PALEO

LOW FODMAP *Replace beets with carrots and almonds with pecans or macadamia nuts.*

SERVES 2

PREP TIME 10 minutes

EQUIPMENT High-speed electric blender

1½ cups filtered water

½ cup coarsely chopped unpeeled carrots

½ cup coarsely chopped peeled beets

¼ cup raw almonds

1½ tablespoons freshly squeezed lemon juice

1 tablespoon minced ginger

1 tablespoon ground flaxseed

1 tablespoon hemp seed (optional)

1 teaspoon ground cinnamon

½ teaspoon vanilla extract

¼ teaspoon ground cloves

Pinch of sea salt

Bacon, Oysters, and Collard Greens Stir Fry

Liver detoxing, estrogen balancing, rich in zinc 🕐 Less than 30 minutes

This is one of my favorite stir-fry dishes as it combines the sweetness of root vegetables, such as sweet potatoes and parsnips, with the saltiness of oysters and the slight bitterness of collard greens. Oysters are very high in zinc, which helps heal the gut, and collard greens help detoxify the liver to keep your estrogen levels in check.

SERVES 2

PREP TIME 10 minutes

COOKING TIME 15 minutes

EQUIPMENT 12-inch skillet with lid

6 bacon slices, cut widthwise into ½-inch pieces

1 cup tightly packed unpeeled grated sweet potato

1 cup tightly packed grated unpeeled parsnip

½ cup raw shucked oysters or raw mussel meat

1 tablespoon oyster brine or fish sauce

1 tablespoon apple cider vinegar

2 cups coarsely chopped, stemmed, tightly packed collard greens

Heat the skillet over medium-high heat. Add the bacon and fry until brown, about 7 minutes.

Reduce the heat to medium and add the sweet potato, parsnip, oysters, oyster brine, and cider vinegar. Cover and cook for 5 minutes or until the sweet potato has softened.

Reduce the heat to low, stir in the collard greens, cover, and cook for another 3 minutes. Serve immediately.

PALEO

AIP

ANTI-CANDIDA *Replace the sweet potato and parsnip with 2 cups grated zucchini.*

LOW FODMAP *Replace sweet potato with more parsnip.*

Zucchini Olive Muffins

Sugar balancing, low in sugar, rich in fiber

This hearty muffin is a convenient guilt-free grab-and-go breakfast, travel snack, or afternoon treat. Teff flour is high in protein and rich in vitamins and minerals.

Preheat oven to 375°F.

In a small bowl, stir the flaxseed into the hot water and let the mixture thicken for about 10 minutes.

In large bowl, combine the teff flour, brown rice flour, baking powder, rosemary, and sea salt.

In another large bowl, combine the zucchini, olives, olive oil, water, lemon juice, and maple syrup. Add the flaxseed mixture.

Add the wet ingredients to the flour mixture and stir until just combined. Do not overmix the batter, as this will make the muffins hard.

Spoon the batter into muffin cups (preferably silicon or paper cups, not aluminum) and bake for 20 to 25 minutes, or until the tops are hard and brown.

The muffins keep well in room temperature for up to 5 days or in the freezer for up to 6 months.

PALEO *Replace the brown rice flour with almond flour (not meal, as it's too moist).*

ANTI-CANDIDA *Replace the brown rice flour with almond flour (not meal, as it's too moist) if you can tolerate nuts.*

LOW FODMAP *If you have SIBO, limit to eating one muffin every other day or omit.*

MAKES 12 muffins

PREP TIME 20 minutes

BAKING TIME 20 minutes

3 tablespoons ground flaxseed

½ cup hot water

1½ cups teff flour

1 cup brown rice flour

2 teaspoons baking powder

1 tablespoon dried rosemary or tarragon

1 teaspoon sea salt

1½ cups firmly packed shredded zucchini

¾ cup pitted black Kalamata olives, coarsely chopped

¾ cup extra virgin olive oil

½ cup room temperature water

2 tablespoons freshly squeezed lemon juice or apple cider vinegar

3 tablespoons Grade B maple syrup

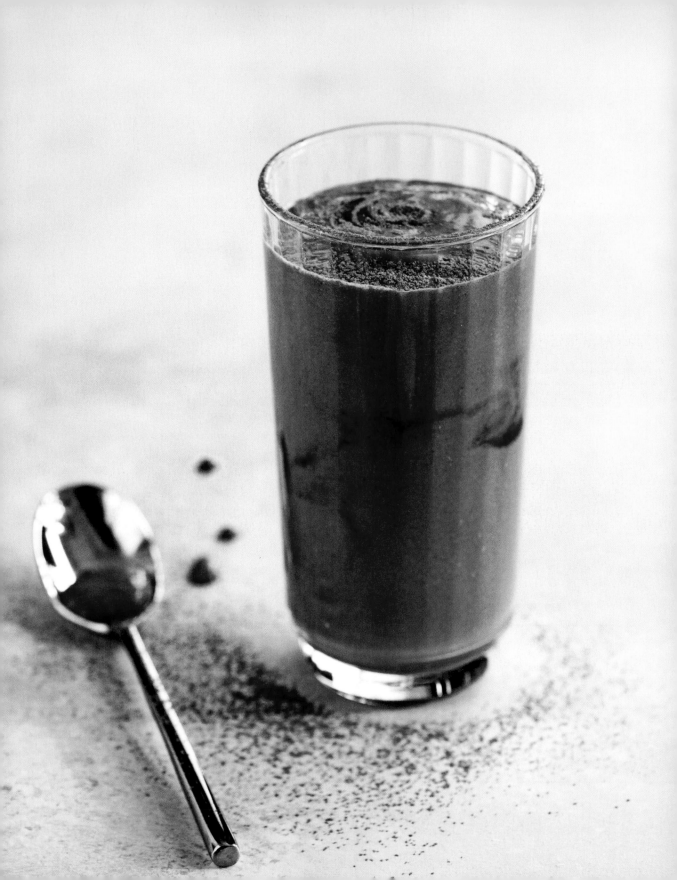

Decadent Chocolate Cherry Smoothie

Low in sugar, energizing, rich in magnesium ⏱ Less than 30 minutes

Need something rich for breakfast? This guilt-free smoothie will satisfy your chocolate cravings and offer plenty of fiber, magnesium, and vitamins A and C. Add some collagen powder to support your digestive health and to add some extra protein.

Add all of the ingredients to a blender and puree until silky smooth.

PALEO

ANTI-CANDIDA *Replace the cherries with an additional four drops of stevia.*

LOW FODMAP *Replace the cherries with blueberries.*

SERVES 2

PREP TIME 10 minutes

EQUIPMENT High-speed electric blender

1½ cups filtered water

½ ripe avocado, peeled, pitted, and sliced

1 cup frozen pitted dark sweet cherries

¼ cup raw pumpkin seeds

¼ cup raw hazelnuts

3 tablespoons raw unsweetened cacao

2 tablespoons collagen powder

1 tablespoon melted coconut oil

1 tablespoon vanilla extract

1 tablespoon freshly squeezed lemon or lime juice

½ teaspoon cinnamon powder

6 drops stevia

Dash of sea salt

Perfect French Crepes

Rich in prebiotics, quercetin, and fiber

These crepes are so light and soft you'd never guess they don't contain wheat and eggs. Mild and neutral in flavor with a fluffy, powdery texture, cassava flour is an excellent 1:1 gluten-free and grain-free replacement for wheat flour. It doesn't contain many nutrients, but the nutritious filling makes up for that. Use a ceramic frying pan to prevent the crepes from sticking.

MAKES 6 crepes

SERVES 2

PREP TIME 7 minutes

COOKING TIME 42 minutes (use two pans to cut the cooking time in half)

EQUIPMENT 11-inch ceramic skillet, whisk, spice grater or microplane

CREPES

2 cups cold water

1 cup cassava flour

¼ cup arrowroot flour

¼ cup ghee, melted

½ teaspoon sea salt

2 tablespoons coconut oil or ghee, divided

FILLING AND TOPPING

¾ cup Homemade Applesauce (page 167)

½ cup Coconut Yogurt (page 164) (optional)

Freshly grated nutmeg

In a large bowl, whisk together the water, cassava flour, arrowroot flour, ghee, and salt until the batter is completely smooth.

In a skillet over medium-high heat, heat 1 teaspoon coconut oil.

Scoop a little less than ½ cup of the batter onto the skillet. Tip and rotate the skillet to spread batter as thinly as possible.

Keep the heat on medium high and cook 4 to 5 minutes or until sides get brown and dry. Flip with a spatula and cook the other side for 1 to 2 minutes. Remove from the pan and keep warm by covering with a hand towel. Repeat the process. If the batter gets too thick, add water to maintain its initial thin consistency.

To serve, spread each crepe with applesauce and roll or fold up. Top each crepe with a dollop of Coconut Yogurt and sprinkle with freshly grated nutmeg.

PALEO

AIP

LOW FODMAP Replace the applesauce with blueberry or raspberry jam or conserve.

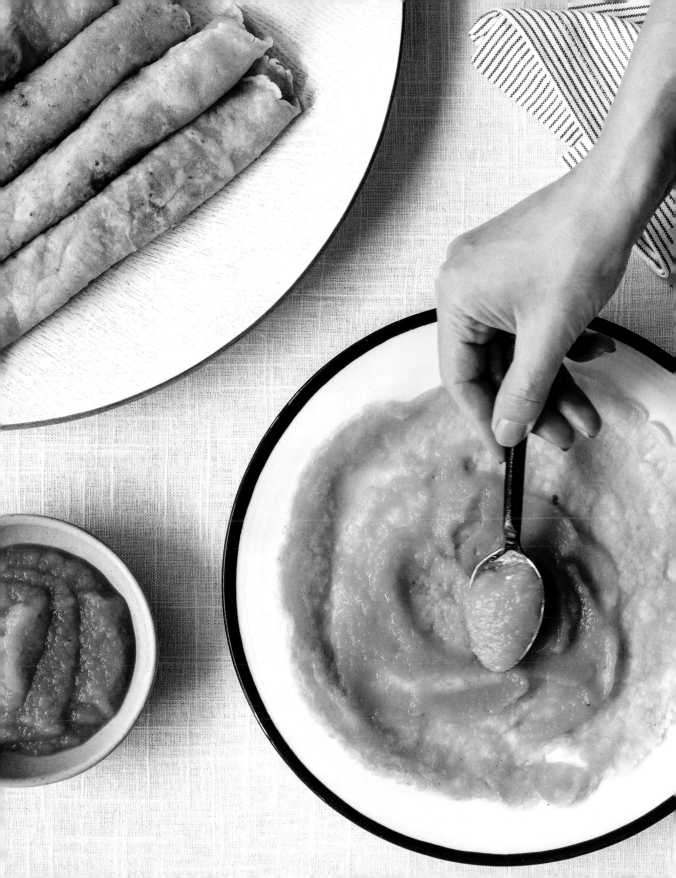

Hearty Beet Stew (Borscht)

Liver detoxing, estrogen balancing, progesterone boosting

6 bacon slices, cut to ½-inch bits

1 tablespoon ghee

1 yellow onion, diced

2 celery stalks, cut into ¼-inch slices

1 large unpeeled parsnip, cut into ¼-inch cubes

2 large unpeeled carrots, cut into ¼-inch cubes

1 leek, white and light green parts, thinly sliced

¾ head Napa cabbage, shredded

1 bay leaf

1 tablespoon dried marjoram

1 tablespoon sea salt

6 cups Mineral Vegetable Broth (page 160) or Healing Bone Broth (page 162)

3 large beets, peeled and grated

1 teaspoon freshly grated lemon peel

2 tablespoons freshly squeezed lemon juice

¼ cup fresh dill, minced, plus extra for garnish

Black pepper, freshly ground, to taste

Whipped Herbal Butter, for garnish (page 173)

The combination of beets and carrots can help alleviate symptoms of estrogen dominance, including PMS pain, mood swings, and irregular periods. This hearty soup is wonderfully warming on a chilly winter night.

SERVES 6 to 8

PREP TIME 10 minutes

COOKING TIME 40 minutes

EQUIPMENT 6-quart Dutch oven or heavy-bottomed pot with lid

In a Dutch oven over medium-high heat, cook the bacon until well browned, about 8 minutes. Add the ghee and onion and cook until translucent, about 5 minutes.

Add celery, parsnip, carrots, leek, cabbage, bay leaf, marjoram, and salt. Reduce the heat to medium, cover, and cook, stirring occasionally, until the vegetables are tender, about 8 minutes.

Add the broth, beets, and grated lemon peel. Bring the soup to a boil, then reduce the heat to a simmer. Cover partly and cook until the vegetables are very tender and the soup is flavorful, about 20 minutes. Turn off the heat, add the lemon juice, and adjust salt, if needed.

Stir in the dill, ladle into individual soup bowls, season with black pepper to taste, and garnish with a dollop of your favorite Whipped Herbal Butter.

Keeps well in the refrigerator for up to 5 days or the freezer for up to 3 months.

PALEO

AIP *Omit the black pepper.*

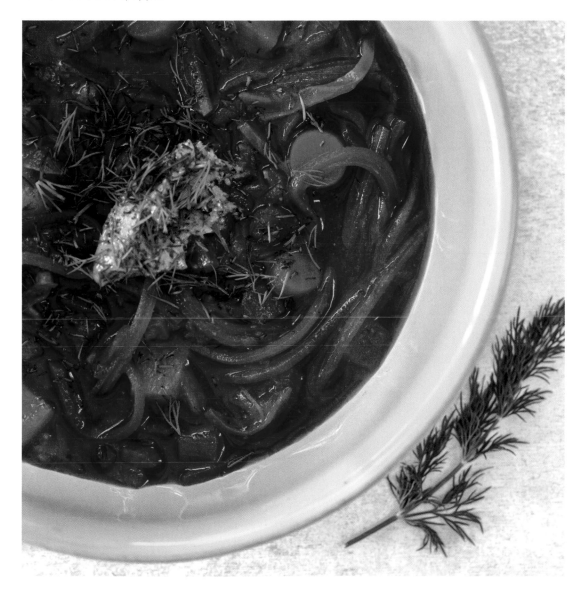

Easy Chicken Curry Stew

Gut healing, sugar balancing, warming

8 bone-in chicken thighs with skin

½ yellow onion, diced

1 13.66-ounce can full-fat coconut milk

1 medium unpeeled parsnip, cut into ½-inch cubes

1 green apple, cut into ½-inch cubes

⅓ cup dried unsweetened cranberries

1½ tablespoons Garam Masala (page 177)

1½ tablespoons freshly grated ginger

1 tablespoon turmeric powder

1 teaspoon sea salt

½ teaspoon freshly ground black pepper

Fresh cilantro, finely chopped, for garnish

PALEO

AIP *Replace the garam masala with ground cinnamon. Omit the black pepper.*

ANTI-CANDIDA *Omit the cranberries.*

LOW FODMAP *Replace the onion with a pinch of asafetida. Omit the apple and replace the cranberries with dried blueberries.*

Sometimes the best recipes are created when the original dinner plan fails. I had a few friends coming over for dinner, the shops were closed early that day, and I had very little food left in the house, apart from some frozen chicken, a can of coconut milk, and of course many spices. Feel free to experiment by adding different vegetables or spices such as ground cinnamon, coriander, or fennel seeds.

SERVES 4

PREP TIME 15 minutes

COOKING TIME, OVEN METHOD 60 minutes

COOKING TIME, SLOW COOKER METHOD 4 to 6 hours

EQUIPMENT 6-quart Dutch oven or large baking dish with lid, or slow cooker

Position a baking rack in the middle of the oven and preheat the oven to 400°F.

Mix all of the ingredients except for the cilantro in the Dutch oven until well combined.

Cook covered for 45 minutes. Remove the lid carefully to avoid being burned by the steam and cook uncovered for another 15 minutes.

Serve on individual plates and sprinkle with cilantro.

Keeps well in the refrigerator for up to 5 days or in the freezer for up to 3 months.

Slow Cooker Version

Mix all of the ingredients except for the cilantro in the slow cooker, cover, and cook on low for 4 to 6 hours or until cooked through.

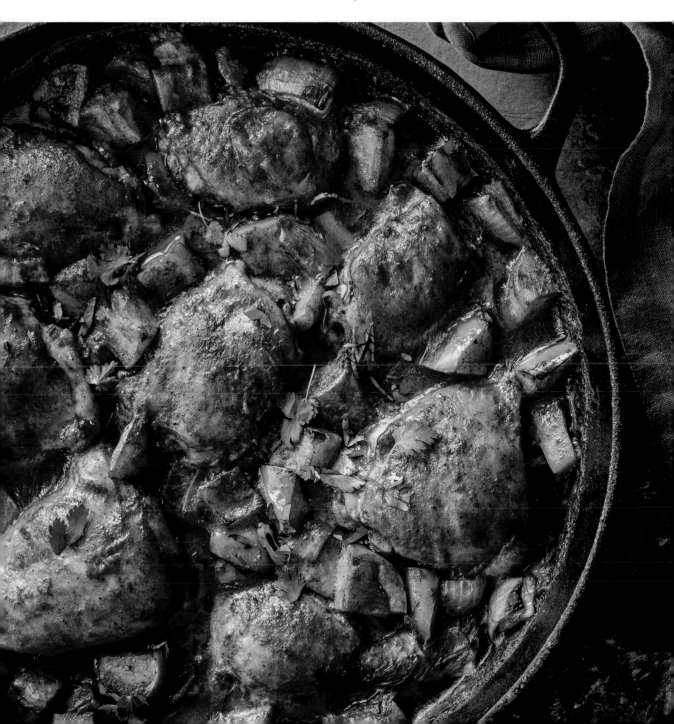

Icelandic Fish Stew

Sugar balancing, liver detoxing, rich in flavonoids

Iceland, this remote, peaceful country, might not have fought many wars, but those that they did fight in the twentieth century, the Cod Wars, were all because of fish! If you ever plan to visit, be prepared to taste some of the best fish and seafood dishes ever. An excellent cook running a middle-of-nowhere inn at the Icelandic East Fjords shared a dairy-based version of this stew with me after our long, rainy, and cold mountain hike. My dairy-free version is just as warming and highly satisfying.

2 tablespoons lard or ghee

½ yellow onion, diced

1 leek, halved, cleaned, and cut into ¼-inch rings

3 celery stalks, cut into ¼-inch pieces

3 medium unpeeled carrots, finely chopped

1 celeriac, cut into ½-inch cubes

4 cups Immune-Boosting Chicken Broth (page 158) or Healing Bone Broth (page 162)

3 cups filtered water

2 tablespoons dried marjoram

1½ tablespoons apple cider vinegar

1½ teaspoons sea salt

1 16.33-ounce can full-fat coconut milk

1 pound halibut or cod, cut into ½-inch cubes

Chives, minced (optional)

SERVES 6 to 8

PREP TIME 10 minutes

COOKING TIME 35 minutes

EQUIPMENT 6-quart Dutch oven or heavy-bottomed pot with lid

In the Dutch oven over medium-high heat, melt the lard.

Add the onion and leek and cook for 5 minutes, or until the onion is translucent.

Add the celery, carrots, and celeriac and cook, stirring once in a while, until softened and brown, about 10 minutes.

Pour in the broth and water. Scrape the bottom of the pot to loosen all the brown bits. Add the marjoram, cider vinegar, and salt; cover and bring to a boil. Reduce to a simmer for 30 minutes or until the vegetables are soft.

Stir in the coconut milk until fully integrated into the soup. Add the fish, cover, and cook for another 3 minutes or until the fish is tender. Adjust salt, if needed.

Ladle into individual bowls and sprinkle with chives.

Keeps well in the refrigerator for up to 3 days or in the freezer for up to 3 months.

PALEO

AIP

ANTI-CANDIDA *Omit the carrots.*

LOW FODMAP *Omit the onion and celery and use only the green parts of the leek. Reduce the liquids (either broth or water) to 5 cups.*

Seriously Mushroom Soup

Gut healing, nutrient dense, immune boosting ⏱ Less than 30 minutes

If you love mushrooms, this intensely earthy and grounding soup will take you to mushroom heaven. Mushrooms have been used medicinally in various cultures for their immune-stimulating properties and high content of B vitamins.

6 bacon slices, cut widthwise into ½-inch pieces

1 large leek, white and light green parts only, thinly sliced

1 celery stalk, finely chopped

1 medium unpeeled carrot, finely chopped

1 pound fresh cremini mushrooms, coarsely chopped

½ pound fresh shiitake mushrooms, coarsely chopped

2 cloves garlic, minced

1 teaspoon dried tarragon

1 teaspoon dried thyme

1 teaspoon sea salt

6 cups Healing Bone Broth (page 162) or Immune-Boosting Chicken Broth (page 158)

2 tablespoons coconut aminos

½ pound fresh oyster mushrooms, coarsely chopped

1 tablespoon freshly squeezed lemon juice, or more to taste

A handful of microgreens, for garnish

PALEO
AIP

SERVES 6 to 8

PREP TIME 30 minutes

COOKING TIME 30 minutes

EQUIPMENT 6-quart Dutch oven or heavy-bottomed pot

In the Dutch oven over medium-high heat, cook the bacon until brown and crisp, about 7 minutes. Remove the bacon bits and set aside. Leave the bacon fat in the pot.

Add the leek, celery, and carrot and cook uncovered until softened, about 10 minutes.

Add the cremini and shiitake mushrooms; cook uncovered until reduced in size by half, about 5 minutes.

Add garlic, tarragon, thyme, and salt and cook until fragrant, about 1 minute.

Add broth and coconut aminos. Scrape the bottom of the pot to loosen any bits of vegetable, and then bring the soup to a boil on high heat. Reduce to medium-high heat, add oyster mushrooms, and cook for 3 more minutes.

Turn off the heat and stir in the lemon juice.

Ladle into serving bowls and garnish with the bacon bits and microgreens.

Keeps well in the refrigerator for up to 5 days and in the freezer for up to 3 months.

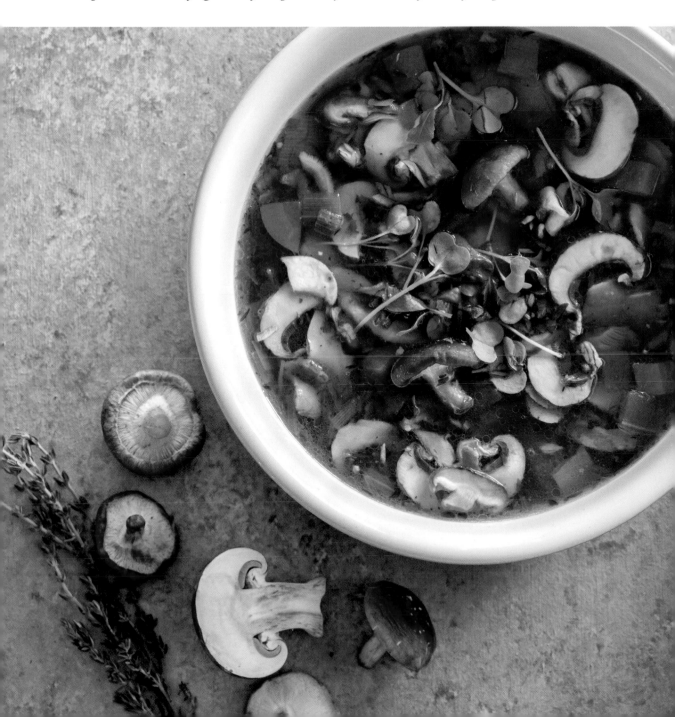

Quick Detoxifying Soup

Liver detoxing, estrogen balancing, rich in iodine 🕐 Less than 30 minutes

I originally created this recipe for my detox program, and many women told me that it became their staple soup for when they have little time to cook and feel like enjoying a healthy meal. The cruciferous vegetables, broccoli and cauliflower, have potent anti-estrogenic properties. Dulse is rich in iodine, an essential mineral for brain and breast health in women. Avoid it, however, if you have Hashimoto's disease.

SERVES 4 to 6

PREP TIME 10 minutes

COOKING TIME 18 minutes

EQUIPMENT Immersion blender or high-speed electric blender

4 cups Healing Bone Broth (page 162), Mineral Vegetable Broth (page 160), or water

4 cups coarsely chopped broccoli

4 cups coarsely chopped cauliflower

1½ teaspoons sea salt

½ teaspoon dried thyme

2 tablespoons apple cider vinegar

1 teaspoon dried turmeric powder

1 tablespoon dulse flakes, for garnish

Handful of flat-leaf parsley, chopped, for garnish

Olive oil, for garnish

In a medium saucepan, bring the broth to a boil. Add the broccoli, cauliflower, salt, thyme, and cider vinegar. Cook covered over medium heat for 7 minutes or until the vegetables are softened but not overcooked. Set aside and cool uncovered for 10 minutes.

Add the turmeric powder and blend the soup with the immersion blender until silky smooth. Adjust taste with salt and cider vinegar, if needed.

Ladle into bowls, sprinkle with dulse and parsley, and drizzle with olive oil. Serve warm.

Keeps well in the refrigerator for up to 1 week and in the freezer for up to 6 months.

PALEO

AIP

ANTI-CANDIDA

LOW FODMAP Replace cauliflower by doubling the broccoli.

Cauliflower and Sweet Potato Soup

Liver detoxing, estrogen balancing, energizing

Sweet potato, the darling of athletes as a source of sustained energy, can be added to your diet in so many ways, including in a soup. Naturally high in sugar, sweet potatoes pair well with the liver-detoxing cauliflower. A perfect duo.

In a Dutch oven over medium-high heat, melt the ghee. Add the onion and cook for 5 minutes, or until translucent.

Add the garlic and cook for another 2 minutes.

Add the sweet potato, cauliflower, broth, cider vinegar, coconut aminos, and salt.

Cover and bring to a boil. Reduce the heat and simmer for 20 minutes or until the vegetables are soft.

Turn off the heat and let the soup cool uncovered for a few minutes. Transfer to a blender in two batches. Add half of the basil leaves to each batch and puree until silky smooth.

Ladle into bowls and top with broccoli sprouts, pumpkin seeds, ground flaxseed, or olive oil.

Keeps well in the refrigerator for up to 5 days or in the freezer for up to 3 months.

PALEO

AIP *Omit the pumpkin seeds and ground flaxseed.*

SERVES 4 to 6

PREP TIME 30 minutes

COOKING TIME 20 minutes

EQUIPMENT 6-quart Dutch oven or heavy-bottomed pot with lid, high-speed electric blender

1 tablespoon ghee

1 small yellow onion, diced

2 cloves garlic, minced

1 medium sweet potato, cut into ½-inch cubes

1 head cauliflower, coarsely chopped

1½ quarts Healing Bone Broth (page 162) or Mineral Vegetable Broth (page 160)

1 tablespoon apple cider vinegar

1 tablespoon coconut aminos

1½ teaspoons sea salt

⅔ cup lightly packed fresh basil leaves

Topping options: Broccoli sprouts, pumpkin seeds, ground flaxseed, and olive oil

Quick Miso Soup

Gut healing, rich in probiotics, rich in iodine ⏱ Less than 30 minutes

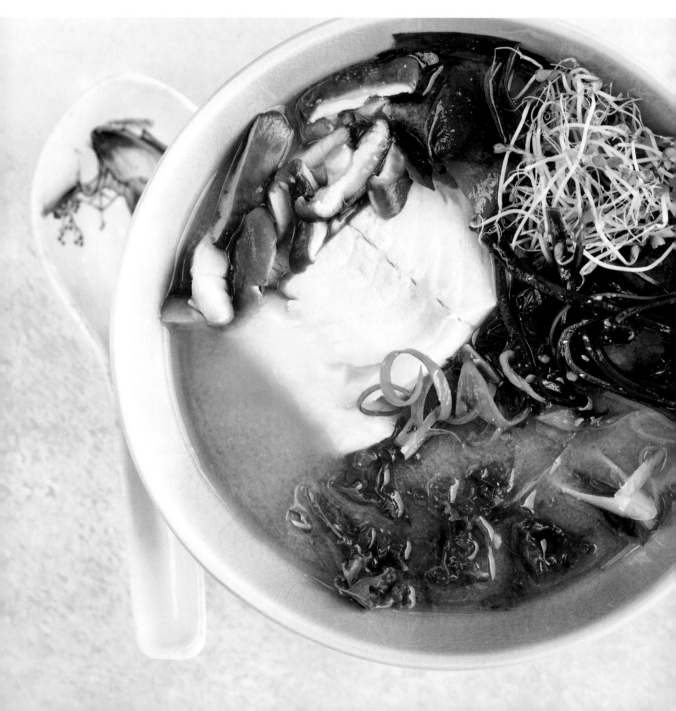

This is the perfect soup for cold winter nights when you crave a home-cooked meal but don't have much time. I ate this warming, strengthening soup a lot when I lived in Shanghai. A nutritional powerhouse full of omega 3 fatty acids, probiotics, iodine, and estrogen-detoxifiers, this miso soup will revitalize you. To retain the probiotic potency of miso, never add it to a boiling broth. Follow my instructions to experience all of miso's benefits.

Even though this recipe contains soy, I decided to make an exception and include it here because fermented soy, such as miso, tends to be well tolerated by most people. If you are doing the Elimination Diet or can't eat soy, use soy-free miso made of chickpeas or adzuki beans. If you suffer from a thyroid condition or Hashimoto's disease, omit this recipe.

In a medium bowl, soak the wakame and arame in the hot water. Set aside.

Place 3 cups of the broth and the mushrooms and kelp in a medium saucepan. Cover, bring to a boil, and simmer for 10 minutes.

In a small bowl, whisk the remaining broth with the miso paste until fully dissolved. Set aside.

Add the cod to the saucepan, turn off the heat, and cover for 3 minutes.

Gently fold the greens into the saucepan and cover again for another 3 to 5 minutes or until the greens have withered.

Gently stir the miso paste into the saucepan.

Remove the kelp sheet before serving. Ladle into bowls and top with the drained wakame and arame and sprouts, scallions, and sesame oil.

Serve and eat right away.

ANTI-CANDIDA *Omit the mushrooms.*

LOW FODMAP *Use soy-based miso if tolerated. If not, skip this dish. Omit the shiitake mushrooms. Use the green part of the scallion only.*

SERVES 2

PREP TIME 7 minutes

COOKING TIME 18 minutes

EQUIPMENT Whisk

2 tablespoons dried wakame

2 tablespoons dried arame

1 cup hot water

1 quart Healing Bone Broth (page 162) or Mineral Vegetable Broth (page 160), divided

1½ cups sliced shiitake mushrooms

1 kelp sheet

3 tablespoons sweet white miso paste

9- to 12-ounce black codfish fillet, cut into 1-inch pieces

2 cups firmly packed leafy greens such as kale, spinach, or collards

½ cup fresh broccoli sprouts, for garnish

2 tablespoons finely chopped scallions, for garnish

2 teaspoons roasted sesame oil, for garnish

Squash, Apple, and Turmeric Soup

Gut healing, anti-inflammatory, alkalizing

There are many butternut squash soup recipes, but often they call for roasting the vegetables, which prolongs the cooking time and increases the effort. This recipe doesn't require that step, and I have found that guests always ask for seconds of this delightful soup, despite its simplicity. I like to cool the soup before transferring it to my high-speed electric blender so that the heat from the soup does not help release toxins from the plastic container. If you have a blender with a glass container, use it!

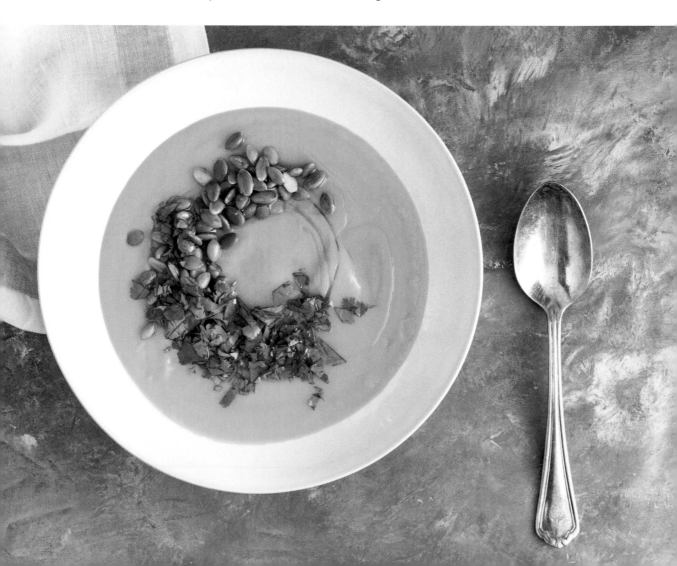

In a large saucepan over medium-high heat, melt the ghee. Add the onion and garlic and cook for 8 to 10 minutes or until brown.

Add the broth, butternut squash, apples, grated lemon peel, ginger, and salt. Cover and bring to a boil. Reduce the heat to medium low and simmer for 40 minutes or until the squash is soft.

Remove from the heat and stir in the coconut butter and lemon juice and cool for 10 minutes. Add the turmeric and pepper. Puree in batches until smooth and creamy.

Pour into individual serving bowls, drizzle with olive oil, and sprinkle with pumpkin seeds and cilantro.

Stores well in the refrigerator for up to 5 days and in the freezer for up to 3 months.

PALEO

AIP *Omit the black pepper and pumpkin seeds.*

ANTI-CANDIDA *Limit to one serving per day.*

SERVES 6

PREP TIME 15 minutes

COOKING TIME 60 minutes

EQUIPMENT High-speed electric blender

2 tablespoons ghee

1 yellow onion, diced

2 cloves garlic, minced

1 quart Immune-Boosting Chicken Broth (page 158) or Mineral Vegetable Broth (page 160)

2 to 2½ pounds peeled butternut squash, cut into 1-inch cubes (about 10 cups)

2 unpeeled Granny Smith apples, cored and cut into ½-inch cubes

Freshly grated peel of ½ lemon

1½ tablespoons grated fresh ginger root

1⅓ teaspoons sea salt

½ cup coconut butter

2 tablespoons freshly squeezed lemon juice

1½ teaspoons turmeric powder

¼ teaspoon freshly ground black pepper

Olive oil, for garnish

Roasted pumpkin seeds, for garnish

Fresh cilantro, finely chopped, for garnish

Porcini Mushroom Beef Stew

Gut healing, rich in selenium, rich in vitamin Bs

My favorite way to serve this woodsy, grounding stew is over the Creamy Celeriac and Cauliflower Mash (page 267). You might be surprised to see anchovies in this stew; they are the secret ingredient that gives it the extra umami, or depth of flavor.

SERVES 6

PREP TIME 40 minutes

COOKING TIME 2 hours

EQUIPMENT 6-quart Dutch oven or heavy-bottomed pot with lid

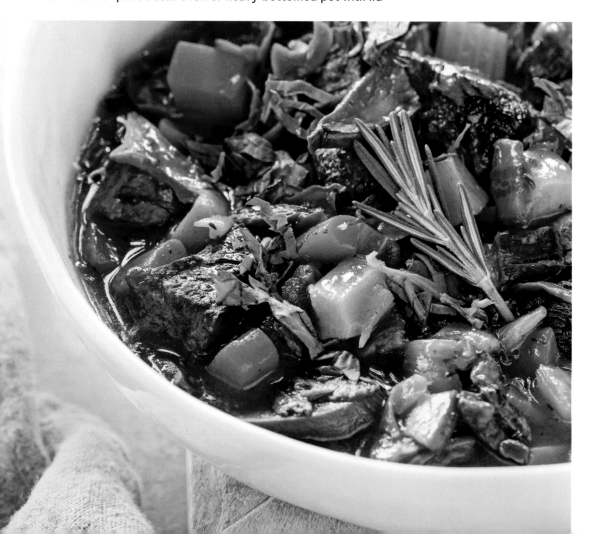

Pat the beef cubes with a paper towel and leave them to dry for 10 to 20 minutes.

In a medium glass bowl, cover the porcini mushrooms with hot water and set aside.

In the Dutch oven over medium-high heat, fry the bacon until brown, about 8 minutes. Remove the bacon bits but leave the fat.

Salt and pepper the beef, then brown on all sides in the bacon fat. Keep the pieces at least ½-inch apart. When brown, remove the beef cubes and set aside. You might repeat the process in three batches, each taking about 10 minutes.

Over medium-high heat, melt the lard in the Dutch oven and add the onion, carrots, and celery. Cook uncovered until soft, about 8 minutes.

Strain the porcini mushrooms, retaining the liquid, and then chop them up.

To the Dutch oven add the beef cubes, bacon, mushrooms, bone broth, parsnip, anchovies, cider vinegar, thyme, bay leaf, rosemary, and salt. Bring the stew to a boil; then reduce the heat and simmer covered for 1 hour and 50 minutes.

Increase the heat to medium and cook uncovered for 10 minutes. Taste and add a pinch of salt or pepper, if needed.

In a small bowl, combine the arrowroot flour and water to form a slurry. Turn the heat off under the stew and slowly stir in the arrowroot slurry to thicken the stew.

Serve warm and garnish with parsley.

Keeps well in the refrigerator for up to 5 days or in the freezer for up to 3 months.

2 pounds beef stew cubes

3 cups broken to pieces dried porcini mushrooms

2 cups hot filtered water

8 bacon slices

1 teaspoon fine sea salt

½ teaspoon freshly ground black pepper

2 tablespoons lard, duck fat, or ghee

1 large yellow onion, chopped

2 medium carrots, cut into ½-inch pieces

2 celery sticks, sliced into ¼-inch pieces

2 cups Healing Bone Broth (page 162)

1 small parsnip, diced

1½ tablespoons minced anchovies

1½ tablespoons apple cider vinegar

½ tablespoon dried thyme

1 bay leaf

1 teaspoon dried rosemary

½ teaspoon sea salt

2 teaspoons arrowroot flour

2 tablespoons cold filtered water

Parsley, finely chopped, for garnish

PALEO

AIP Omit the black pepper.

Honey Glazed Tarragon Chicken

High in vitamin B3, high in good fats

When you need a no-fuss delicious dinner, this is your go-to recipe. The tartness of the mustard and the sweetness of the honey are a match made in heaven. You can replace the chicken thighs with drumsticks or breasts.

SERVES 4

PREP TIME 10 minutes

COOKING TIME 30 minutes

EQUIPMENT whisk, 13 × 9-inch baking pan

8 bone-in, skin-on chicken thighs

1½ tablespoons Dijon mustard

1½ tablespoons raw honey

1½ tablespoons melted ghee or brown butter

1½ teaspoons dried tarragon

¾ teaspoon salt

¼ teaspoon freshly ground black pepper

Preheat the oven to 400°F.

Place the chicken in the baking pan, skin up.

In a small bowl, whisk mustard, honey, ghee, tarragon, salt, and pepper. Coat the chicken with the mixture.

Bake uncovered for 30 minutes or until the juices run clear and the skins are brown.

Let rest for 10 minutes before serving.

Keeps well in the refrigerator for up to 1 week.

PALEO

AIP *Replace Dijon mustard with 1 tablespoon freshly squeezed lemon juice. Omit black pepper.*

ANTI-CANDIDA *Omit the honey or replace it with four drops of liquid stevia.*

LOW FODMAP

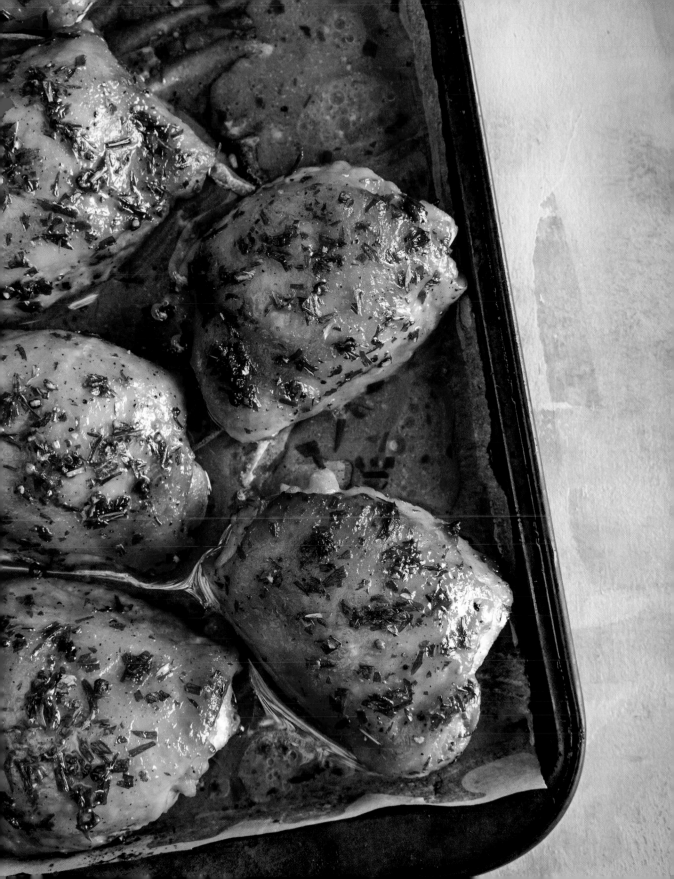

Grain-Free Pizza—Two Ways

Immune boosting, rich in fiber

I was determined to find a pizza recipe that does not depend on grains, nuts, yeast, eggs, or tomatoes and still tastes good. After exactly two full days and sixteen attempts, I found it. Made with medicinal Herbal Pesto (page 288), both toppings are loaded with liver-supporting herbs. The Medicinal Mushroom Topping has a wonderfully earthy taste and helps to boost the immune system.

I cut parchment paper into a 10-inch circle to guide me on how much to spread the crust dough. To save time, buy cashew meal or grind the nuts or seeds in larger quantities and freeze them for future use.

MAKES One 10-inch pizza

PREP TIME 15 minutes

COOKING TIME 25 minutes

EQUIPMENT Parchment paper, high-speed electric blender or food processor

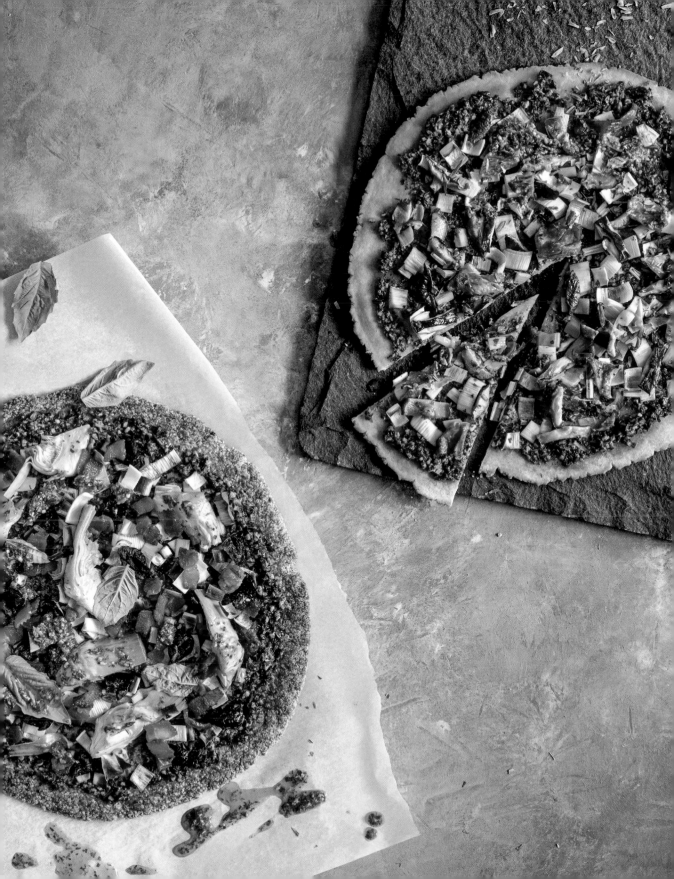

Crust option 1: Sunflower Seed (or Cashew)

1 cup raw sunflower seeds or raw cashew nuts

½ cup filtered room temperature water

2 tablespoons whole psyllium husk

1½ tablespoons extra virgin olive oil

¼ teaspoon sea salt

PALEO
ANTI-CANDIDA

Preheat the oven to 400°F.

Pulse the sunflower seeds in the blender until the consistency of flour.

In a large bowl, combine the pulsed sunflower seeds with the water, psyllium husk, olive oil, and salt and knead with your hands. The dough will be runny.

Line a baking tray with the parchment paper, place the dough on the parchment paper, and spread it using your fingertips to form a round 10-inch crust. If the dough sticks to your fingers, dip them in water and continue.

Bake for 10 minutes. Remove from the oven and finish with the topping of your choice.

Crust option 2: Cassava Flour

½ cup cassava flour

⅓ cup filtered lukewarm water

2 tablespoons extra virgin olive oil

¼ teaspoon baking powder

Dash of sea salt

PALEO
AIP

Preheat the oven to 400°F.

In a medium bowl, combine all of the ingredients and knead to develop a dough.

Line a baking tray with the parchment paper, place the dough on the parchment paper, and spread it using your fingertips to form a round 9- to 10-inch crust.

Bake for 10 minutes. Remove from the oven and finish with the topping of your choice.

Topping option 1: Medicinal Mushroom Topping

In a circular motion, spread the pesto onto the crust.

In a medium bowl, add all of the remaining ingredients and toss to combine.

Spread the mushroom mixture evenly over the crust. Bake 15 to 20 minutes.

Serve right away.

2 tablespoons Herbal Pesto (page 288)

¾ cup sliced shiitake mushrooms

¾ cup sliced maitake or oyster mushrooms

½ cup thinly sliced leek, white part only

1½ teaspoons dried tarragon

2 tablespoons coconut aminos

1 tablespoon extra virgin olive oil

2 teaspoons rice vinegar or apple cider vinegar

PALEO
AIP

Topping option 2: Bacon and Artichoke Topping

In a circular motion, spread the pesto onto the crust.

Scatter the bacon pieces, olives, leek, and artichoke over the crust, and bake for 20 minutes.

Garnish with basil leaves and serve right away.

2 tablespoons Herbal Pesto (page 288)

2 bacon slices, cut to ½-inch pieces

10 pitted Kalamata olives, coarsely chopped

½ cup thinly sliced leek, white part only

4 marinated artichoke hearts, quartered

10 fresh basil leaves, for garnish

PALEO

AIP Replace baking powder with an AIP baking powder (page 143).

ANTI-CANDIDA

Nutritious Quick Bowls—Two Ways

Liver detoxing, estrogen balancing, nutrient dense ⏱ Less than 30 minutes

You know when you are tired and making dinner feels like too much of a chore? Ordering takeout is an easy option, but it never sits well with you. Quick Bowls are my answer. I created these because I needed quick, nutritious dinners that take very little effort to pull together. The idea is simple: Precook a larger batch of the base (see below) ahead of time, add some protein and vegetable toppings, and sprinkle with a dressing of your choice. Many of the ingredients will keep well in the refrigerator for days. Reheat the base on the stove, if needed.

BASE OPTIONS

Grains: Cooked rice, buckwheat, millet, quinoa, or amaranth

Nongrains: Roasted spaghetti squash, zucchini noodles, kelp noodles

TOPPING OPTIONS

Proteins: Leftover dinner meats like fish, lamb, or beef. Smoked fish, smoked oysters, canned sardines, or eggs (if tolerated)

Fermented vegetables: Sauerkraut, dill pickle, cultured beets or kimchi (if nightshades are tolerated)

Grated vegetables: Carrot, radish, butternut squash, zucchini, or beets

Fresh vegetables: Arugula, heart of romaine, or broccoli sprouts

Crunch: Roasted nuts or seeds such as almonds, pumpkin seeds, or sesame seeds

DRESSING OPTIONS

Any of the Salad Dressings—Five Ways (page 285)

Extra virgin olive oil

Freshly squeezed lemon juice

SERVES 1

PREP TIME 10 to 15 minutes

COOKING TIME 0 to 4 minutes

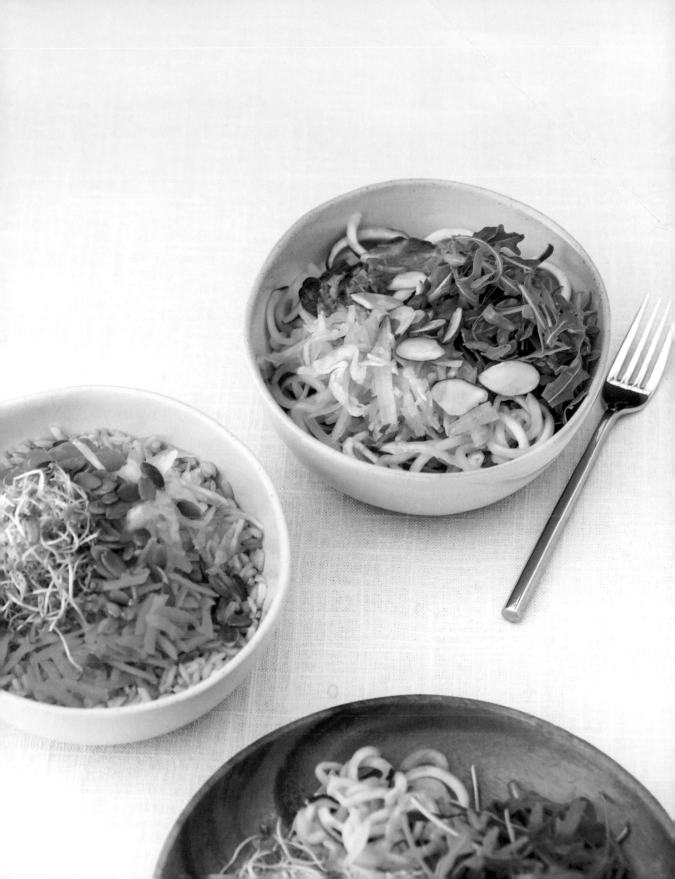

Salmon Rice Bowl

BASE

¾ to 1 cup cooked quinoa, brown rice, or spaghetti squash, reheated

TOPPING

1 piece smoked salmon

½ cup grated unpeeled carrots

½ cup lacto-ferments like Kohlrabi Kraut (page 275), Cultured Vegetable Medley—Four Ways (page 277), or store-bought lacto-fermented sauerkraut

½ cup firmly packed broccoli sprouts

DRESSING AND CRUNCH

2 tablespoons homemade dressing or extra virgin olive oil

Roasted pumpkin seeds, for garnish

Place the quinoa in a serving bowl. Top with salmon, carrots, kraut, and sprouts.

Drizzle with a dressing of your choice and sprinkle with pumpkin seeds. Serve right away.

ANTI-CANDIDA
LOW FODMAP

Paleo Lamb Bowl

Place the zucchini noodles in a serving bowl. Top with lamb chop, kraut, and arugula.

Drizzle with a dressing of your choice. Serve right away.

PALEO *Avoid grains.*

AIP *Avoid grains, nuts, seeds, and seed-based spices.*

ANTI-CANDIDA *Avoid grains and fermented foods during the first 4 weeks of the diet. Replace root vegetables such as carrots with cucumbers, zucchinis, or fennel bulb.*

LOW FODMAP *Limit grains to ½ to 1 cup per serving; use only approved vegetables found on page 88. Eat no more than 1 tablespoon fermented vegetables per day.*

BASE

1½ to 2 cups store-bought or homemade zucchini noodles, sautéed for 3 minutes in a splash of olive oil and a dash of sea salt.

TOPPING

1 cooked lamb shoulder chop, reheated

½ cup lacto-ferments like Kohlrabi Kraut (page 275), Cultured Vegetable Medley—Four Ways (page 277), or store-bought sauerkraut

Handful of baby arugula

DRESSING

2 tablespoons homemade dressing or extra virgin olive oil

Lamb with Collard Greens and Radishes

Liver detoxing, estrogen balancing, rich in iodine ⏱ Less than 30 minutes

Fennel, cumin, and lamb remind me of the many Moroccan classics that can be simple yet so tasty. Fish sauce adds umami flavor and depth. Be careful not to overcook collard greens, which makes them taste bitter and lose their nutritional potency. I often make this dish for breakfast.

SERVES 4

PREP TIME 5 minutes

COOKING TIME 13 minutes

EQUIPMENT Large heavy-bottomed skillet with lid

1 tablespoon ghee or lard

1 yellow onion, diced

1 pound ground lamb

1 tablespoon ground fennel seeds

1 tablespoon ground cumin seeds

2½ tablespoons fish sauce or 1 teaspoon sea salt

2 bunches of collard greens, about 20 small leaves, stemmed and cut into ½-inch strips

15 radishes, sliced thinly

⅔ cup dried dulse

1 tablespoon freshly squeezed lemon juice

Life-Giving Sprouts (page 163), for garnish

In a large skillet over medium-high heat, melt the ghee. Add the onion and cook until translucent, about 5 minutes.

Stir in the lamb, fennel, cumin, and fish sauce and cook uncovered on medium high until the meat is thoroughly cooked, about 7 minutes.

Stir in the collard greens, radishes, dulse, and lemon juice. Cook covered until collard greens turn bright green, about 3 minutes.

To serve, garnish with broccoli sprouts.

Keeps well in the refrigerator for up to 5 days.

PALEO

AIP *Replace the fennel and cumin with AIP-compliant herbs such as 1 tablespoon oregano or sage.*

ANTI-CANDIDA

LOW FODMAP *Omit the onions or replace with the green part of two leeks.*

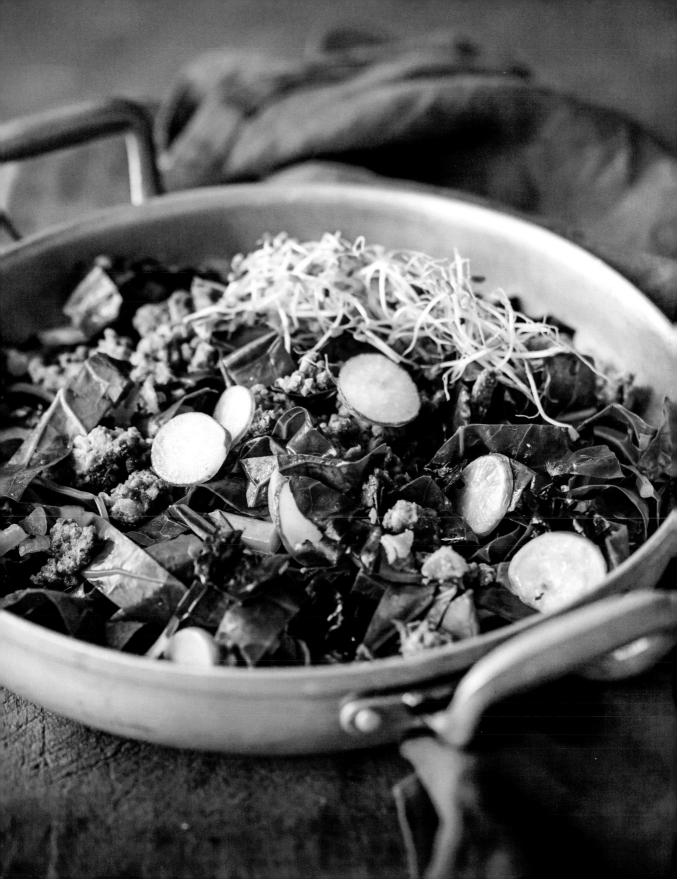

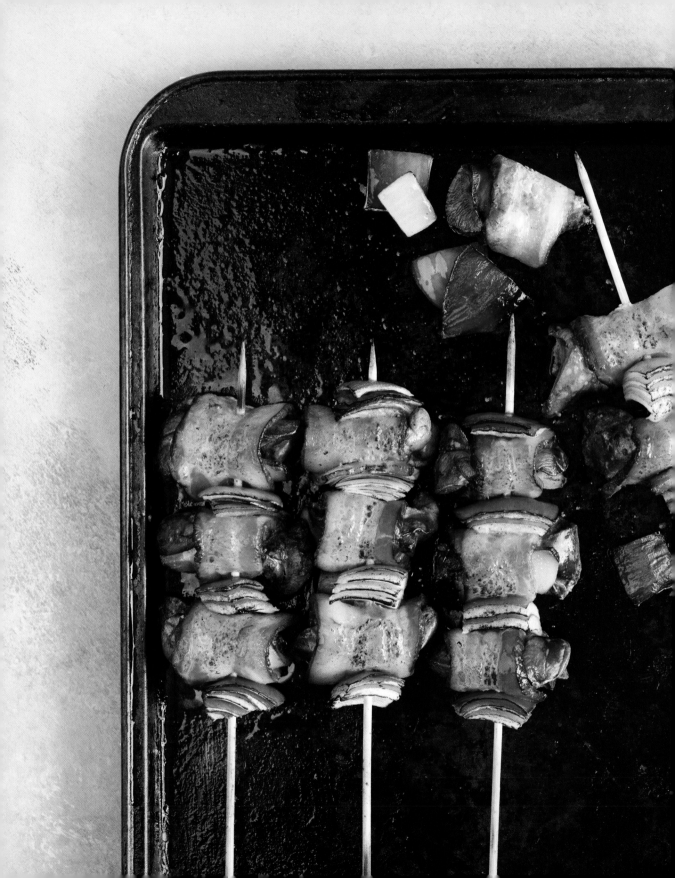

Nomad's Kebabs (Liver and Bacon)

Rich in iron, selenium, vitamins A and B12 ⏱ Less than 30 minutes

When we arrived at the Saharan nomads' camp, they had just slaughtered a sheep. With no refrigeration, the liver was the first part we needed to eat. We sat around the campfire, dicing the sheep's liver, wrapping the bits in fat, and grilling it with much anticipation. We didn't speak the same language, but we were connected through the food. The nutrient-dense liver in this simple dish will help you to get your vitality back. For maximum iron absorption, serve these kebabs with foods high in vitamin C, such as steamed broccoli or sauerkraut, drizzled with your favorite homemade dressing (page 285).

Preheat the oven on the broil setting. If using wooden skewers, soak them in water for 15 minutes.

Wash the livers and pat them dry with a paper towel. Cut them in half and remove the membranes.

In a medium bowl, toss the liver pieces with cumin powder, coriander powder, and salt.

Wrap each piece of liver with one slice of bacon. Thread each piece onto the skewers, alternating pieces of liver with pieces of onion.

Rest the ends of the skewers on the sides of the baking pan, so the fat drips into the pan.

Broil 3 to 4 inches from the heat for 6 to 8 minutes, or until the bacon is cooked and crisp on one side. Turn and cook for another 6 to 8 minutes.

Serve and eat immediately.

MAKES 16 kebabs

SERVES 4

PREP TIME 13 minutes

COOKING TIME 16 minutes

EQUIPMENT Four wooden or metal skewers, 11 × 7-inch baking pan

8 chicken livers

1 teaspoon cumin powder

1 teaspoon coriander powder

½ teaspoon sea salt

16 bacon slices

½ red onion, quartered, layers separated

PALEO

AIP *Replace cumin and coriander with any AIP-compliant spices of your choice, such as sage, rosemary, or thyme.*

ANTI-CANDIDA

LOW FODMAP *Replace the onion with the green parts of a leek or omit.*

Butter Cod with Gremolata

Liver detoxing, estrogen balancing, rich in vitamins C and K ⏲ Less than 30 minutes

Fresh from the water and prepared simply with butter and salt, the fish I've eaten on camping trips stands out as the most delicious. Be sure to get the freshest fish and cook it right away. Parsley is loaded with vitamins K and C, garlic contains antimicrobial and liver-supporting sulfur, and the grated lemon peel adds liver-cleansing d-limonene. My favorite gremolata variation is made with parsley, cilantro, and orange peel.

SERVES 4

PREP TIME 15 minutes

COOKING TIME 6 minutes

EQUIPMENT 21-inch skillet

2 tablespoons brown butter or ghee, divided

4 cod fillets, with or without skin

½ teaspoon sea salt

¼ teaspoon freshly ground black pepper

GREMOLATA

½ cup loosely packed fresh parsley, finely chopped

1 small clove garlic, finely chopped

Peel of 1 lemon, finely grated or thinly sliced

In a large skillet over medium-high heat, melt 1 tablespoon of the butter.

Season the cod fillets with salt and pepper.

Fry the fish skin down for 4 minutes on one side and 2 minutes on the other, or until the flesh easily flakes away when tested with a fork. Place on serving plates.

Melt the remaining butter and drizzle it over the cod fillets.

To make the gremolata, combine the parsley, garlic, and grated lemon peel on a cutting board and chop together finely.

Sprinkle the cod fillets with gremolata, drizzle with leftover butter from the pan, and serve immediately.

PALEO

AIP Omit the black pepper.

ANTI-CANDIDA

LOW FODMAP Omit the garlic.

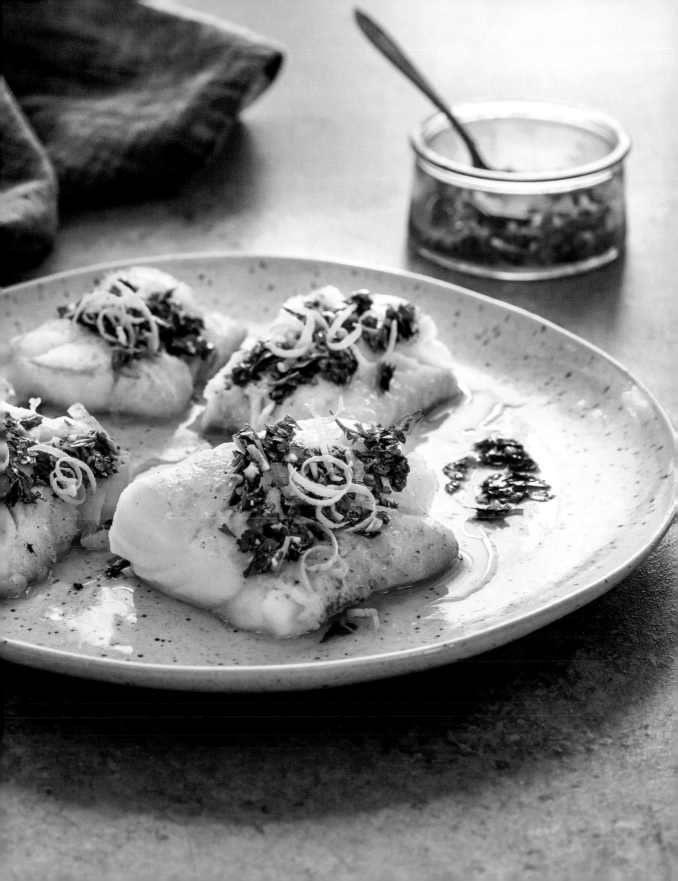

Sticky Spare Ribs Casserole

Liver detoxing, rich in vitamin K, rich in potassium and iron

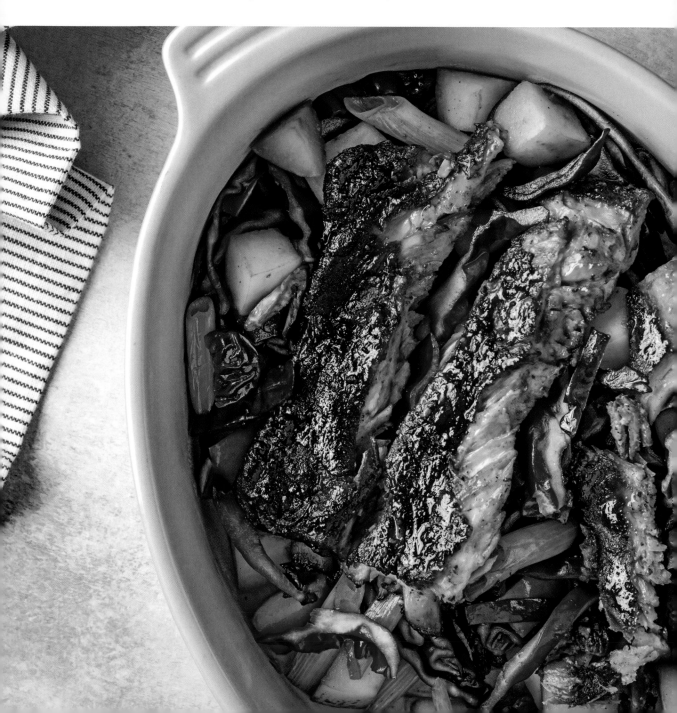

This is a warm, comforting dish for a cold winter night. I love one-pot meals because they take the fuss out of cooking and reduce the wash-up time. Packed with healing foods such as red cabbage, apples, and green onions, this is one medicinal dish for the whole family.

Preheat the oven to 400°F.

In a medium bowl, make the marinade by whisking together the mustard, molasses, Five-Spice Mix, and salt.

Pat the ribs dry, remove the membrane, and cut the rack in half. Place the ribs in a baking pan and rub with the marinade on both sides.

In the Dutch oven, toss the cabbage, apples, green onions, cherries, cider vinegar, ghee, and salt.

Place the ribs on top of the vegetables, meaty side up, cover, and cook for 1 hour.

Carefully remove the lid so the steam does not burn you, and switch the oven to broil; broil the ribs for another 10 minutes or until they are brown.

Remove from the oven and let the ribs rest for 10 minutes before serving.

Keeps well in the refrigerator for up to 5 days or in the freezer for up to 3 months.

PALEO

AIP *Replace mustard with apple cider vinegar. Replace Five-Spice Mix with ground cinnamon and ground cloves.*

LOW FODMAP *Replace apples and cherries with kumquats or grapes. Omit green onions. Molasses has not been tested for FODMAPs, so if you want to be safe, replace it with maple syrup.*

SERVES 4

PREP TIME 30 minutes

COOKING TIME
1 hour 20 minutes

EQUIPMENT 6-quart Dutch oven or a large casserole with lid

2 tablespoons Dijon mustard

2 tablespoons blackstrap molasses

1½ tablespoons Five-Spice Mix (page 174)

1 teaspoon smoked salt or sea salt

2½ to 3 pounds pork spare ribs rack

1 small head of red cabbage (about 2 pounds), shredded

2 unpeeled Fuji apples, cut into ½-inch cubes

6 to 8 green onions, diced

¼ cup dried unsweetened cherries (optional)

¼ cup apple cider vinegar

¼ cup ghee or lard, melted

½ tablespoon sea salt

Walnut Crusted Salmon

Progesterone boosting, rich in omega 3, rich in magnesium

This quick and easy recipe makes an ideal weeknight dinner. This dish is high in vitamin B6 (from the salmon and walnuts), and I recommend eating it during the luteal phase of the menstrual cycle to help build up progesterone levels. High levels of selenium, magnesium, and vitamin B12 make this dish a nutritional powerhouse. High levels of alpha-linolenic acid (ALA) found in walnuts have been shown to have anticarcinogenic and anti-inflammatory properties.

SERVES 2

PREP TIME 20 minutes

COOKING TIME 15 minutes

EQUIPMENT Spice grinder or small food processor

2 4-inch-long daikon radishes, thinly sliced

Extra virgin olive oil

Dash of smoked salt

2 wild salmon fillets, 6 to 8 ounces each

¾ cup raw walnuts or pecans

2 tablespoons pomegranate molasses

1 teaspoon ground anise seed or ground star anise

¾ teaspoon sea salt

Cilantro, chopped, for garnish

PALEO

LOW FODMAP Replace pomegranate molasses with honey and a dash of lemon juice.

Place oven rack in the middle position and preheat oven to 350°F.

In a baking dish, toss the radishes with a drizzle of olive oil and smoked salt.

Place the salmon on top of the radishes, skin down.

Pulse the walnuts in a grinder until finely ground.

In a medium bowl, whisk molasses, anise seed, and salt to create a smooth glaze. Stir in the ground walnuts to form a thick paste.

Spoon the paste over the salmon, distributing it evenly.

Bake uncovered for 15 minutes or until the salmon easily flakes away when tested with a fork.

Place on serving plates and sprinkle with cilantro. Serve right away.

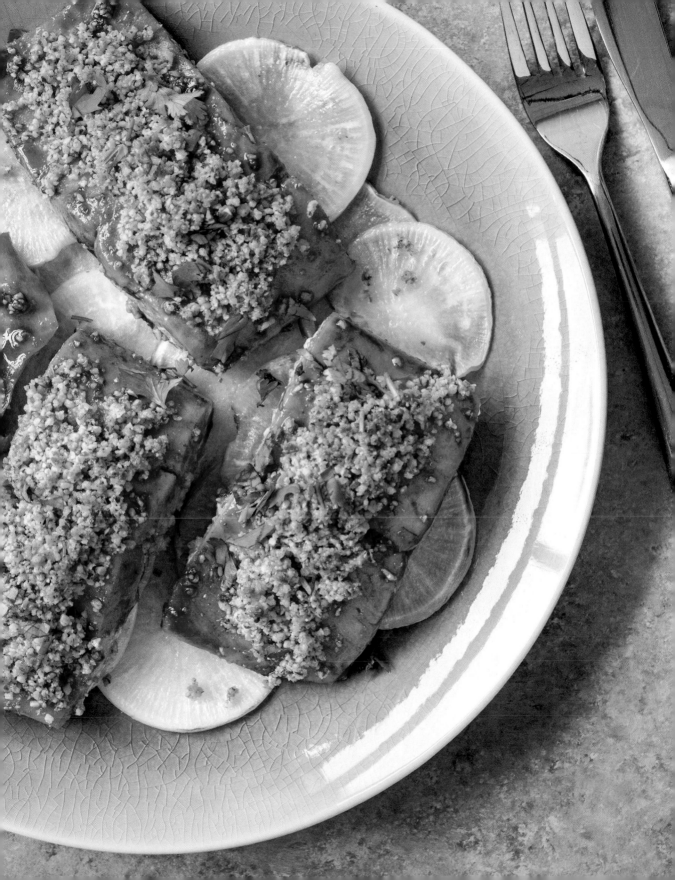

Fennel and Coriander Crusted Liver

Liver detoxing, nutrient dense, rich in vitamin B12 and selenium

When I lived in New York City, I used to buy veal or lamb livers at the Union Square Farmers' Market. One day, the farmer told me he had run out of livers, even though it was still early in the day. The same thing happened the following week. He explained that so many people had been eating liver medicinally and seeing such significant health improvements that his livers were beginning to sell out immediately.

As annoying as this was, I was thankful that more people were appreciating the healing powers of liver. It can really taste good if you know how to cook it. Using spices such as fennel, coriander, and cumin reduces the gaminess of this otherwise creamy and rich meat. If you are worried about livers not being clean, see Chapter 8 for more information on this superfood.

SERVES 4

PREP TIME 20 minutes

COOKING TIME 15 minutes

EQUIPMENT Spice grinder or mortar and pestle, 10-inch skillet (or larger)

1 tablespoon fennel seeds

2 teaspoons coriander seeds

1 teaspoon cumin seeds

1 teaspoon smoked sea salt

1 pound beef, veal, lamb, or pork liver

2 tablespoons ghee, divided

PALEO
ANTI-CANDIDA
LOW FODMAP

Grind the fennel, coriander, cumin, and sea salt. Spread the blend on a large, flat plate.

Rinse the liver, remove all of the membranes, and pat it dry with a paper towel. Transfer it to the plate with the spice blend and gently press down. Turn the liver over and repeat on the other side. Slice the liver into ½-thick pieces.

In a large skillet over medium-high heat, heat 1 tablespoon of the ghee. Place as many slices of liver as will fit into the skillet without overcrowding. Reduce the heat to medium and fry the liver for 4 minutes on one side. Turn the pieces over and fry for another 2 minutes. Do not overcook. Pink juices should flow out when you cut into a piece of the liver.

Repeat using the remaining ghee until all slices are cooked.

Remove the liver from the skillet and let it rest for 10 minutes before serving.

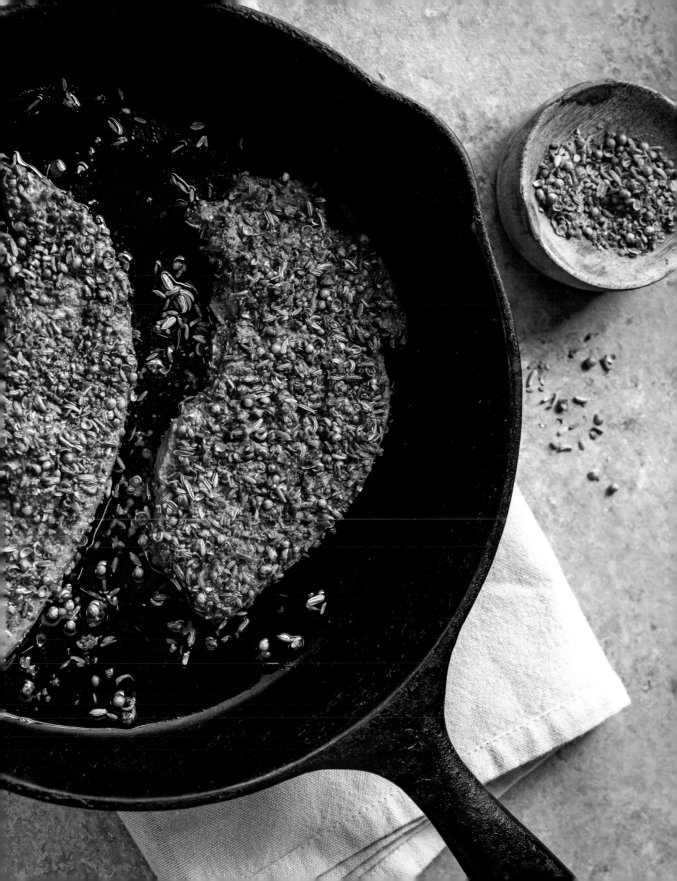

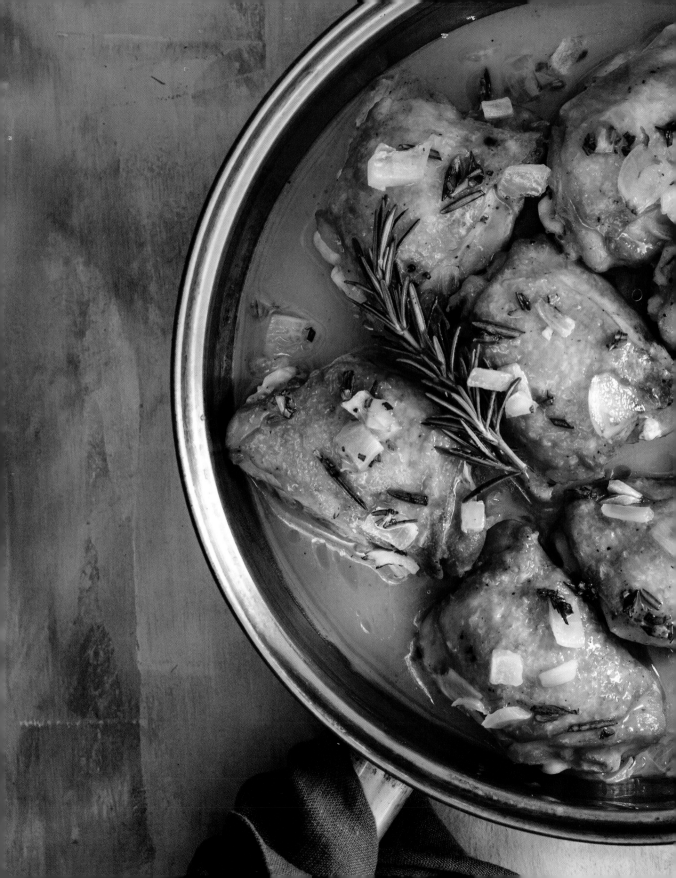

Creamy Rosemary Chicken

Rich in vitamin B6, high in good fats and protein

You do not need eggs and dairy cream to make a rich, decadent dish. With a few tweaks I transformed this classic French recipe for rabbit into a dairy-free dream that is sure to satisfy and impress. If you want to eat something closer to the French classic, replace the chicken in this recipe with rabbit.

In a skillet over medium-high heat, heat 1 tablespoon ghee. Fry the chicken, skin down, for 3 minutes. Turn over and fry for another 3 minutes. Remove from the skillet and set aside.

Add the remaining ghee to the skillet, raise the heat to high, and fry the onion for 3 minutes.

Transfer the chicken back to the skillet and add the stock, wine, mustard, rosemary, salt, and pepper.

Cover and simmer for 40 minutes or until the chicken is nearly falling off the bone.

Remove the chicken and place in a serving dish. Cover to keep warm.

Over high heat, boil the liquid remaining in the skillet until reduced by half, about 10 minutes.

Remove from the heat and whisk in the coconut cream until fully dissolved.

In a small bowl, whisk the arrowroot flour and water. Slowly whisk the arrowroot slurry into the sauce to thicken it.

SERVES 4

PREP TIME 20 minutes

COOKING TIME 1 hour

EQUIPMENT 11-inch skillet with lid, whisk

2 tablespoons ghee, divided

8 bone-in, skin-on chicken thighs

1 onion, diced

1 cup Immune-Boosting Chicken Broth (page 158) or water

1 cup dry white wine such as Sauvignon Blanc

2 teaspoons Dijon mustard

1 tablespoon chopped fresh rosemary or ½ tablespoon dried rosemary

1 teaspoon sea salt

½ teaspoon freshly ground black pepper

2 tablespoons coconut cream from full-fat coconut milk

1 teaspoon arrowroot flour

2 teaspoons water

Drizzle the sauce over the chicken and serve.

Keeps well in the refrigerator for up to 5 days or in the freezer for up to 3 months.

PALEO

AIP *Replace the mustard with freshly squeezed lemon juice. Replace the wine with chicken stock. Omit the black pepper.*

ANTI-CANDIDA *Replace the wine with chicken stock.*

LOW FODMAP *Replace the onions with the green parts of a leek, or omit.*

Rosemary and Garlic Stuffed Lamb Roast

Antibacterial, rich in protein, high in good fats

I created this recipe in a pinch when the dish I planned to serve my dinner guests failed. Simple and quick to prepare, this leg of lamb will fill your house with the mouthwatering smells of rosemary and garlic.

Preheat the oven to 400°F.

Place the garlic, rosemary, salt, and olive oil in the mortar and pound with the pestle until a paste is formed.

Make deep cuts to the meat in several places and stuff them with ¾ of the paste. Rub the remaining paste on the outside of the shank.

Place the meat in the roasting pan. Glaze the legs with 1 teaspoon ghee.

Roast for 30 minutes. Remove from the oven and glaze with the remaining 1 teaspoon ghee. Roast for another 10 minutes or until the internal temperature reaches 135°F.

Keeps well in the refrigerator for up to 5 days or in the freezer for up to 6 months.

SERVES 4

PREP TIME 15 minutes

COOKING TIME 40 minutes

EQUIPMENT Roasting pan, mortar and pestle or spice grinder, meat thermometer

2 large cloves garlic, crushed

2 tablespoons minced fresh rosemary

1 tablespoon smoked sea salt

2 teaspoons extra virgin olive oil

1 to 1½ pounds lamb shanks

2 teaspoons melted ghee or brown butter, divided

PALEO

AIP

ANTI-CANDIDA

LOW FODMAP *Omit the garlic or use garlic-infused oil to replace the olive oil and ghee.*

Detoxing Beet and Carrot Salad

Liver detoxing, estrogen balancing, progesterone boosting ⏱ Less than 30 minutes

This recipe is the result of an Aha! moment I had when I overheard a friend, Dr. Jolene Brighten, a naturopath who also helps women rebalance their hormones, say that she detoxes her PMS patients with carrots and beets five days before the start of their periods. Which makes complete sense. Beets support the liver's methylation pathway by helping detox excess estrogen, dopamine, histamine, and heavy metals. Carrots help produce more progesterone and bind the antagonistic estrogen metabolites. This salad is high in natural sugars, so be sure to eat it with a piece of protein like chicken, fish, or lamb.

SALAD

2 cups shredded peeled beets

2 cups shredded unpeeled carrots

1 cup chopped raw walnuts

¼ cup chopped scallions

¼ cup chopped fresh flat-leaf parsley

DRESSING

½ cup extra virgin olive oil

Freshly grated peel of 1 orange

¼ cup freshly squeezed orange juice

2 tablespoons apple cider vinegar

1 teaspoon ground cumin

1 teaspoon salt

SERVES 4 to 6

PREP TIME 25 minutes

EQUIPMENT Grater, jar with lid

To make the salad, combine all of the salad ingredients in a large bowl.

To make the dressing, place all the dressing ingredients in a jar. Seal the lid and shake until well combined.

Pour the dressing over the salad and toss until well coated.

Serve at room temperature or chilled.

Keeps well in the refrigerator for up to 4 days.

PALEO

AIP *Omit the walnuts and replace the cumin with an AIP-compliant spice of your choice.*

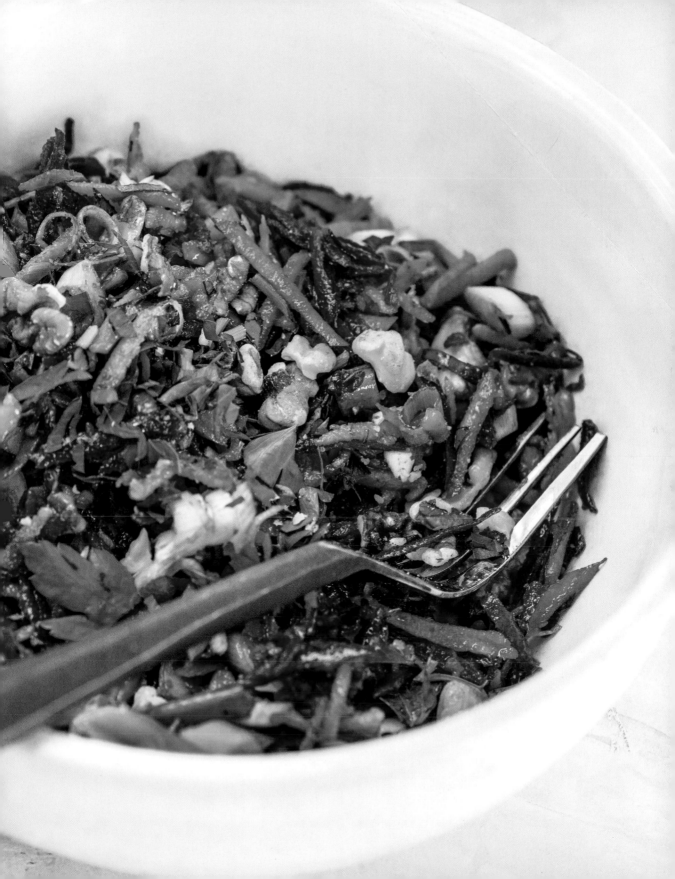

Quick Salads—Four Ways

Liver detoxing, estrogen balancing, anticarcinogenic ⏱ Less than 30 minutes

Salads are a quick and easy way to get fresh vegetables and nutrients into your diet. Pay attention to how your body feels after having a salad—do you feel nourished and light? or cold and unsatisfied, with an achy tummy? As much as salads have been pronounced a healthy food, they might not be for everyone. I, for one, can't eat salads in winter but cherish them on warmer days. Many people with digestive issues find cooked vegetables to be a better choice, so tune in to your body to be the judge.

Time-saving tip: Have salad dressings ready ahead of time.

SERVES 2 to 4

PREP TIME 15 minutes

Classic Italian

3 cups firmly packed mixed greens

2 roasted chicken thighs, skin-on, deboned and sliced (optional)

1 ripe avocado, pitted, peeled, and cut into chunks

½ cup pitted black olives, coarsely chopped

1 small zucchini, thinly sliced

½ fennel bulb, thinly sliced

¼ cup Classic Balsamic Dressing (page 285)

Creamy Radishes and Pear

3 cups variety of thinly sliced radishes; I like red, white, and daikon radishes

1 cup firmly packed chopped frisée

1 ripe unpeeled Bartlett pear, cut into ½-inch cubes

2 roasted chicken thighs, skin-on, deboned and sliced

¼ cup Thick and Cheesy Dressing (page 286)

2 tablespoons roasted pumpkin seeds (optional)

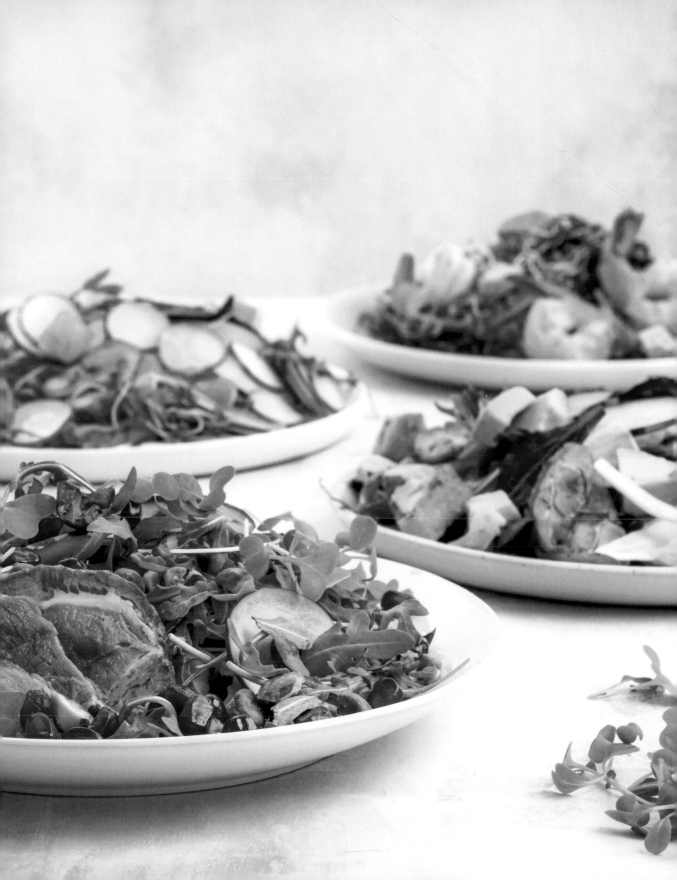

The Persian

3 cups lightly packed arugula

4 ¼-inch slices of roasted lamb

Seeds from one small pomegranate

1 medium zucchini, thinly sliced

10 Kalamata olives, coarsely chopped

⅓ cup walnuts or pistachio nuts, coarsely chopped

3 tablespoons Persian Delight Dressing (page 287)

Sea Vegetable Salad

2 tablespoons arame or wakame, soaked for 5 minutes in 1 cup room temperature water, then strained

¼ cup firmly packed dulse, cut with scissors into small pieces and dipped in water

2 cups firmly packed baby mizuna leaves

½ cup loosely packed broccoli sprouts

1 medium unpeeled carrot, grated

2-inch daikon radish, cut into matchsticks

1 ripe avocado, peeled, pitted, and cut into chunks

10 precooked shrimps or oysters

⅓ cup Japanese Miso Dressing (page 287)

Combine all of the ingredients in a large bowl, toss, and serve immediately.

PALEO

*To make the salads **AIP**, **LOW-FODMAP**, and **ANTI-CANDIDA** compliant, please modify them using the allowed foods shown in the respective guides in Chapter 5.*

Do-It-Your-Way
Salad Guide

DRESSING
For flavor: Pick from page 285

CRUNCH
For fun: Nuts, seeds, bacon bits, sprouts

FATS
For comfort: Avocado, nuts

PROTEINS
For sustenance: Chicken, lamb, beef, fish, seafood, eggs

SHREDDED VEGGIES AND FERMENTS
For health: Carrots, beets, radishes, sauerkraut

BASE
Leafy greens such as arugula, spinach, lettuce, etc.

Parsnip and Apple Coleslaw

Supports breast health, rich in iodine

Living in Iceland, where root vegetables like the parsnip are available all year, inspired me to develop this recipe. If you have Hashimoto's disease, omit the dulse flakes.

SERVES 4 to 6

PREP TIME 20 minutes

CHILLING TIME 1 hour

EQUIPMENT Food processor or grater

2 cups lightly packed shredded peeled parsnip

2 medium unpeeled Royal Gala apples, cored and shredded

1½ cups cooked and peeled shrimp

⅓ cup chopped scallions

¼ cup dulse flakes

¾ cup Classic Mayo (page 168)

In a medium bowl, toss the parsnip, apples, shrimp, scallions, and dulse flakes.

Fold in the mayo and chill for an hour before serving.

Keeps well in the refrigerator for up to 3 days.

PALEO

AIP *Replace the Classic Mayo with Creamy Peruvian Dressing (page 286) or Classic Balsamic Dressing (page 285)*

ANTI-CANDIDA *Do not eat more than ½ cup at a time.*

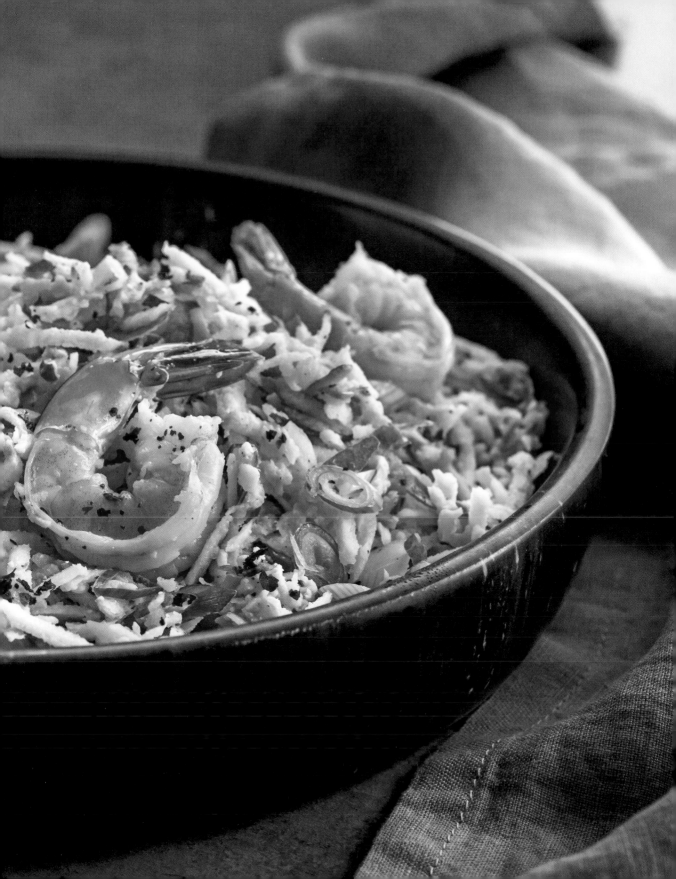

Steam 'n Toss Veggies and Proteins on the Run

Liver detoxing, nutrient dense, alkalizing ⏱ Less than 30 minutes

When you find yourself with little time and craving a healthy meal, give a go to steamed vegetables and protein such as fish or seafood tossed with your favorite dressing. Steamed veggies are a great meal if raw salads do not agree with you (many people with digestive issues don't feel good after eating raw food).

STEAM TIME: 2 TO 5 MINUTES	STEAM TIME: 5 TO 7 MINUTES	STEAM TIME: 8 TO 10 MINUTES
Arugula (2 minutes)	Broccoli (florets)	Asparagus
Beet greens	Brussels sprouts (quartered)	Butternut squash (¼-inch cubes)
Dandelion leaves	Collard greens (destemmed)	Green beans
Green peas	Endive	Carrots (¼-inch slices)
Kale (destemmed)	Kohlrabi (¼-inch cubes)	Cauliflower (florets)
Spinach	Leeks, white parts (¼-inch slices)	Celeriac (¼-inch cubes)
Swiss chard (destemmed)	Zucchini (¼-inch slices)	Daikon and other radishes (¼-inch slices)
		Parsnip (¼-inch slices)
		Sweet potato (¼-inch slices)
	Fresh shrimp, fish chunks (my favorite is black cod)	Fresh scallops, frozen shrimp, frozen fish chunks

Toss with a dressing or dollop of your choice, such as Herbal Pesto (page 288), Salad Dressing—Five Ways (page 285), or Whipped Herbal Butter—Two Ways (page 173). A drizzle of olive oil, a splash of lemon juice, and a dash of sea salt work very well, too.

Zesty and Creamy Collard Greens

Liver detoxing, estrogen balancing, rich in fiber ⏲ Less than 30 minutes

The healing power of this dish resides in the potent liver detoxifiers: collard greens, dandelions, onions, and freshly grated lemon peel.

In the Dutch oven over high heat, melt the ghee, then add the onion and fry until translucent, about 7 minutes.

Reduce the heat to medium high, add the garlic, and cook for 2 minutes.

Add the collard greens, cover, and cook until softened, about 5 minutes.

Add the coconut milk, grated lemon peel, fennel, and salt. Stir in the dandelion leaves, reduce the heat to medium, and cook uncovered for 3 minutes or until the dandelion leaves are softened.

Stir in the lemon juice, sprinkle with walnuts, and serve.

PALEO

AIP *Omit the fennel and walnuts.*

ANTI-CANDIDA

LOW FODMAP *Replace the onion and garlic with a pinch of asafetida. Since dandelion leaves have not been tested for FODMAP, it's best to replace them with the same amount of arugula.*

SERVES 4 to 6

PREP TIME 15 minutes

COOKING TIME 18 minutes

EQUIPMENT 6-quart Dutch oven or heavy-bottomed pot with lid

2 tablespoons ghee or coconut oil

1 small yellow onion, diced

2 cloves garlic, minced

Collard greens, 20 medium leaves, stemmed and cut into ½-inch strips

1 13½-ounce can full-fat coconut milk

Freshly grated peel of 1 lemon (about 1 teaspoon)

1 teaspoon ground fennel seed

1 teaspoon sea salt

4 cups firmly packed ½-inch strips of dandelion leaves

1 tablespoon freshly squeezed lemon juice, plus more if needed

Raw walnuts, chopped, for garnish (optional)

Tuscan Shredded Fennel and Orange Salad

Liver detoxing, estrogen balancing, kidney cleansing ⏱ Less than 30 minutes

I learned a version of this recipe in Tuscany at a traditional foods culinary workshop. The brilliance of this dish lies in marrying the bitter but oh-so-good-for-you dandelion and the sweet orange, making it a highly refreshing and delicious salad.

SERVES 4

PREP TIME 20 minutes

½ teaspoon freshly grated orange peel

⅓ cup freshly squeezed orange juice

⅓ cup extra virgin olive oil

1 teaspoon ground fennel seeds

½ teaspoon sea salt

2 cups firmly packed arugula, coarsely chopped

1 cup firmly packed dandelion leaves, coarsely chopped to ½-inch strips

1 fennel bulb, thinly sliced

1 navel orange, peeled and cut into ½-inch pieces

⅓ cup finely chopped parsley

½ cup coarsely chopped walnuts

Place the orange peel, orange juice, olive oil, fennel seeds, and salt in a jar, close the lid, and shake vigorously until the mixture is well emulsified.

In a large mixing bowl, place the arugula, dandelion, sliced fennel bulb, orange, and parsley.

Add the dressing and toss until the leaves are well coated. Sprinkle with the walnuts.

Serve immediately.

PALEO

AIP Omit the fennel seeds and walnuts.

ANTI-CANDIDA Omit the orange and replace the orange juice with 2 tablespoons lemon juice.

LOW FODMAP Replace the dandelion leaves with an additional cup of arugula.

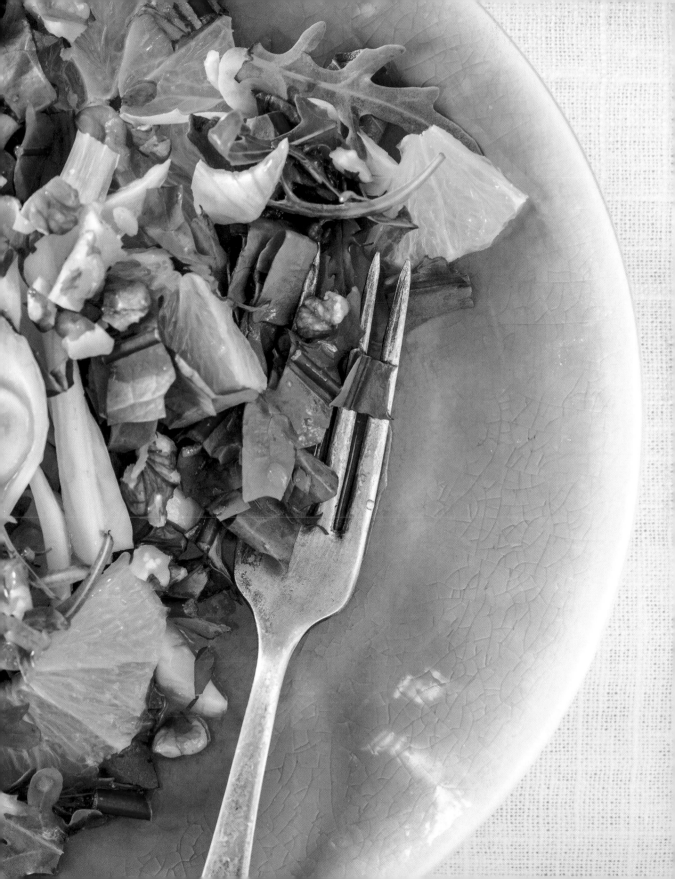

Sauerkraut Carrot Salad

Gut healing, estrogen balancing, immune boosting ⏱ Less than 30 minutes

If sauerkraut is not your best friend yet because of its sour taste, this recipe might help you learn to like it. Adding carrots and fat such as the olive oil will take the edge off this highly healing food. Sauerkraut is very high in probiotics, vitamins C and K, and glucosinolates—an anticarcinogenic agent. As a cruciferous vegetable, it also helps detoxify from harmful estrogens.

SERVES 2

PREP TIME 10 minutes

EQUIPMENT Grater

1½ cups sauerkraut

1 cup grated unpeeled carrots

3 tablespoons Creamy Peruvian Dressing (page 286) or olive oil

½ teaspoon cumin seeds

½ teaspoon caraway seeds

TOPPINGS

1 ripe avocado, peeled, pitted, and sliced

Pick from: Broccoli sprouts, microgreens, young cilantro shoots

½ cup chopped walnuts

Bacon bits (optional)

Place sauerkraut and carrots in a medium bowl. Add the dressing or olive oil, cumin, and caraway seeds and toss until well combined.

Divide the salad and place in individual bowls. Garnish with the avocado and broccoli sprouts, then sprinkle with walnuts and bacon bits.

Keeps well in the refrigerator for up to 5 days without the toppings.

PALEO

AIP *Omit the cumin, caraway seeds, and walnuts. Soak the broccoli sprouts to remove the seeds.*

ANTI-CANDIDA *Eat only after the first 4 weeks of the anti-Candida diet. Replace the carrots with zucchini.*

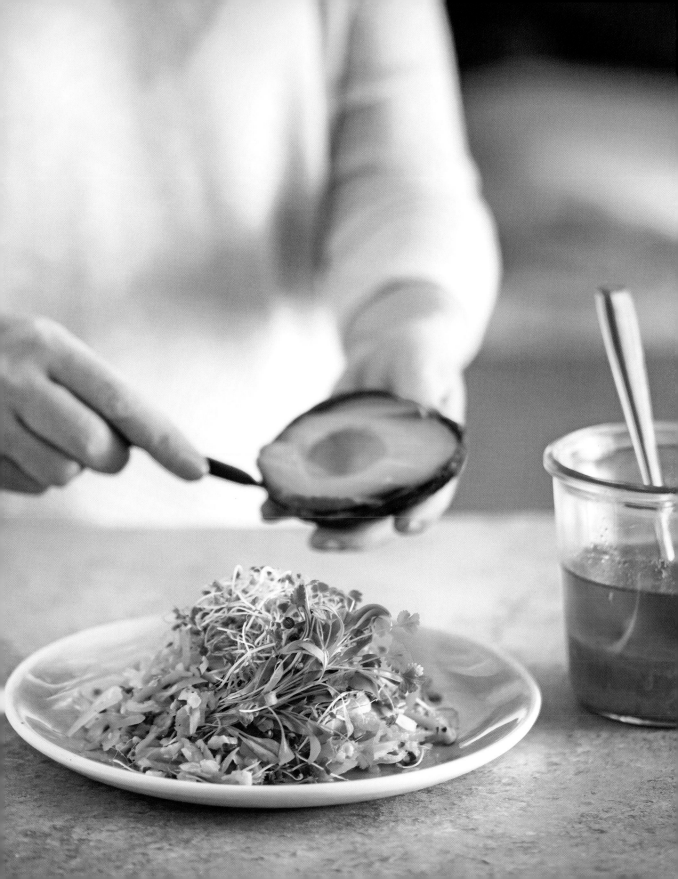

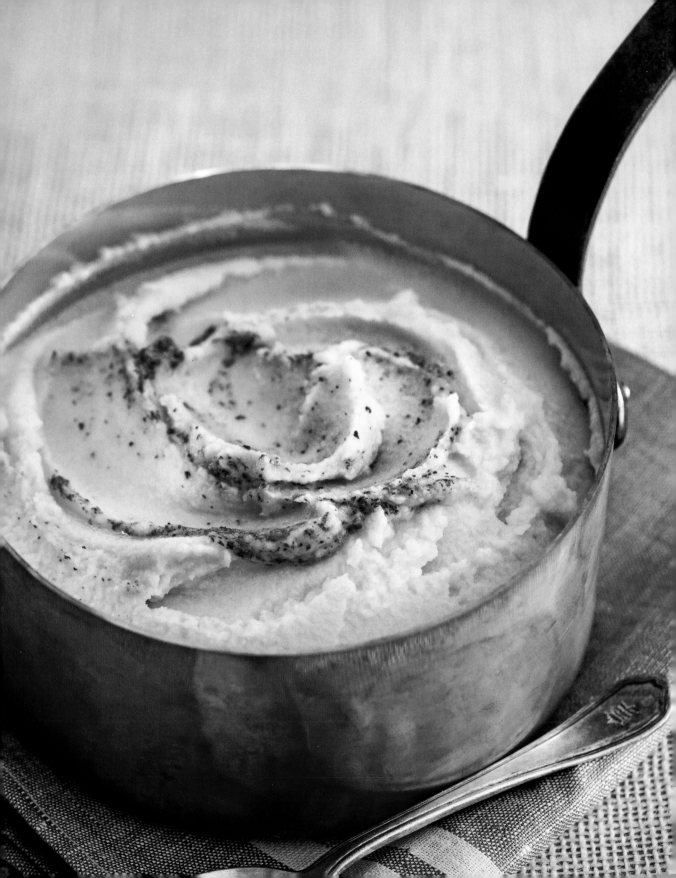

Creamy Celeriac and Cauliflower Mash

Estrogen balancing, immune boosting, comforting 🕐 Less than 30 minutes

If you can't tolerate nightshades, such as potatoes, this dish is a wonderful replacement. In fact, it's richer in flavor than regular potatoes. This silky smooth mash is full of vitamin C and phytoestrogens to rebalance your estrogen levels. It contains about 17 percent protein, and with its starch content, it will sustain you for hours. Celeriac is also known as celery root.

Place the cauliflower, celeriac, and bone broth in the Dutch oven. Cook covered over medium-high heat for 15 minutes or until the vegetables are soft.

Remove from heat and allow to cool for a few minutes. Transfer to the blender. Add the ghee, cider vinegar, and salt. Puree until silky smooth.

Keeps well in the refrigerator for up to 5 days.

PALEO

AIP

ANTI-CANDIDA

LOW FODMAP *Replace cauliflower with two medium-size parsnips.*

SERVES 6

PREP TIME 12 minutes

COOKING TIME 15 minutes

EQUIPMENT Dutch oven or a large pot with lid, high-speed blender or food processor

1 medium head cauliflower, coarsely chopped

1 medium head celeriac, cut into ½-inch cubes

½ cup Healing Bone Broth (page 162) or filtered water

⅓ cup ghee or brown butter

1 tablespoon apple cider vinegar

½ tablespoon truffle salt or smoked sea salt

Jicama and Pomegranate Slaw

Gut healing, estrogen balancing, immune boosting ⏱ Less than 30 minutes

You see jicama in most health stores but probably wonder what to do with it. This crunchy and yummy root gets its sweet flavor from inulin, which is a prebiotic, or food for the probiotics in your gut. This salad couples jicama with the mighty phytoestrogenic pomegranate; I hope it becomes one of your favorites.

SERVES 6 to 8

PREP TIME 10 minutes

CHILL TIME 20 minutes

SALAD

1 2½- to 3-pound jicama, peeled and cut into ⅛-inch sticks

1 medium pomegranate, seeds removed

½ red onion, sliced thinly

1 cup loosely packed fresh cilantro, finely chopped

½ cup loosely packed fresh mint, finely shredded

DRESSING

½ cup extra virgin olive oil

⅓ cup freshly squeezed lime juice

2 tablespoons pomegranate molasses (optional)

½ teaspoon sea salt

Place the jicama, pomegranate seeds, onion, cilantro, and mint in a large salad bowl.

In a small bowl make the dressing by whisking together the olive oil, lime juice, pomegranate molasses, and salt.

Pour the dressing over the salad and toss until the jicama is well coated.

Chill for 20 minutes before serving.

PALEO

AIP Omit the pomegranate seeds.

ANTI-CANDIDA Use half the pomegranate or omit.

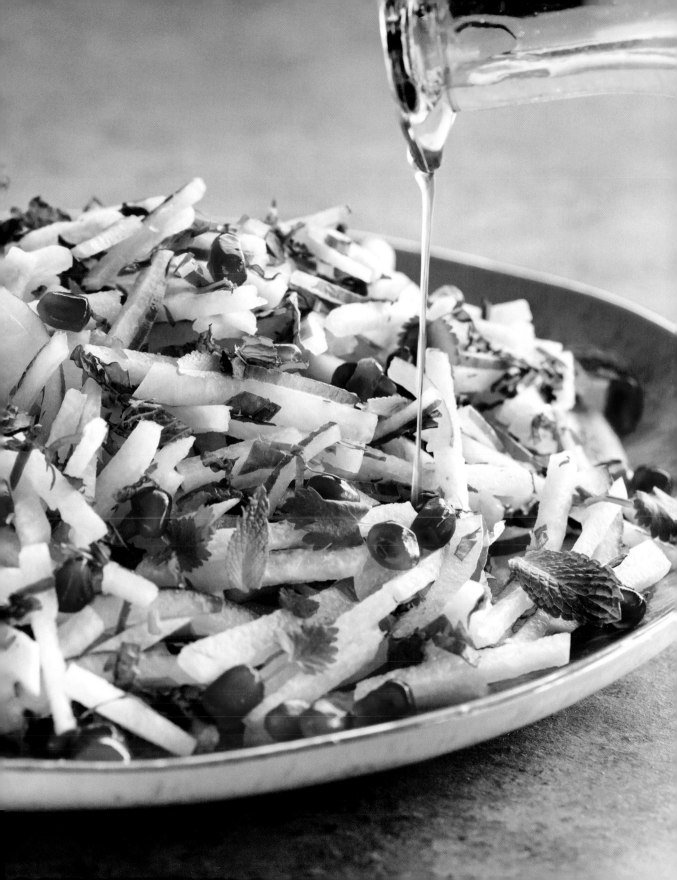

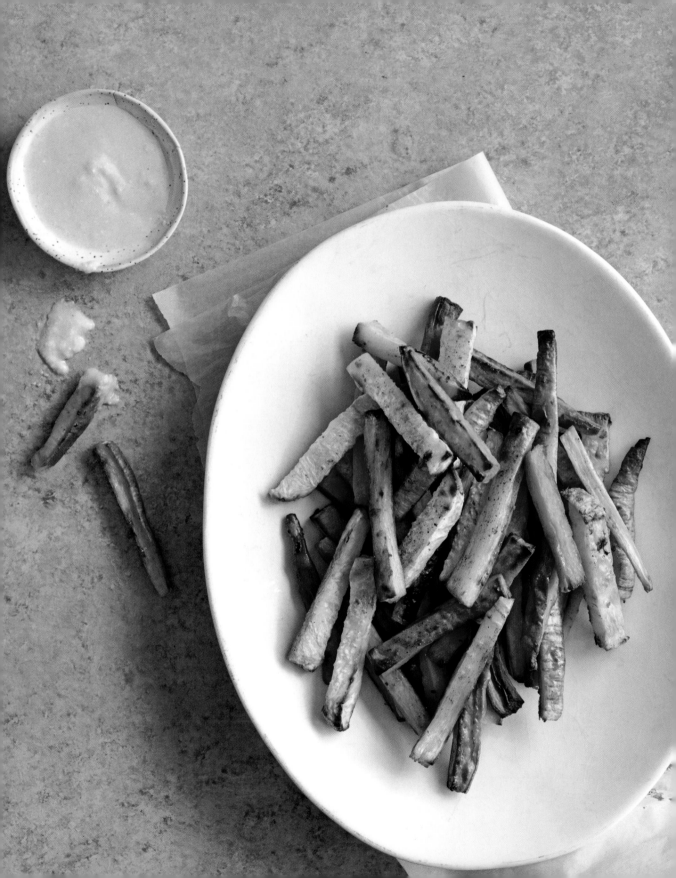

Fries Baked in Duck Fat

Rich in antioxidants, vitamin A, and fiber

Root vegetables are a great source of sustained energy. Cooked in duck fat, these fries will become a favorite of the whole family. The arrowroot flour helps the fries turn crispy.

Place the oven rack in the middle of the oven and preheat the oven to 425°F.

In a large zipper bag, toss the vegetables with the arrowroot flour until well coated. Add salt and Five-Spice Mix and toss again. Add the duck fat and toss until the sticks are well coated.

Line a baking pan with the parchment paper and spread the vegetables so they don't touch each other much.

Bake for 25 minutes or until fries are brown and crispy.

Open the oven door and let the fries cool for 20 minutes.

Place on a serving platter and sprinkle with salt flakes.

Serve with a mayo of your choice on the side.

SERVES 2 to 4

PREP TIME 15 minutes

COOKING TIME 45 minutes

EQUIPMENT Parchment paper, large zipper bag

1 small sweet potato, washed and dried, cut into ⅓- to ½-inch sticks

½ celeriac, peeled, washed and dried, cut into ⅓- to ½-inch sticks

1 medium parsnip, peeled, washed and dried, cut into ⅓- to ½-inch sticks

2 tablespoons arrowroot flour

½ teaspoon smoked sea salt or truffle salt

½ tablespoon Five-Spice Mix (page 174), Ras el Hanout (page 175), or Garam Masala (page 177)

2 tablespoons duck fat, bacon fat, or ghee, melted

Sea salt flakes, for garnish

Creamy Egg-Free Mayo of your choice (page 168)

PALEO

AIP *Replace Garam Masala or Five-Spice Mix with ground cinnamon.*

ANTI-CANDIDA *Limit to 10 fries, no more than twice per week.*

LOW FODMAP *Replace the sweet potato with an additional ½ celeriac or a large parsnip.*

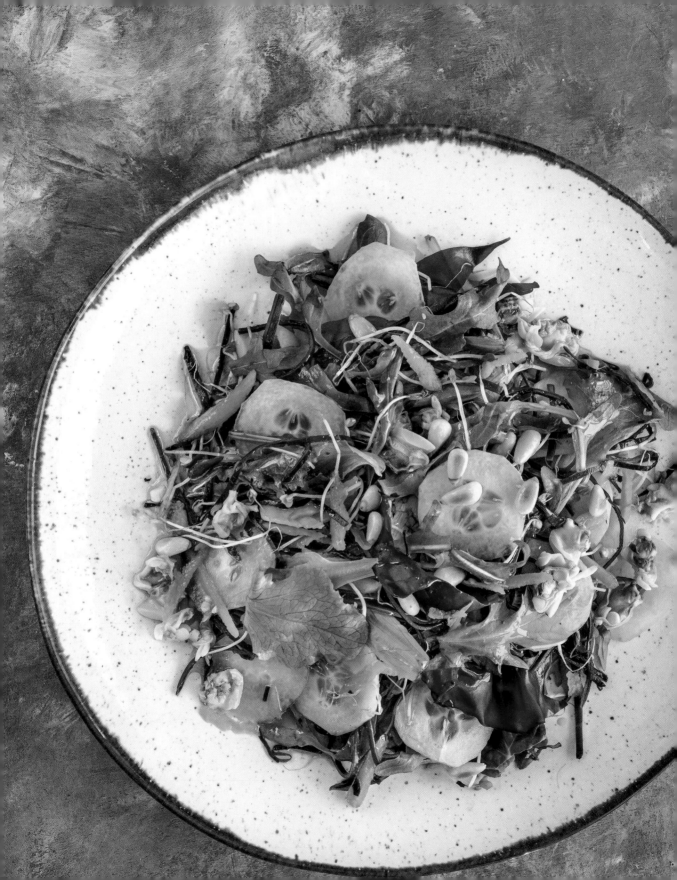

Japanese Seaweed and Cucumber Salad

Estrogen balancing, rich in iodine and magnesium, supports breast health ⏱ Less than 30 minutes

This light, energizing salad can be a quick lunch or addition to a fish or seafood dish. Seaweed is rich in iodine, calcium, iron, and magnesium. One serving contains more vitamin C than an orange. Research also points to the ability of seaweed and broccoli sprouts to regulate estrogen and estradiol, the aggressive form of estrogen, helping to reduce the risk of breast cancer.

SERVES 4

PREP TIME 20 minutes

To soften the arame, place it in a bowl and cover with hot water for 5 minutes. Drain and set aside.

In a large serving bowl, place all of the salad ingredients except the pine nuts.

Place all the dressing ingredients in a jar with a lid, seal the lid, and shake to combine.

Pour the dressing over the salad and toss. Sprinkle with pine nuts.

Serve immediately, as the salad does not keep well.

PALEO

AIP Omit the pine nuts and soak the broccoli sprouts to remove the seeds.

ANTI-CANDIDA Replace the carrots with shredded zucchini, or omit. Replace the rice vinegar with lime juice.

LOW FODMAP

SALAD

½ cup dried arame seaweed

4 cups lightly packed mixed greens

4 cups lightly packed arugula

2 cups peeled and sliced cucumber

1 cup grated unpeeled carrots

1 cup lightly packed broccoli sprouts

1 6½-ounce can chopped clams

4 tablespoons dried dulse seaweed flakes

¼ cup pine nuts, roasted

DRESSING

⅓ cup avocado oil

2½ tablespoons rice vinegar

2 tablespoons roasted sesame oil

1 tablespoon coconut aminos

1 tablespoon fish sauce

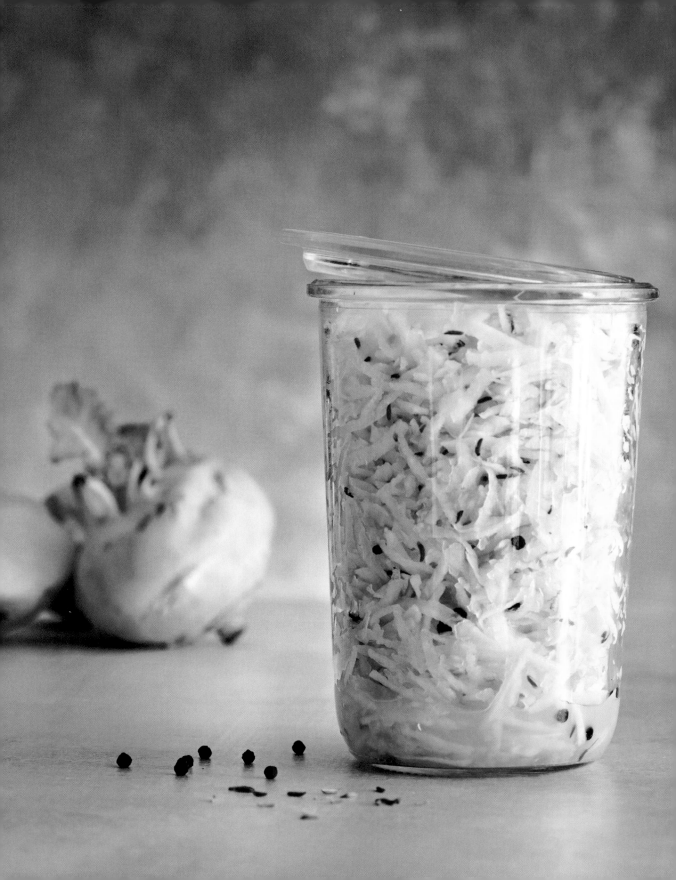

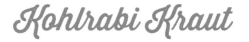

Kohlrabi Kraut

Gut healing, liver detoxing, estrogen balancing

Kohlrabi is a delicious vegetable that is often overlooked. Come fall and spring, keep your eyes open for this odd-looking bulb. As a crucifer, kohlrabi will help to balance your estrogen levels and support your liver health. It is also very high in vitamin C. Crunchy and sweet, kohlrabi is a perfect vegetable to ferment. If you prefer a traditional sauerkraut, just replace the kohlrabi in this recipe with shredded cabbage. Feel free to replace the caraway seeds with cumin, coriander seeds, fennel seeds, or juniper berries. If you want to make your own signature kraut using cabbage or other vegetables, take a look at the chart on page 276 for an inspiration, choosing from the various salts, starters, herbs, spices, and seaweed.

In a large bowl, combine the shredded kohlrabi and salt. Knead for a few minutes and then let it rest for about 10 minutes to allow the juices to develop. Mix in the caraway seeds and peppercorns.

Transfer the kohlrabi mixture to a mason jar and pack it down so that the kohlrabi is completely submerged in juice. Add water, if needed, to create at least 1 inch of brine over the shredded kohlrabi, but leave 1 inch headspace.

If the kohlrabi floats to the top, weigh it down under the brine, using weight stones or a small glass jar.

Cover the mason jar with a tight lid, airlock lid, or coffee filter secured with a rubber band.

Culture at room temperature, preferably at 60°F to 70°F, for 14 days or until the kraut becomes tart and soft. If using a tight lid, burp it daily to release excess pressure.

MAKES 2 pounds

PREP TIME 15 minutes

FERMENTATION TIME 14 days

EQUIPMENT 1-quart mason jar (with lid, or coffee filter and rubber band)

2 pounds kohlrabi, washed, peeled, and shredded

2 teaspoons salt

1 teaspoon caraway seeds

½ teaspoon black peppercorns

Once the kraut tastes good to you, remove the weight, seal with a tight lid, and refrigerate. The flavor will continue to develop.

Keeps well in the refrigerator for up to 2 years.

Customized Kraut

Want to make your own signature kraut?

You can make your own kraut with vegetables other than cabbage or kohlrabi. Use this guide to make your signature recipe that your family and friends will love.

1. SHREDDED VEGETABLES	2. SALT	3. STARTER (OPTIONAL)	4. HERBS, SPICES, AND SEAWEED
Cabbage	Celtic salt	Body Ecology Culture Starter	Pickling mix
Turnips (sauerruben)	Pink Himalayan salt	2 tablespoons juice of a previous batch of sauerkraut	Caraway
Zucchinis	Utah salt		Cumin
Carrot and ginger	Unrefined sea salt	Whey, fresh (if tolerated)	Dill seeds
Root mix: turnips, beets, carrots, and daikon radish	Smoked salt		Garlic
			Ginger
			Allspice
			Bay leaves
			Orange peel
			Lemon peel
			Seaweed

PALEO

AIP Replace seed-based spices such as caraway or peppercorns with any AIP-compliant spices such as garlic, ginger, thyme, or dulse flakes.

ANTI-CANDIDA Eat only after the first 4 weeks of the anti-Candida diet.

LOW FODMAP Eat no more than 1 tablespoon per day.

Vegetable-to-salt ratio: 5 pounds vegetables to 3 tablespoons salt

BEST TEMPERATURE

Day 1–14: 70°F
Day 14 forward: below 60°F

Cultured Vegetable Medley— Four Ways

Gut healing, liver detoxing, sugar balancing

Discover the nutritional and flavorful richness of fermented vegetables. This traditional pickling method uses lacto-fermentation, which over time develops beneficial bacteria for your gut, as opposed to vinegar pickling, which offers no medicinal benefit. For maximum nutritional value, use unpeeled root vegetables (such as carrots and parsnips), but make sure they are organic. Using the vegetable starter is optional; the fermentation will happen without it, but the starter inoculates the ferments with additional bacteria.

The ideal fermentation temperature for these medleys is between 68°F and 74°F. Open the jars once a day during the first three days to release the naturally occurring gas. Check the vegetables after 14 days for readiness—they should taste tart and be softened. You can easily keep the fermentation going for up to 30 days to allow a richer bacterial profile to develop.

MAKES Two 1-quart jars

PREP TIME 20 minutes

FERMENTATION TIME 14 to 30 days

EQUIPMENT Two 1-quart glass mason jars with screw-top or airlock lids

Cauliflower and Broccoli Medley

2 packets Body Ecology Culture Starter (optional)

5 cups Salt Brine for Cultured Vegetables (page 178)

2 medium heads broccoli, cut into small florets

1 medium head cauliflower, cut into small florets

1 bay leaf

2 sprigs of dill

½ teaspoon coriander seeds

1 large clove garlic, crushed

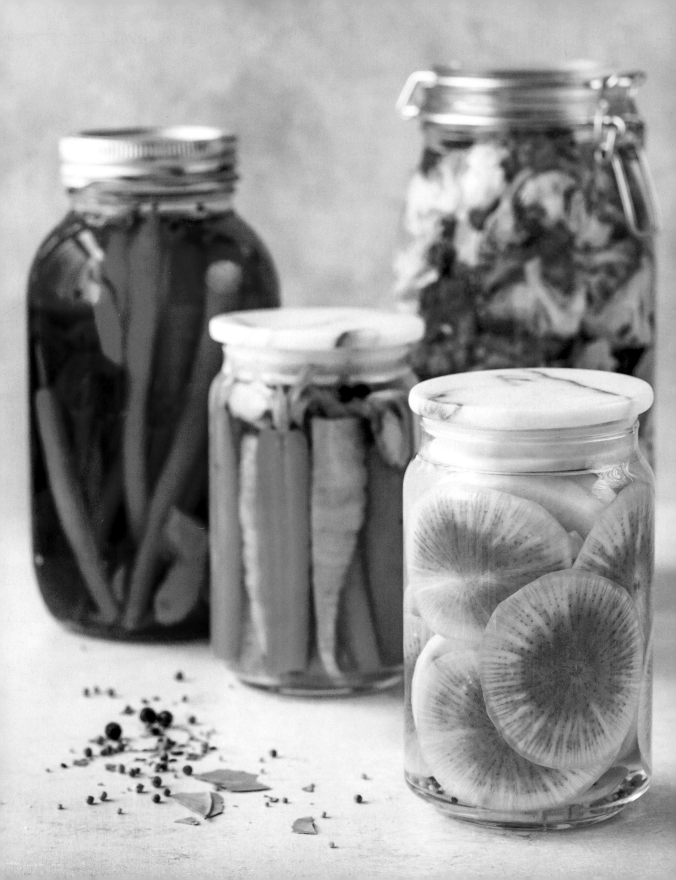

Carrot, Parsnip, and Orange Medley

2 packets Body Ecology Culture Starter (optional)

4 to 6 cups Salt Brine for Cultured Vegetables (page 178)

6 medium young unpeeled carrots, cut into ½-inch matchsticks and trimmed to fit the jar

2 medium unpeeled parsnips, cut into ½-inch matchsticks and trimmed to fit the jar

Freshly grated peel of 1 orange

2-inch ginger knob, sliced

1 teaspoon juniper berries

Radish Medley

2 packets Body Ecology Culture Starter (optional)

4 to 6 cups Salt Brine for Cultured Vegetables (page 178)

6-inch daikon radish, peeled and cut into ¼-inch slices

3 medium watermelon radishes, peeled and cut into ¼-inch slices

2 cloves garlic, crushed

2 teaspoons pickling spice (containing cinnamon, bay leaves, mustard seed, allspice berries, cloves, and black peppercorns)

Beet and Carrot Medley

2 packets Body Ecology Culture Starter (optional)

4 to 6 cups Salt Brine for Cultured Vegetables (page 178)

2 small beets, peeled, quartered, and cut into ¼-inch slices

4 medium unpeeled carrots, cut into ½-inch matchsticks and trimmed to fit the jar

2 teaspoons pickling spice (containing cinnamon, bay leaves, mustard seed, allspice berries, cloves, and black peppercorns)

2-inch ginger knob, sliced

In a large pitcher or bowl, dissolve the vegetable starter in the brine by whisking it vigorously.

Divide the vegetables and spices between two jars, leaving 1 inch of headspace.

Cover the vegetables with the brine, fully submerging them. Secure each jar with a lid.

Ferment at room temperature for 14 to 30 days. Release the gas by loosening the lid once a day for the first 4 days.

Keeps in the refrigerator for up to 12 months.

PALEO

AIP *Replace seed-based spices with AIP-compliant herbs and spices such as garlic, horseradish, or bay leaf.*

ANTI-CANDIDA *Avoid if you're on the first 4 weeks of the diet. Replace root vegetables such as beet and carrots with cauliflower, turnips, or radishes.*

LOW FODMAP *Pick low-FODMAP vegetables such as turnips, radishes, carrots, or parsnips. Eat no more than 1 tablespoon per day.*

Homemade Seed Butter (for Seed Rotation)—Two Ways

Estrogen balancing, progesterone boosting, rich in fiber ⏱ Less than 30 minutes

You can use seed rotation to rebalance your hormones, and seed butters can help you do that. To learn more about this easy and effective technique, see page 104. To improve digestibility, soak and dehydrate the pumpkin and sunflower seeds before blending. You can roll 2 tablespoons of each butter into a ball and use it as your daily hormone booster. Do not refrigerate because it will make the butters rock hard.

SERVES 14 (2 tablespoons per serving)

PREP TIME 15 minutes per butter

EQUIPMENT Spice grinder and food processor

Flaxseed and Pumpkin Seed Butter

Estrogen boosting

1¼ cups firmly packed freshly ground golden flaxseed

1⅓ cups pumpkin seeds

2 teaspoons ground coriander seeds

Pinch of sea salt

⅔ cup melted coconut oil, or more if needed

2 tablespoons Grade B maple syrup

Sesame and Sunflower Seed Butter

Progesterone boosting

1⅓ cups firmly packed ground white sesame seeds

1⅓ cups sunflower seeds

1 tablespoon vanilla powder

1 tablespoon ground cinnamon

1 teaspoon ground cardamom

Pinch of sea salt

½ cup melted coconut oil

2 tablespoons Grade B maple syrup

Pulse the seeds in the food processor until crumbly. Add the spices and salt.

With the food processor running, slowly drizzle in the coconut oil and the maple syrup, scraping down the sides as needed.

Blend until the butter reaches a smooth consistency. If the mixture is crumbly, add 2 tablespoons melted coconut oil at a time until the batter is smooth.

The butters keep well at room temperature for up to 2 weeks.

PALEO

ANTI-CANDIDA *Replace the maple syrup with five drops of liquid stevia and add 2 tablespoons coconut oil to the Flaxseed and Pumpkin Seed Butter.*

LOW FODMAP

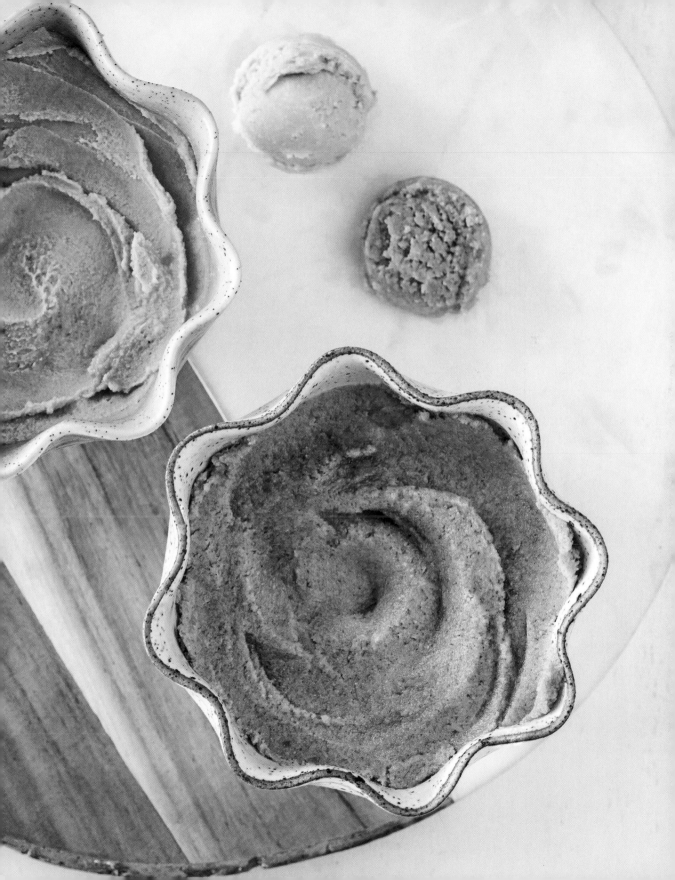

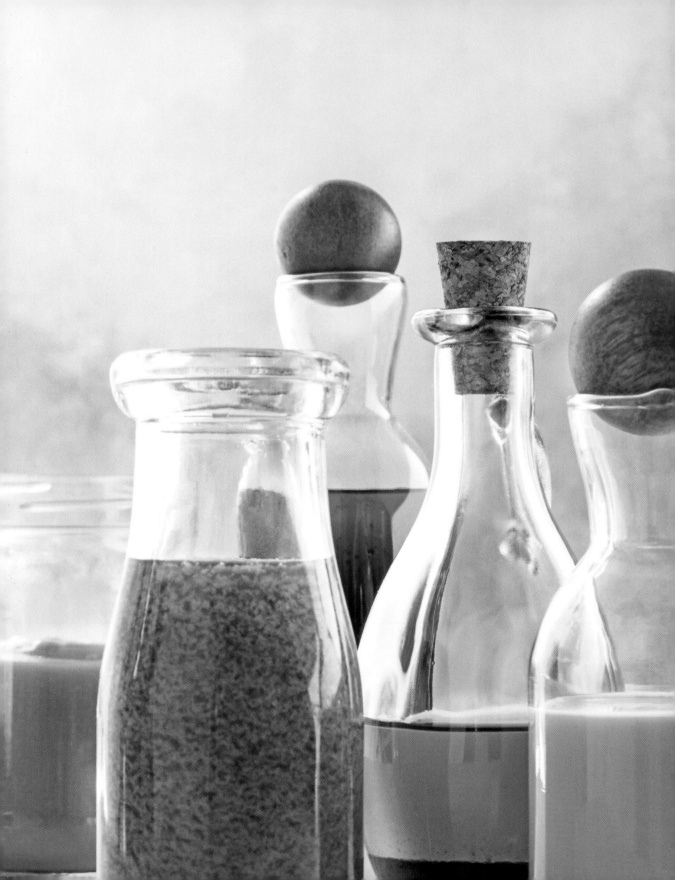

Salad Dressing—Five Ways

⏱ Less than 30 minutes

Keep a few salad dressings in your kitchen already made so that you can create a quick weeknight meal. Add them to salads or drizzle on top of steamed vegetables. A good dressing can transform a plain meal into a culinary explosion of flavors.

PALEO

*To make the dressings **AIP**, **LOW-FODMAP**, or **ANTI-CANDIDA** compliant, please modify them using the allowed foods shown in the respective guides in Chapter 5.*

Classic Balsamic

1 cup extra virgin olive oil
¼ cup balsamic vinegar
1 teaspoon dried garlic
¾ teaspoon sea salt
½ teaspoon dried oregano
½ teaspoon dried basil
1 tablespoon raw honey or Grade B maple syrup

Place all of the ingredients in a 16-ounce jar, close the lid, and shake until well combined. Keeps well at room temperature for up to 30 days.

Creamy Peruvian

1½ medium ripe avocados, peeled, pitted, and cut into chunks

¾ cup avocado oil

½ cup extra virgin olive oil

Freshly grated peel of 1 lime

2 tablespoons freshly squeezed lime juice

1½ tablespoons minced green onions

½ tablespoon raw honey

½ teaspoon sea salt

½ cup lightly packed cilantro

Place all of the ingredients except the cilantro in a high-speed electric blender and puree until smooth. Add the cilantro and pulse. Transfer to a 16-ounce jar and refrigerate for up to 10 days.

Thick and Cheesy

1 cup filtered water

⅔ cup tahini (sesame paste)

½ cup nutritional yeast

⅓ cup extra virgin olive oil

2 tablespoons freshly squeezed lemon juice

½ tablespoon raw honey or Grade B maple syrup

1 teaspoon sea salt

Place all of the ingredients in a high-speed electric blender and puree until smooth. Transfer to a 16-ounce jar and refrigerate for up to 10 days.

Japanese Miso

1 cup avocado oil

½ cup sweet white miso

⅓ cup roasted sesame oil

3 tablespoons rice vinegar

1 tablespoon coconut aminos

1½ tablespoons minced green onions

1 tablespoon raw honey or Grade B maple syrup

Place all of the ingredients in a high-speed electric blender and puree until smooth. Transfer to a 16-ounce jar and refrigerate for up to 10 days.

Persian Delight

¾ cup extra virgin olive oil

¼ cup hazelnut, walnut, or macadamia oil

⅓ cup pomegranate molasses

½ tablespoon blackstrap molasses

¾ teaspoon sea salt

Place all of the ingredients in a 16-ounce jar, close the lid, and shake until well combined. Store at room temperature for up to 30 days.

Herbal Pesto

Liver detoxing, nutrient dense 🕐 Less than 30 minutes

This leafy powerhouse packs all of the flavor of a conventional pesto without the dairy and with more nutrient-dense ingredients. Cilantro binds heavy metals; basil is packed with vitamin K (for bone support); and parsley and dandelion are liver detoxifiers loaded with vitamins A, C, and K and folate. Use this herbal pesto alongside grilled or fried meat or fish, on top of steamed vegetables, on toast, as a pizza topping, or as a pasta sauce. Sprinkle the pesto with roasted pine nuts for added texture and a nutty flavor.

MAKES 2 cups

PREP TIME 15 minutes

EQUIPMENT Food processor, two 12-ounce mason jars

2 cups firmly packed fresh cilantro, coarsely chopped

1 cup firmly packed fresh basil, coarsely chopped

1 cup firmly packed fresh parsley, coarsely chopped

2 cups firmly packed dandelion leaves, coarsely chopped

1 cup extra virgin olive oil, or more if needed

Freshly grated peel of 1 lime

¼ cup freshly squeezed lime juice

1 large clove garlic, crushed

1 teaspoon sea salt

Pack the cilantro, basil, parsley, and dandelion into the food processor.

Add all remaining ingredients to the food processor and pulse. You may need to stop the food processor a few times and use a spatula to clean the sides, pushing down some of the unprocessed herbs. Pulse until the pesto is smooth but not runny. Add more olive oil if the mixture is too dry or not getting processed.

Transfer the pesto to the mason jars.

Keeps well in the refrigerator for up to 10 days and the freezer for up to 3 months.

PALEO

AIP

ANTI-CANDIDA

LOW FODMAP Omit the garlic. Replace dandelion leaves with ½ cup more basil and ½ cup cilantro or parsley.

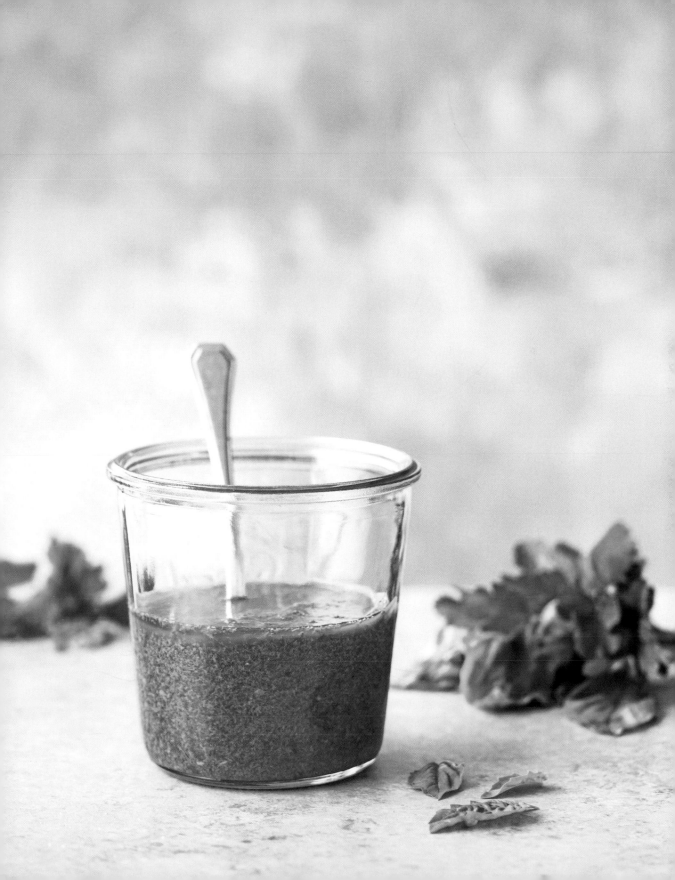

Easy French Pate

Liver detoxing, rich in vitamins A and B12, rich in iron and selenium ⏱ Less than 30 minutes

This creamy, rich pate has turned liver haters into liver lovers and is a delicious way to incorporate liver into your diet. The French know the secret to a delicious pate: Do not overcook the liver. Overcooking results in the strong gamey taste that many people find unappetizing. My favorite way to serve pate is on Flaxseed Crackers (page 327) with a fermented vegetable, such as Sauerkraut Carrot Salad (page 264) or dilled pickles.

MAKES Four 6-ounce jars

PREP TIME 30 minutes

EQUIPMENT Food processor or high-speed electric blender, four 6-ounce glass jars

1 pound chicken livers

1 cup plus 2 tablespoons ghee

1 large shallot, diced, or ½ yellow onion, diced

1 tablespoon fresh sage, coarsely chopped, or 1 teaspoon dried sage, plus 4 extra fresh leaves, for garnish

1 tablespoon fresh tarragon, coarsely chopped, or 1 teaspoon dried tarragon

¾ teaspoon sea salt

½ cup sherry or bourbon

2 teaspoons freshly squeezed lemon or lime juice

4 tablespoons melted lard

Rinse the chicken livers and pat them dry with a paper towel.

In a skillet over medium-high heat, heat 2 tablespoons ghee. Add the shallots and cook for about 4 minutes, or until lightly browned.

Add the chicken livers. They will release a significant amount of liquid. Simmer for about 4 minutes, or until brown, stirring occasionally. The livers will be breaking up, which is appropriate.

Increase to high heat, add the sage, tarragon, salt, and sherry, scraping the bottom of the pan to loosen and dissolve the brown bits. Continue to cook for 3 minutes, or until the sherry is mostly evaporated and you can no longer smell the alcohol. Remove from the heat and cool for 10 minutes.

In a food processor, puree the liver mixture, 1 cup ghee, and the lemon juice until smooth.

Spoon the pate into the glass jars. "Seal" each jar by pouring 1 tablespoon lard on top and garnishing with a sage leaf. Chill in the refrigerator for 4 hours or overnight to set before serving.

Keeps well in the refrigerator for up to 5 days and in the freezer for up to 3 months.

PALEO

AIP *Omit the sherry.*

ANTI-CANDIDA *Omit the sherry.*

LOW FODMAP *Omit the shallots/onions, or replace with the green part of six scallions.*

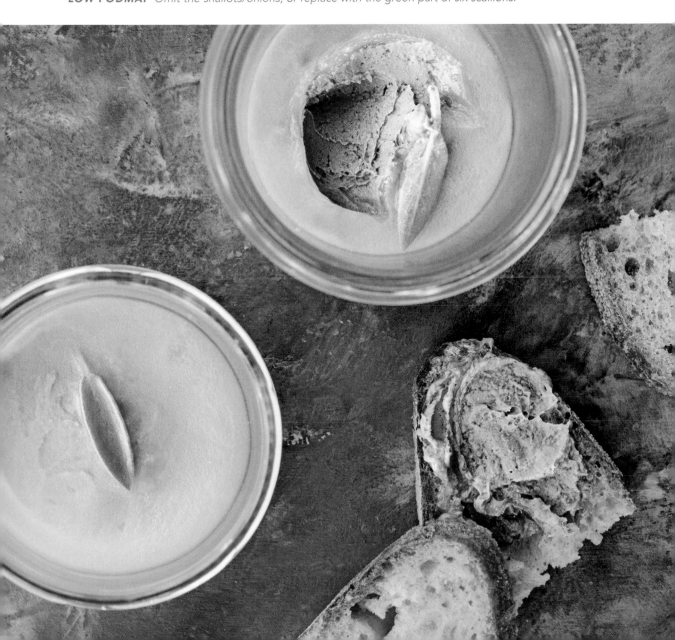

Olive and Preserved Lemon Tapenade

Liver detoxing, estrogen balancing 🕐 Less than 30 minutes

This savory Mediterranean tapenade makes a wonderful dip, spread, or salad dressing. My favorite way to serve it is as a topping for pan-fried cod or salmon. The rind of the preserved lemon is full of d-limonene, which supports liver detoxification.

MAKES 16 servings

PREP TIME 10 minutes

EQUIPMENT Food processor, one 16-ounce mason jar

2 cups pitted Kalamata olives, coarsely chopped

1 Preserved Lemon (page 170), deseeded and chopped

2 anchovy fillets (optional)

½ cup extra virgin olive oil

PALEO

AIP

ANTI-CANDIDA *Eat only after the first 4 weeks of the anti-Candida diet.*

LOW FODMAP

Place the olives, preserved lemon, and anchovies in the food processor and pulse until well combined.

With the engine running, drizzle in the olive oil and blend until the mixture becomes a coarse paste. Transfer to a mason jar and serve.

Keeps well in the refrigerator for up to 3 months.

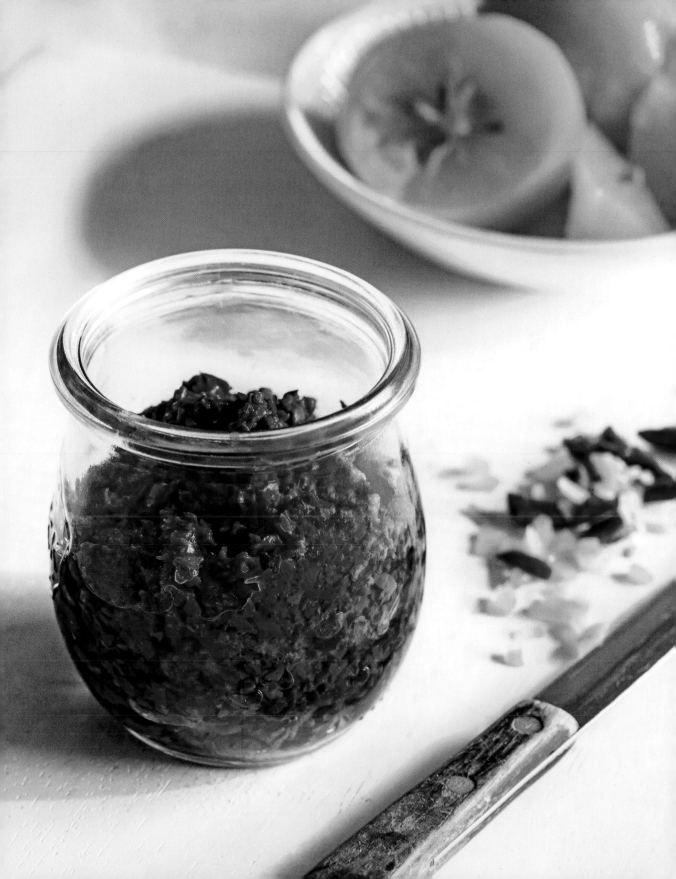

Spiced Nut Butter—Two Ways

Rich in protein, fiber, and vitamin Bs ⏱ Less than 30 minutes

Making your own nut butter is quick and easy. Add your favorite spices to make a signature butter: I've experimented with orange peel, star anise, nutmeg, and lavender with outstanding results.

To improve the digestibility of nuts, I recommend buying sprouted nuts whenever possible or soaking and dehydrating them yourself. Do not soak macadamia nuts as they become mushy. Note that frequently consuming large amounts of nuts can cause you to develop a sensitivity to them.

SERVES 12

PREP TIME 15 minutes

EQUIPMENT Food processor or high-speed electric blender, one 12-ounce jar

PALEO

ANTI-CANDIDA *Replace the maple syrup with six drops of liquid stevia.*

LOW FODMAP *Limit consumption of the almond butter to ½ tablespoons per day.*

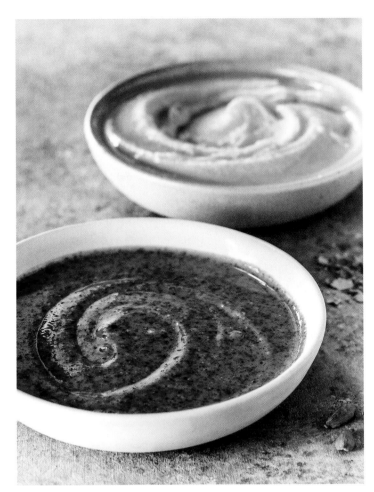

Cardamom and Clove Almond Butter

3 cups sprouted almonds

½ tablespoon ground cardamom

½ tablespoon vanilla powder

1 teaspoon ground cloves

¼ teaspoon sea salt

¾ cup avocado oil

1 tablespoon Grade B maple syrup

Vanilla and Rose Macadamia Butter

3 cups raw macadamia nuts

½ tablespoon vanilla powder

½ teaspoon rose water

Pinch of sea salt

¼ cup macadamia oil

2 tablespoons Grade B maple syrup

Pulse the nuts in the food processor until crumbly. Add the spices and salt.

With the food processor running, slowly drizzle in the oil and the maple syrup, scraping down the sides as necessary.

Blend for 10 minutes or until the butter reaches the desired consistency.

Keeps well in the refrigerator for up to 6 months.

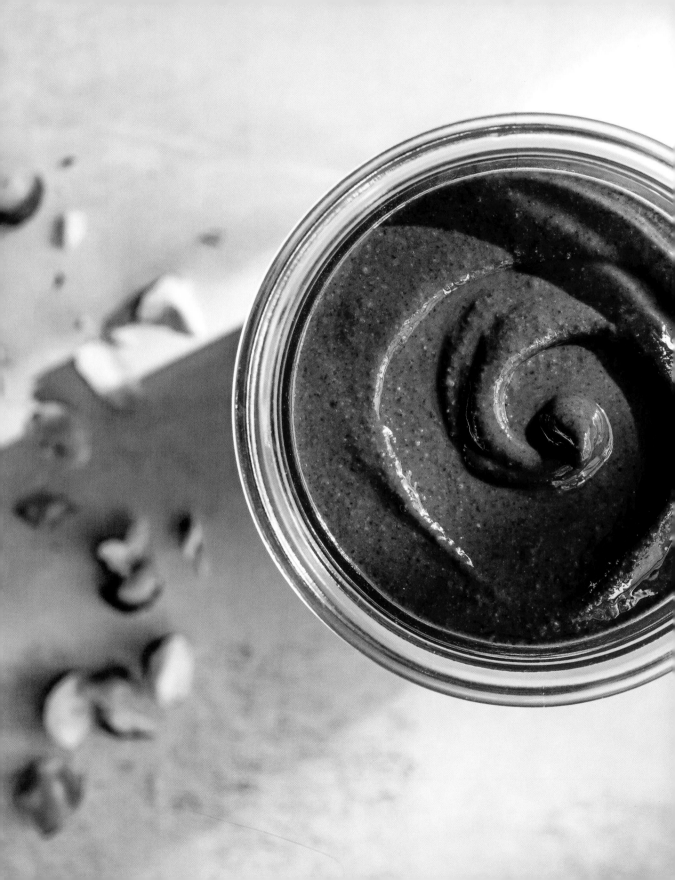

Silky Chocolate Hazelnut Butter

High in good fats, rich in magnesium and thiamine (a mood and immunity booster)

⏱ Less than 30 minutes

How can such an indulgent food be healthy? This butter is packed with nutrients like magnesium (craved by most women) and thiamine, or vitamin B1, which helps boost metabolism, energy, mood, and the immune system. To save time, I do not soak and dehydrate the hazelnuts in this recipe. However, if you are suffering from digestive issues and plan to serve this butter frequently in your household (kids love it!), I recommend soaking and dehydrating the nuts before making the butter.

Place the hazelnuts in the food processor. Pulse until crumbly. Add the cacao, coconut butter, vanilla powder, and salt and pulse until well combined.

With the food processor running, slowly drizzle in the hazelnut oil, coconut oil, and maple syrup, scraping down the sides as necessary.

Blend for 5 minutes or until the butter reaches a silky consistency.

Store in an airtight container at room temperature for up to 2 months.

MAKES 2 cups, about 24 servings

MAKING TIME 15 minutes

EQUIPMENT Food processor or high-speed electric blender

1 cup raw hazelnuts

½ cup raw unsweetened cacao powder

¼ cup coconut butter

1 tablespoon vanilla powder or extract

Dash of sea salt

¾ cup hazelnut or macadamia oil

¼ cup melted coconut oil

¼ cup Grade B maple syrup

PALEO

LOW FODMAP Limit consumption to 2 tablespoons per day.

Salmon and Avocado in Nori Sheets

Estrogen balancing, rich in omega 3, rich in iodine ⏱ Less than 30 minutes

This simple and yummy snack will bring lots of nutritional goodness to your diet. Chilling is optional; I often skip it and just dig right in.

MAKES 6 nori rolls

SERVES 2

PREP TIME 15 minutes

CHILLING TIME 1 hour (optional)

EQUIPMENT Twelve toothpicks

1 6-ounce cooked salmon steak, deboned, or 1 6-ounce can pink salmon

2 ripe avocados, peeled, pitted, and sliced

3 tablespoons fresh dill, finely chopped, or 1 tablespoon dried dill

2 tablespoons minced scallions

3 tablespoons melted coconut oil or extra virgin olive oil

1 tablespoon freshly squeezed lemon juice

¼ teaspoon sea salt

6 nori sheets

3 cups lightly packed fresh arugula leaves or mixed greens, such as baby kale, mizuna, or lettuce

Handful of broccoli sprouts

In a large bowl, place the salmon, avocado, dill, scallions, coconut oil, lemon juice, and salt. Mash with your hand or a fork. Chill for 1 hour.

Place a nori sheet on a serving plate, and spoon 3 tablespoons of the mashed salmon on the nori sheet, about 2 inches from the edge.

Place ½ cup of the arugula leaves and some of the broccoli sprouts on top, roll up the nori sheet, and cut it diagonally in half. Secure each half with a toothpick. Repeat the process five more times.

The mashed salmon mixture keeps well in the refrigerator for up to 5 days. Wrap in nori sheets when ready to serve.

PALEO

AIP *Soak the broccoli sprouts to remove the seeds.*

ANTI-CANDIDA

LOW FODMAP *Use only the green parts of the scallions. Limit to 2 tablespoons per serving.*

Matcha Frappe

Energizing, anticarcinogenic, antioxidant ⏱ Less than 30 minutes

A wonderful morning or afternoon pick-me-up, this beverage will give you a sustained boost of energy for the rest of the day. Matcha was my replacement beverage when I quit coffee, and I loved it for the gentle kick it offers. This ceremonial Japanese tea has some special super powers; it is alkalizing, detoxifying, rich in antioxidants, anti-inflammatory, anticarcinogenic, calming and energizing at the same time. To retain its antioxidant properties, do not bring hot water into direct contact with matcha tea.

Put all of the ingredients in the blender, adding the hot water last.

Blend for 30 seconds.

Sprinkle with cinnamon and serve as a warm drink or over ice.

SERVES 2

PREP TIME 5 minutes

EQUIPMENT Electric blender

1 cup room temperature water

2 teaspoons matcha tea

½ cup canned full-fat coconut milk

1 tablespoon Grade B maple syrup

¼ teaspoon vanilla powder

1 cup hot water

¼ teaspoon cinnamon powder (optional)

PALEO

AIP

ANTI-CANDIDA *Replace the maple syrup with six drops of stevia.*

LOW FODMAP

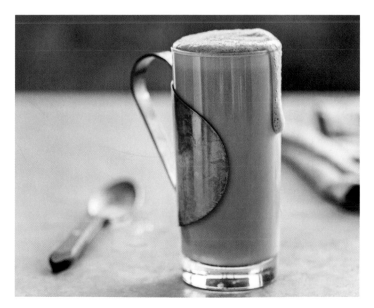

Nut and Seed Milks

Estrogen balancing, nutrient dense ⏱ Less than 30 minutes

Making your own milk without the preservatives and additives of store-bought brands is easier than you think and so much healthier. Note that despite its name, tigernut is not a nut or a seed; it's a tuber that can be consumed by people who have nut and seed sensitivities.

Make nut milks from almonds, hazelnuts, macadamia nuts, pecans, walnuts, or shredded coconut. Make seed milks from sunflower seeds, pumpkin seeds, or hemp seeds. Make a tuber milk from tigernuts.

MAKES 1 quart

MAKING TIME 10 minutes

EQUIPMENT High-speed electric blender, nut bag or cheesecloth (100 percent cotton) folded in multiple layers, one 1-quart mason jar

4 cups lukewarm filtered water

1 cup raw nuts, seeds, or tubers of your choice

2 to 3 pitted dates (optional)

1 teaspoon vanilla extract or powder (optional)

Dash of sea salt

To the blender container, add the water; nuts, seeds, or tubers; dates; vanilla; and salt.

Puree on high for 1 to 2 minutes. Tigernuts need 2 to 3 minutes.

Strain through a nut bag if using almonds, hazelnuts, coconut, pumpkin seeds, or tigernuts. There is no need to strain walnuts, pecans, macadamia nuts, hemp seeds, or sunflower seeds.

Transfer to a 1-quart mason jar.

Keeps well in the refrigerator for up to 5 days or in the freezer for up to 6 months.

PALEO

AIP Use only tigernuts and coconut.

ANTI-CANDIDA Omit dates.

LOW FODMAP Use macadamia nuts, pecans, walnuts, sunflower seeds, pumpkin seeds, or hemp seeds. Replace the dates with maple syrup.

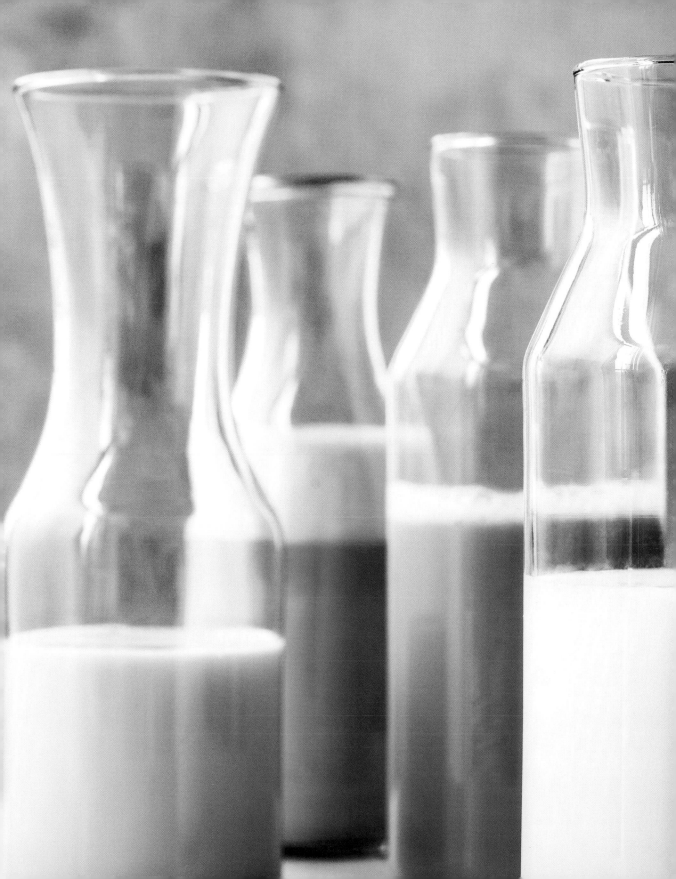

HEALING TEA INFUSIONS AND DECOCTIONS

Making your own tea is not only fun but empowering, giving you the opportunity to use your favorite herbs and spices to support your body and mind. I've studied herbs for years and continue to be enchanted by the possibilities they create for healing and making extraordinary flavor combinations that delight the senses. I encourage you to work with herbs in your own kitchen.

Even though ready-made herbal teas are widely available for purchase, the blends you make yourself will be more flavorful and personalized to your tastes and needs. You can be much more creative when you make your own. You can decide which herbs to use and adjust the amounts on the basis of your own newly developed intuition. If an herb does not resonate with you, do not use it. If you crave it, add it to more teas.

Also, the bags used to contain ready-made tea blends raise health safety concerns. Many of them are bleached and infused with anti-tear chemicals, and some contain plastic. I've also found that when packed in paper, herbs quickly lose their fragrant essential oils and their healing potency. So I invite you to start buying herbs in bulk (online or at your local health store), which will save you money and open a world of new herbal and culinary possibilities.

There are two ways of making herbal teas: *Infusions* are made by steeping soft plant material, such as leaves and flowers, in hot water for 10 to 15 minutes. *Decoctions* are made by simmering harder plant materials, such as roots, barks, dried berries, and seeds, for 20 to 40 minutes.

These teas are made with dried herbs and spices. If you prefer to use fresh herbs, double the amount used in the recipe. The yield for these teas is low (1 quart) so that you can try a tea without worrying about too much waste if you don't like it. Each of these recipes can be scaled up to yield a gallon (quadruple the recipe). Store your dried herbal teas in airtight containers. All the infusions and decoctions keep well in the refrigerator for up to a week.

The first two or three ingredients have the strongest healing qualities, so if you do not have one of them, go ahead and make the tea anyway, and you will still get many benefits from it. I recommend drinking one to two cups of tea per day for a couple of weeks to experience health improvements.

As much as these teas can bring wonderful relief, remember to always focus on resolving the root cause of your health issues and rebalancing your body. If you drink these teas while binging on sugar or gluten, you won't feel much relief.

These teas taste wonderful without any sweeteners, but a touch of honey, for example, opens up their flavors so you can appreciate them more deeply. If you are pregnant, nursing, or taking any medication, please consult your doctor before trying them.

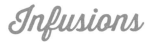

Infusions

Place ingredients in 1 quart hot water.

Steep covered for 10 to 20 minutes.

Strain and add sweetener to taste, if desired.

MAKES 1 quart

PALEO

AIP Omit seed-based herbs such as peppercorns, fennel, cardamom, milk thistle seed, and fenugreek.

ANTI-CANDIDA

LOW FODMAP Omit fennel seed, dandelion, and burdock root. Slippery elm and marshmallow have not been tested, so it is best to omit them or test them in small quantities and check for digestive upset such as bloating or gas.

Immune Booster

Feel like you're coming down with something? This tea will kick your immune system into a higher gear and provide plenty of vitamin C.

1 tablespoon elderberry or elderflower

1 tablespoon lemon balm

1 tablespoon ginger root

1 tablespoon rosehip

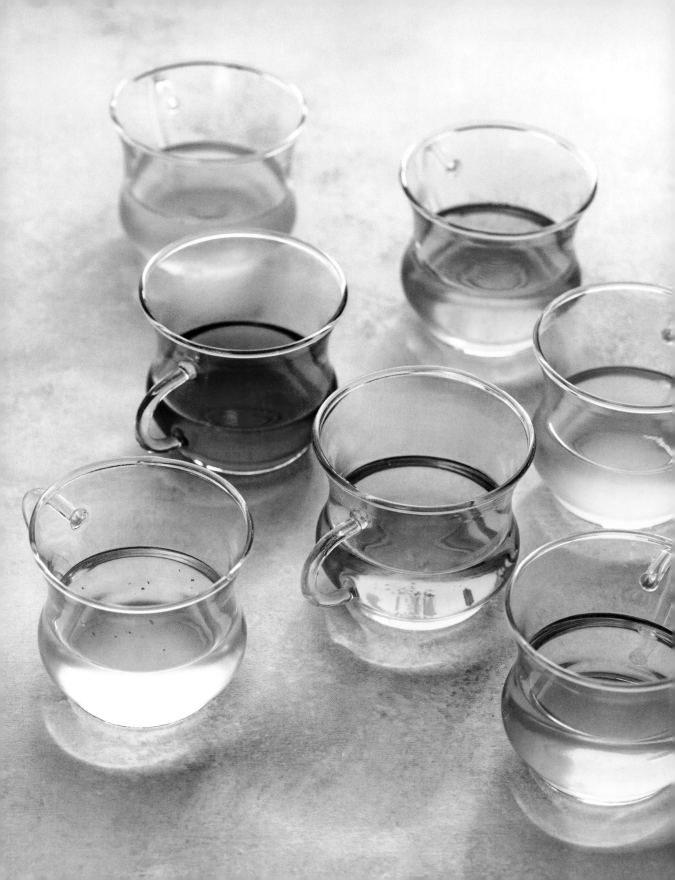

Regular Cycle

Chasteberry is a natural progesterone booster. Progesterone is often low in women who have irregular cycles and PMS. With the mighty raspberry leaf and rose petals combined, this makes a potent women's tonic.

1 tablespoon rose petals

1 tablespoon raspberry leaf

½ tablespoon chasteberry (vitex), crushed

½ tablespoon hibiscus

½ tablespoon ginger

Adrenal Love

Herbs such as rhodiola and tulsi are renowned adrenal adaptogens. Rosehip, high in vitamin C, nourishes the adrenals. Schisandra berry, another adaptogen, has been consumed in Russia and China for centuries to overcome fatigue and boost energy.

1 tablespoon rhodiola

1 tablespoon tulsi (holy basil)

½ tablespoon rosehip

½ tablespoon schisandra berry

Easy Digestion

Drink this after a heavy dinner to help stimulate your digestion.

1 tablespoon ginger root

1 tablespoon fennel seeds, crushed

1 tablespoon peppermint

½ tablespoon lemongrass

Everyday Nourishing

Here's a wonderful pick-me-up you can sip every day. Raspberry leaf is an all-time women's super herb in Western herbalism.

1 tablespoon rose petals

1 tablespoon red raspberry leaf

1 tablespoon oat straw

1 tablespoon lemon balm

1 cardamom pod, crushed

Daily Balancer

Tulsi, an all-around remedial herb used in Ayurveda medicine, is a key ingredient in the tea I drink to start my day. Oat straw can help with focus and concentration. Feel free to add any other of your favorite herbs such as rose buds or lavender to make it your own.

2½ tablespoons tulsi (holy basil)

1½ tablespoons oat straw

Easy Move

If you struggle with constipation, drink one cup of this tea before bedtime to get things moving. It takes about 12 hours to work. I do not recommend drinking it regularly; instead, investigate the root causes of your constipation.

1 tablespoon senna pods or leaves

1 tablespoon lemon balm

1 tablespoon spearmint

Decoctions

To a large pot, add the recipe ingredients and 1 quart cold water.

Cover and bring to a boil. Reduce the heat and simmer for 20 to 40 minutes. For the best extraction of nutrients, let the decoction infuse overnight in the refrigerator.

Strain, warm up if previously refrigerated, and add a sweetener to taste, if desired.

MAKES 1 quart

PALEO

AIP *Omit seed-based herbs such as peppercorns, fennel, cardamom, milk thistle seed, and fenugreek.*

ANTI-CANDIDA

LOW FODMAP *Omit fennel seed, dandelion, and burdock root. Slippery elm and marshmallow have not been tested, so it is best to omit them or test them in small quantities and check for digestive upset such as bloating or gas.*

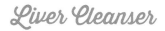

Liver Cleanser

This potent decoction of herbs was used for centuries in Western herbalism as a liver and blood tonic. You can also turn this tea into a latte (see Nourishing Lattes, page 309). Drink 1 to 2 cups per day for 3 months to support and cleanse your liver.

1½ tablespoons dandelion root

¾ tablespoon burdock root

¾ tablespoon milk thistle seed

½ tablespoon sassafras

Sugar Balancer

Here's an ideal tea for women with insulin resistance and fluctuating sugar levels. Research has shown that both cinnamon and fenugreek can bring down sugar levels. Drink any time during the day, two cups per day. This tea is not suitable for pregnant women.

1½ tablespoons cinnamon chips
1½ tablespoons fenugreek
½ tablespoon ginger root
½ tablespoon turmeric root

Gut Repair

This gut-soothing tea will reduce gastrointestinal inflammation and pain. It's great for people with leaky gut, IBS, gastritis, or acid reflux. Precaution: Take any medications 1 hour before or a few hours after you drink this tea.

1 tablespoon slippery elm powder
1 tablespoon marshmallow powder

Add the elm powder and marshmallow powder to 1½ cups hot water, stir, and drink. Add sweetener to taste, if desired.

Nourishing Lattes

These nourishing, warming, and comforting lattes will help you to reduce or eliminate your dependence on caffeine and commercial lattes, which are loaded with sugar and chemicals.

These lattes are potent medicinal concoctions, so start with a small quantity first to see how they agree with you. One herb may help one person but not another. Lattes are a great way of masking the medicinal flavors of some of the herbs, making them a delightful and delicious experience.

The herbs used in these recipes are dried. If you prefer to use fresh herbs, double the amount used in the recipe. Store the dried herbal blends in airtight containers. If you like a latte, quadruple the recipe to yield a gallon and keep it in the refrigerator. Find the herbs online or in the bulk section of your local health store. The lattes keep well for up to a week in the refrigerator unless you use tigernut milk, which keeps for only 3 days.

I encourage you to modify these recipes and make them even better—and most importantly, to have fun making them.

MAKES 1 quart

To a large pot, add the recipe ingredients and 1 quart cold water.

Cover and bring to a boil. Reduce the heat and simmer for 20 to 40 minutes.

Place a strainer over a blender and pour in the liquid.

Add ½ cup homemade coconut milk, almond milk, cashew milk, or tigernut milk (page 300). (Alternatively, use ¼ cup coconut butter and sweetener, such as two to three dates, 2 to 3 tablespoons maple syrup, or coconut syrup). If using honey, let the latte cool before adding.

Blend for 1 minute or until a thick foam forms on top.

PALEO

AIP Omit any seed-based spices such as star anise and peppercorns. Use only coconut or tigernut milk.

ANTI-CANDIDA Use nut-based milks only if you can tolerate nuts; otherwise, pick coconut or tigernut milk. For a sweetener, use stevia.

LOW FODMAP Omit carob, chicory, and dandelion root. Reishi, chaga, chasteberry (vitex), maca, dong quai, and black cohosh have not been tested, so it is best to omit them or test them in small quantities and check for digestive upset such as bloating or gas. Use only coconut, tigernut, pumpkin seed, or macadamia nut milk. For sweeteners, only use maple syrup.

Immune-Boosting Latte

Reishi and chaga are strong immune-regulating mushrooms. Together with turmeric, this is a real power drink to start the day. Unleash your imagination and add spices such as cinnamon, cardamom, star anise, cloves, or ginger to create your own favorite morning beverage.

3 tablespoons reishi mushrooms

3 tablespoons chaga mushrooms

1 tablespoon turmeric

Warming Chai Latte

This is an old-time favorite of friends and guests. The warming and delicious spices in this latte will help you get off caffeine, sugar, and commercial lattes to honor your body's desire to heal. Rooibos, an exquisite, sweet-tasting, caffeine-free tea made from the leaves of a South African shrub, is cited to have 50 percent more antioxidants and phytophenols than green tea.

1½ tablespoons rooibos

1 tablespoon cinnamon

½ tablespoon ginger root

½ tablespoon spearmint

½ tablespoon star anise

6 black peppercorns

5 cloves

2 cardamom pods, crushed

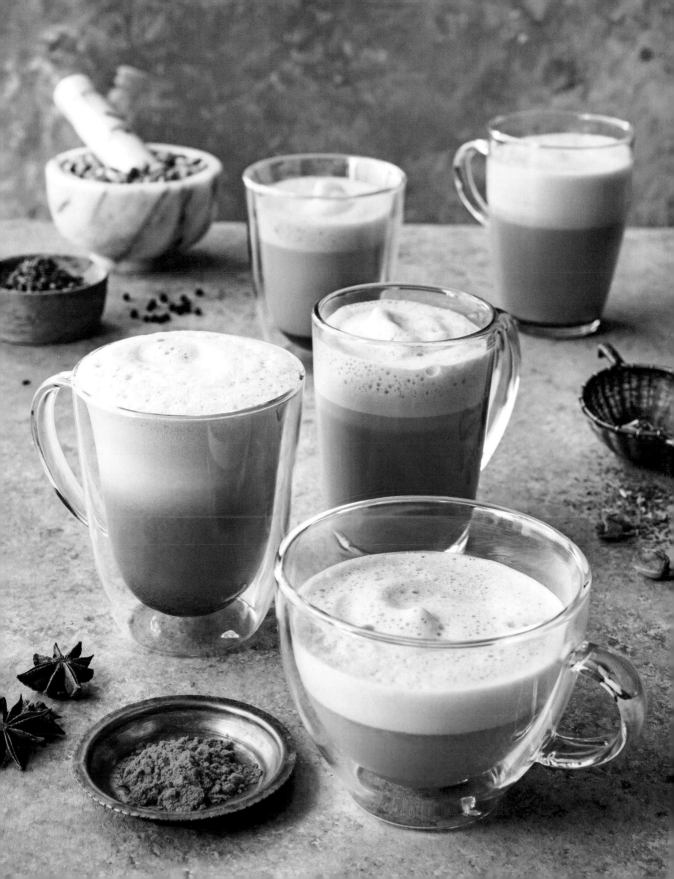

PMS Tamer

Start drinking this tea three to five days before your period. It will help with cramping and mood swings. Drink 2 cups per day.

2 tablespoons cramp bark

1 tablespoon cinnamon chips

1 tablespoon rose petals or buds

½ tablespoon chasteberry (vitex)

½ tablespoon lavender

1 teaspoon lemon peel

Easy Menopause Latte

Dong quai and black cohosh in Chinese medicine have a long history of relieving menopausal discomfort, from hot flashes to irritation. Drink 2 cups per day for no longer than 6 months.

1½ tablespoons dong quai (*Angelica sinensis*)

1½ tablespoons black cohosh

1 tablespoon spearmint

1 tablespoon orange peel

Better Than Coffee Latte

Liver detoxing, sugar balancing ⏱ Less than 30 minutes

If you are dealing with adrenal problems, fluctuating sugar levels, or you intuitively feel that coffee undermines your hormonal balance, try this caffeine-free drink made with chicory and dandelion roots, which have been used medicinally in Western herbalism for centuries. Chicory root is rich in inulin, a prebiotic, and is known to stimulate bile production, which facilitates the liver's detoxification process and keeps hormones in check. Dandelion root has a long history of being used to detoxify and restore liver function. Chaga mushroom boosts the immune system when necessary and slows it down when it is overactive.

You will find that this beverage tastes surprisingly close to coffee. Many people who have tried it report feeling rejuvenated, which I attribute to the positive effect it has on the liver.

In a saucepan over high heat, bring the water to a boil. Add the chicory, dandelion root, and chaga mushroom. Remove from heat, cover, and steep for 10 minutes.

Using a sieve, strain the liquid into the blender. Add the ghee, dates, and maca powder. Blend on high for 1 minute or until froth builds on top.

Pour into serving glasses and sprinkle with nutmeg. Serve warm.

For a cold beverage, chill before adding the nutmeg.

PALEO

AIP

ANTI-CANDIDA *Replace the dates with two to four drops of liquid stevia.*

SERVES 2

PREP TIME 20 minutes

EQUIPMENT High-speed electric blender, sieve

3 cups filtered water

2 teaspoons roasted chicory root

1 teaspoon dried chaga mushroom (optional)

1 teaspoon roasted dandelion root

1 tablespoon ghee or coconut butter

2 pitted dates

1 teaspoon maca powder

Freshly grated nutmeg

Hot Chocolate with Pink Roses

Energizing, rich in magnesium and fiber ⏲ Less than 30 minutes

There is great comfort in hugging a steaming cup of hot chocolate on a cold, dreary day. High in magnesium, this beverage brings both added energy and deep relaxation. Make the pink rose powder by grinding pink roses or rose petals in a spice grinder. The roses add a delightful floral scent and romantic feel. If you don't have roses on hand, don't let that stop you from making this comforting drink. Instead, use your favorite spices such as ground nutmeg, cloves, star anise, or lavender.

MAKES 1 drink

PREP TIME 10 minutes

1½ cups homemade coconut milk (page 300) or ½ cup canned full-fat coconut milk combined with 1 cup filtered water

2 to 3 tablespoons raw unsweetened cacao powder

2 teaspoons raw honey

½ teaspoon ground cinnamon

½ teaspoon vanilla extract

½ teaspoon pink rose powder

In a small pot over medium heat, warm the coconut milk until it starts to steam.

Turn off the heat and whisk in the cacao, honey, cinnamon, and vanilla extract.

Pour into a mug and sprinkle with the rose powder. Serve hot.

Keeps well in the refrigerator for up to 3 days.

PALEO

AIP *Replace cacao with carob powder.*

ANTI-CANDIDA *Replace honey with two to three drops of liquid stevia.*

LOW FODMAP *Replace honey with Grade B maple syrup.*

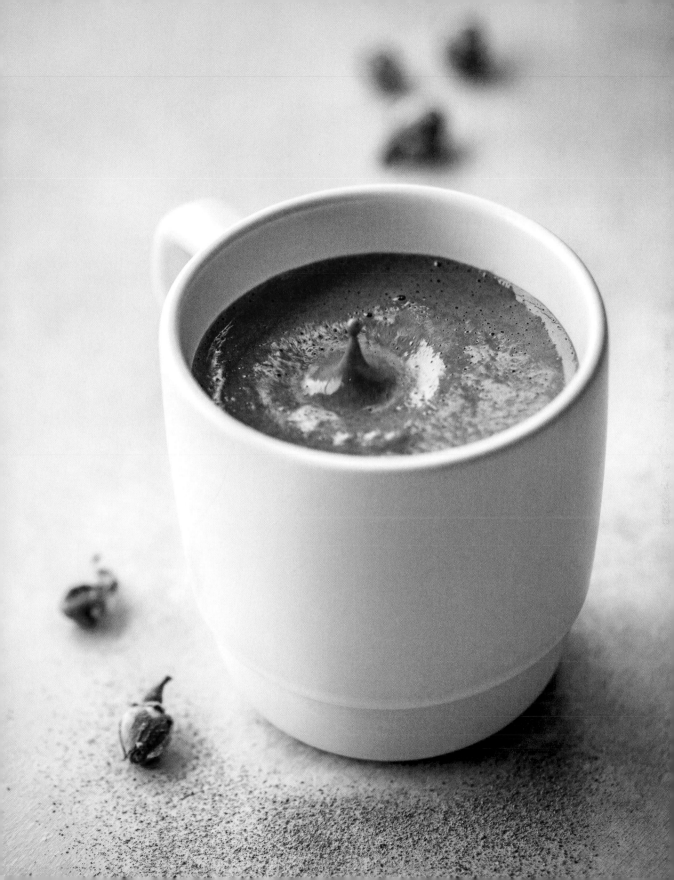

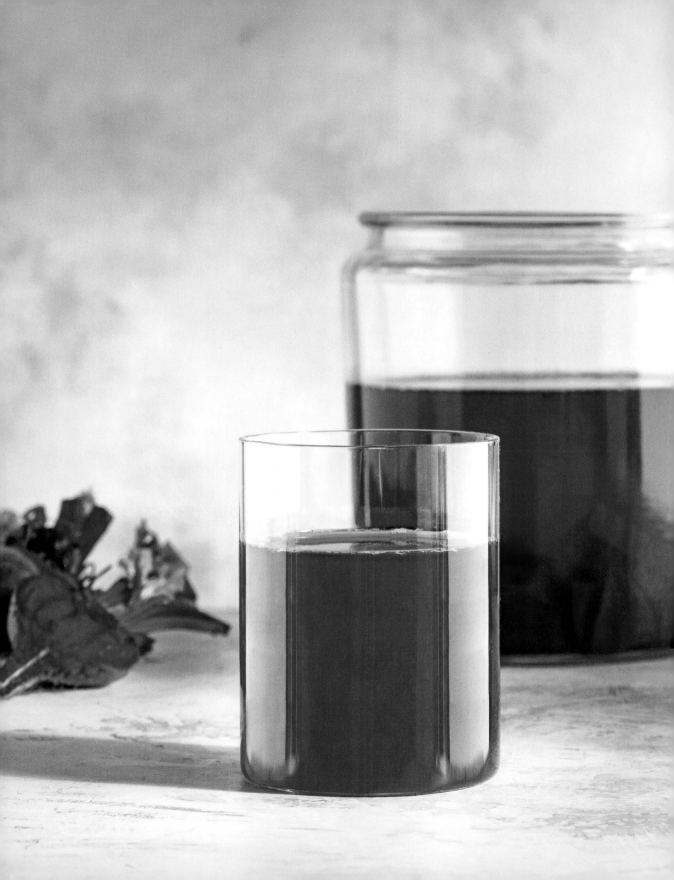

Ginger Beet Kvass

Liver detoxing, estrogen balancing, blood cleansing

Kvass in Russian means "acid." Originally, kvass was made from stale rye bread crumbs; instead of being thrown away, the bread was kept in salted water until it developed a tart flavor.

Kvass has evolved, and today's common way of making it is with beets. I personally find kvass made with beets alone to be too earthy and bland. I've found that by adding zesty ginger, lemons, oranges, kumquats, or tangerines, this drink becomes rather addictive. If you can't find organic beets, peel them for this recipe; otherwise, leave the skin on. The culture starter is optional, but I like to use it to inoculate the drink with more beneficial bacteria.

In the jar, dissolve the salt in the water.

Add all of the remaining ingredients to the jar and weigh the food down with a weighing stone or a small glass jar so the food does not float to the top and get moldy. If using the 1-quart mason jars, divide the ingredients equally.

Keep the jar covered with cheesecloth and secured with a rubber band, or place an airlock over it.

Ferment at room temperature for 4 to 5 days.

Strain and transfer to the fliptop bottles. Refrigerate for a week.

When ready to drink, if you want extra carbonation, leave the kvass out for a few hours at room temperature. Serve at room temperature or chilled.

Keeps well in the refrigerator for up to a month.

MAKES 3 quarts

PREP TIME 15 minutes

EQUIPMENT One 1-gallon jar or four 1-quart mason jars, cheesecloth (100 percent cotton), rubber band, strainer, three 32-ounce fliptop bottles

1 tablespoon sea salt

3 quarts water

3 medium unpeeled organic beets, coarsely chopped

2 oranges, quartered

2 limes with peel, quartered

2-inch fresh unpeeled ginger knob, shredded

1 tablespoon turmeric powder

1 packet Body Ecology Culture Starter (optional)

PALEO
AIP

Strawberry Ginger Ale

Gut healing, low in sugar, rich in probiotics

Do not be alarmed by the amount of sugar in this recipe. The sugar is not for you; it feeds the kefir grains to produce the beneficial bacteria. Fermenting fruit drinks can be fun and easy, but be careful when opening the bottle. I have had unopened bottles explode in the past, making an annoying mess. Depending on the fruit variety, sugar content, and room temperature, the fermentation time can be as short as 24 hours or as long as 4 days. A longer fermentation time will reduce the sugar content and make the drink more bubbly and tart and higher in beneficial bacteria. Pop the bottle open over a kitchen sink every day to release the carbon dioxide.

MAKES 1 quart

PREP TIME 15 minutes

FERMENTATION 1 to 4 days

EQUIPMENT Electric blender, whisk, one 32-ounce fliptop bottle

2½ cups water

2 cups chopped fresh strawberries

⅓ cup freshly squeezed orange juice

¼ cup cane sugar

2 tablespoons minced fresh ginger

1 packet Body Ecology Kefir Starter

Place all of the ingredients except the kefir starter in the blender and puree until smooth.

In a medium bowl, whisk the kefir starter into the pureed strawberry mixture. Pour into the fliptop bottle.

Place in a warm corner of the kitchen, ideally between 70°F and 73°F.

After 24 hours, open the bottle over the sink and taste for tartness. Continue fermenting or, if you like the flavor, transfer to the refrigerator. Serve chilled.

Keeps well in the refrigerator for up to 2 weeks.

PALEO

AIP

LOW FODMAP Always use freshly squeezed orange juice because reconstituted orange juice is high in FODMAP. Fermented ginger ale has not been tested; try it in small quantities and check for digestive upset such as bloating or gas.

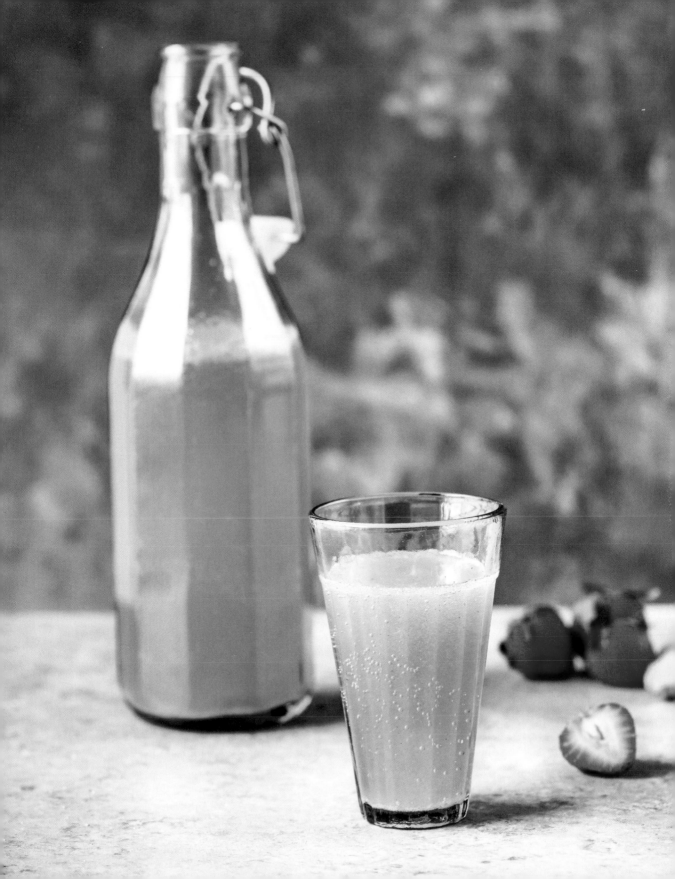

Fizzy Orange, Carrot, and Beet Soda

Gut healing, low in sugar, rich in probiotics

The carrot and beet pairing will help with PMS symptoms if you start drinking this soda 4 to 5 days before your period. Carrots support progesterone production, and beets help with estrogen detoxification. Depending on the fruit variety, sugar content, and room temperature, the fermentation time can be as short as 24 hours or as long as 3 days. Taste the soda every day to decide whether it's ready. Ideal soda is tart and effervescent. Longer fermentation will reduce the sugar content and make the drink more bubbly and tart and higher in beneficial bacteria. Pop the bottle open over a kitchen sink every day to release the naturally occurring carbon dioxide. I have had unopened bottles explode in the past, making an annoying mess.

MAKES 1 quart

PREP TIME 15 minutes

FERMENTATION TIME
24 hours to 3 days

EQUIPMENT Electric juicer,
1-quart fliptop bottle

4 medium red beets, peeled
and cut into chunks

4 navel oranges, peeled
and quartered

8 medium unpeeled carrots,
cut into chunks

1 packet Body Ecology
Kefir Starter

Juice the beets, oranges, and carrots. In the juice bowl, whisk in the kefir starter.

Transfer to the fliptop bottle, lock it, and place it in a warm corner of the kitchen, ideally at 72°F to 75°F.

After 24 hours, open the bottle over the sink and taste for tartness. Continue fermenting or transfer to the refrigerator. Serve at room temperature or chilled.

Keeps well in the refrigerator for up to 2 weeks.

PALEO
AIP

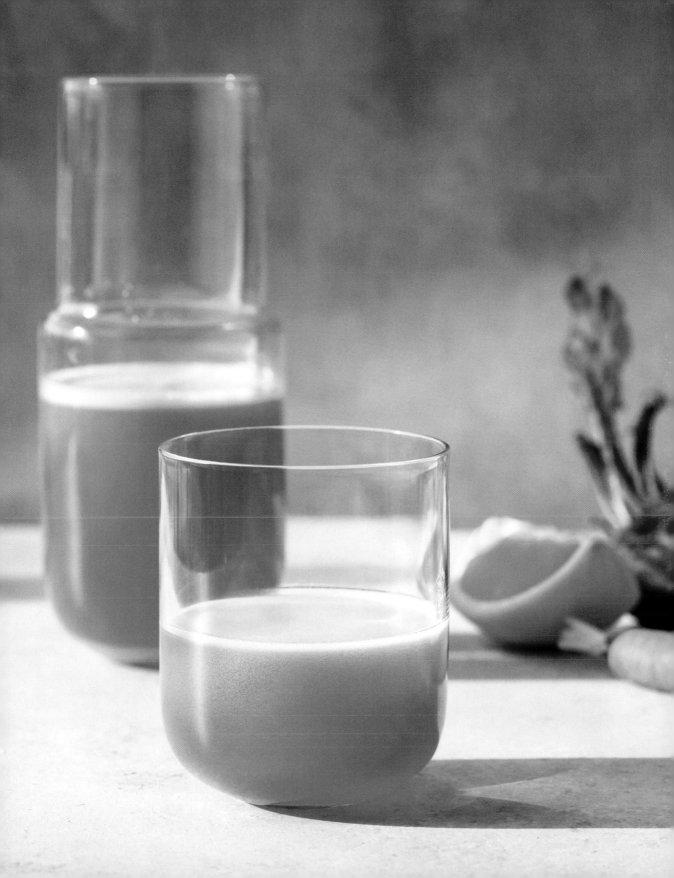

Rustic Olive Bread

Rich in fiber, comforting

Many store-bought gluten-free breads are full of preservatives and stabilizers and are low in fiber. This simple, hearty bread is a wonderful alternative. I use xanthan gum to give the bread a soft and bouncy feel. However, if you suffer from serious digestive issues, skip it and the bread will still turn out perfectly well.

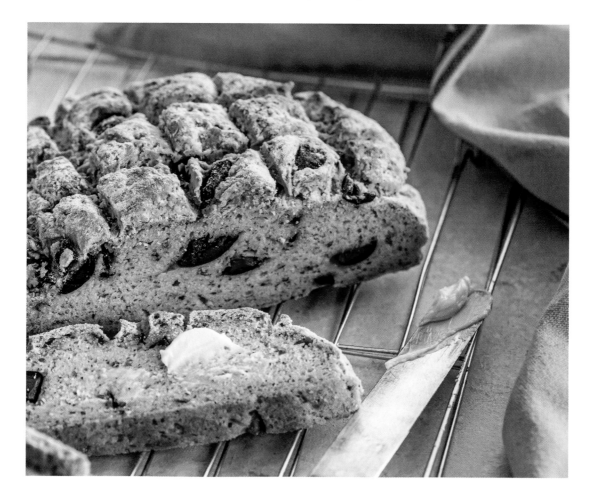

Preheat the oven to 400°F.

Line a baking sheet with parchment paper and drizzle with a small amount of olive oil.

In a small bowl, whisk the flaxseeds with the hot water and set aside.

In a large bowl, combine the brown rice flour, white rice flour, arrowroot flour, baking powder, baking soda, xanthan gum, and salt.

In a medium bowl, combine the room temperature water, olive oil, maple syrup, lemon juice, and olives. Mix in the flaxseed slurry.

Add the wet ingredients to the dry and stir to combine.

Heap the dough on the baking sheet and gently mold into a 7-inch-diameter dome. If the dough sticks to your hands, wet your fingers and continue shaping it. Sift a light dusting of rice flour on top of the loaf. With a sharp knife, slash a diagonal grid pattern on top of the loaf, making five ½-inch-deep cuts each way. Wipe the knife between cuts.

Bake until brown and crusty, 35 to 40 minutes. Cool before slicing.

Keep in an airtight container for up to 3 days. If freezing, slice and wrap each slice in parchment paper. Keep frozen for no longer than 3 months.

ANTI-CANDIDA *Eat only after the first 4 weeks of the anti-Candida diet. Replace maple syrup with six drops of liquid stevia. Limit to one slice every other day.*

LOW FODMAP *If you have SIBO, limit to one slice per day or omit.*

MAKES 1 loaf

PREP TIME 20 minutes

COOKING TIME 40 minutes

EQUIPMENT Parchment paper

2 tablespoons ground flaxseeds

⅓ cup hot filtered water

¾ cup brown rice flour

½ cup white rice flour

⅔ cup arrowroot or tapioca flour

1 teaspoon baking powder

½ teaspoon baking soda

1 teaspoon xanthan gum (optional)

1 teaspoon sea salt

⅔ cup room temperature filtered water

3 tablespoons extra virgin olive oil

1 tablespoon Grade B maple syrup or raw honey

1 teaspoon freshly squeezed lemon juice

12 pitted Kalamata olives, coarsely chopped

Pomegranate Crackers (Progesterone Boosters)

Estrogen balancing, rich in fiber

The sesame and sunflower seeds in these crackers can bring up your progesterone levels, which helps menstruating and menopausal women alike. Eat one 2 × 2-inch cracker per day as part of the Seed Rotation Method (page 104).

If using the oven method for baking, keep the oven temperature in the ideal range of 120°F to 150°F by leaving the oven door ajar or even wide open (most ovens do not offer temperatures lower than 150°F). This will prevent the crackers from burning and will create air circulation to dry them.

MAKES Twenty 2 × 2-inch crackers

SOAKING TIME 15 minutes

PREP TIME 15 minutes

DEHYDRATION TIME 2½ to 3 hours (oven method), 8 hours (dehydration method)

EQUIPMENT Thermometer and 17 x 13-inch baking tray (for oven method), dehydrator (for dehydration method), parchment paper, whisk

PALEO

LOW FODMAP *Replace the pomegranate molasses with maple syrup, coconut nectar, or blackstrap molasses. Replace the dried cherries with unsweetened cranberries.*

In a medium bowl, whisk the chia seeds in the hot water and soak for 15 minutes or until the seeds form a gelatinous mixture.

If using the oven method, preheat the oven to the lowest temperature possible, not higher than 150°F.

In a large bowl, combine the hazelnuts, sunflower seeds, sesame seeds, cranberries, pomegranate molasses, cardamom powder, and salt. Mix in the chia mixture until well combined.

OVEN METHOD

Line the baking tray with parchment paper and spread the mixture evenly, about ¼ inch in thickness. Place the thermometer in the oven to monitor the temperature.

Place the baking tray on one of the upper racks of the oven and bake for 2½ to 3 hours or until fully dried. Check the thermometer regularly to make sure the oven temperature does not rise above 150°F and the crackers don't burn.

Cut the crackers into squares and cool until hardened, about 2 hours, before storing.

DEHYDRATION METHOD

Spread the cracker mixture on dehydrator trays, about ¼ inch in thickness.

Dehydrate for 4 hours at 120°F, then cut into squares, turn over, and dehydrate for another 4 hours at 120°F.

Keep in an airtight container at room temperature for up to 2 weeks.

⅓ cup chia seeds

¾ cup hot water

1 cup raw chopped hazelnuts or spouted almonds

1 cup raw ground sunflower seeds, lightly packed

1 cup raw ground sesame seeds, lightly packed

½ cup unsweetened dried cranberries or dried tart cherries

½ cup pomegranate molasses

2 teaspoons cardamom powder

½ teaspoon sea salt

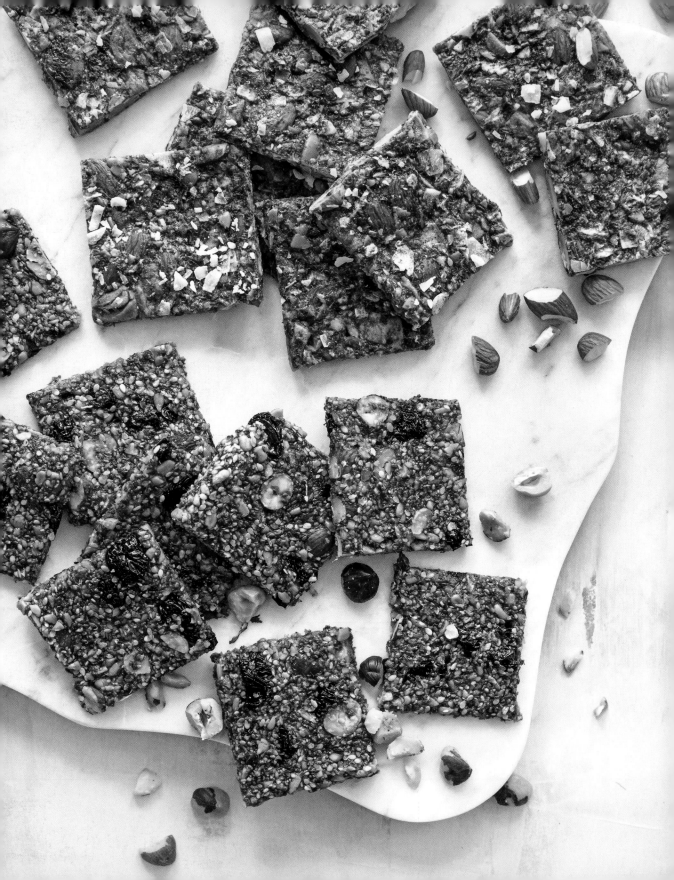

Flaxseed Crackers (Estrogen Boosters)

Estrogen balancing, rich in fiber

Try the Seed Rotation Method (page 104) by adding flaxseeds and pumpkin seeds to your diet to rebalance your estrogen levels. Eat one 2 × 2-inch cracker per day for the first 14 days of your cycle. If you have a sensitivity to nuts, omit the almonds. I use sprouted almonds for better digestibility, but if you can't find them at your local health store, presoak the almonds for 12 hours before starting the recipe.

If using the oven method, keep the oven temperature in the ideal range of 120°F to 150°F by leaving the oven door ajar or even wide open (most ovens do not offer temperatures lower than 150°F). This will prevent the crackers from burning and will create air circulation to dry them.

MAKES Twenty 2 × 2-inch crackers

SOAKING TIME 15 minutes

PREP TIME 15 minutes

DEHYDRATION TIME 2½ to 3 hours (oven method), 8 hours (dehydration method)

EQUIPMENT Thermometer and 17 x 13-inch baking tray (for oven method), dehydrator (for dehydration method), parchment paper, whisk

PALEO

ANTI-CANDIDA Replace the dried apples with ½ cup pitted Kalamata olives.

LOW FODMAP Replace the dried apples with 1 cup of dried bananas. Limit to no more than two crackers per day.

1 cup ground flaxseed, lightly packed

1 cup hot water

1 cup raw chopped sprouted almonds

1 cup raw ground pumpkin seeds, lightly packed

½ cup dried apples, coarsely chopped

1 cup coconut flakes

1 tablespoon apple cider vinegar

1 tablespoon Garam Masala (page 177)

1 teaspoon sea salt

In a medium bowl whisk the flaxseed with the water and let it rest for 15 minutes.

If using the oven method, preheat the oven to the lowest temperature possible, not higher than 150°F.

In a large bowl, combine the almonds, pumpkin seeds, apples, coconut flakes, cider vinegar, garam masala, and salt. Mix in the flaxseed mixture until well combined.

OVEN METHOD

Line the baking tray with parchment paper and spread the mixture evenly, about ¼ inch in thickness. Place the thermometer in the oven to monitor the temperature.

Place the baking tray on one of the upper racks of the oven and bake for 2½ to 3 hours or until fully dried. Check the thermometer regularly to make sure the oven temperature does not rise above 150°F and the crackers don't burn.

Cut the crackers into squares and cool until hardened, about 2 hours, before storing.

DEHYDRATION METHOD

Spread the cracker mixture on dehydrator trays, about ¼ inch in thickness.

Dehydrate for 4 hours at 120°F, then cut into squares, turn over, and dehydrate for another 4 hours at 120°F.

Keep in an airtight container at room temperature for up to 2 weeks.

Grain-Free Sourdough Flatbread

Estrogen balancing, rich in fiber and proteins

This simple recipe of a spongy, satisfying flatbread is a great substitute for focaccia. The sourdough develops through fermentation and naturally raises the bread without the need for yeast or baking powder. I get the best sourdough when fermenting it at a consistent room temperature of 75°F for 12 to 24 hours or until the batter thickens and starts to bubble. A practical tip: On cooler days, leave the batter in a warm place, such as in an oven with the light on or under a microwave light, to achieve a consistent temperature of 75°F.

In a large bowl, mix chickpea flour and water to form a smooth batter. Cover with a cloth and let it sit on the kitchen counter for 12 to 24 hours, or until it becomes thick and bubbly.

Preheat the oven to 400°F.

Whisk the olive oil, rosemary, and salt into the chickpea batter.

Line the baking pan with parchment paper and grease it with a small amount of olive oil.

Bake for 40 minutes or until the top becomes solid and a toothpick comes out clean.

Remove the bread from the pan by lifting the sides of the parchment paper. Let it cool before slicing and serving. It's best served warm with a dollop of Whipped Herbal Butter (page 173) or a drizzle of olive oil.

Cool completely and then store in an airtight container at room temperature for up to 3 days.

SERVES 6 to 8

FERMENTATION TIME
12 to 24 hours

PREP TIME 10 minutes

COOKING TIME 50 minutes

EQUIPMENT 9 × 5¾ × 2-inch baking pan, parchment paper

2 cups sprouted or regular chickpea flour

2½ cups filtered water

2 tablespoons olive oil

1 teaspoon dried rosemary

½ teaspoon sea salt

Coconut Banana Bread (Grain-Free)

Gut healing, estrogen balancing, rich in prebiotics

Going grain-free can be challenging when you crave comfort food from your "previous life." But this hearty, dense bread, which is rich in nutrients, will hit the spot. Tigernut flour, available now in many health stores or online, is very high in fiber and prebiotics. Bananas add a good dose of vitamin B6, which helps mitigate PMS symptoms, high cholesterol, and homocysteine levels (an inflammation marker in the body).

MAKES 1 loaf

SERVES 8

PREP TIME 20 minutes

COOKING TIME 50 minutes

EQUIPMENT Hand mixer, or food processor or blender, 9 × 5 × 2½-inch baking pan, parchment paper

PALEO

LOW FODMAP According to several flour manufacturers, tigernut flour is low in FODMAPs but it has not been tested by Monagh University, developer of the Low FODMAP diet.

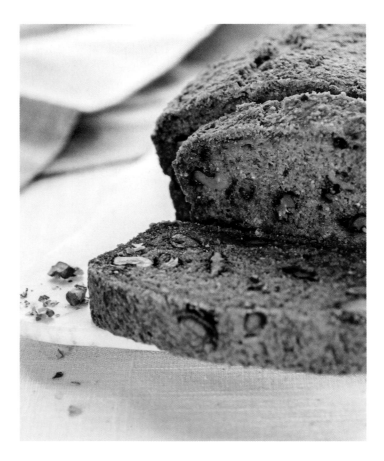

Preheat the oven to 350°F.

In a small bowl, combine the psyllium husk and water and set aside to thicken.

In a large bowl cream the bananas, coconut oil, vanilla, grated orange peel, orange juice, salt, and the psyllium husk slurry with a hand mixer. You can also use a food processor or a high-speed blender. (If using a food processor or a high-speed blender, transfer the mixture to a large bowl when done).

Stir in the tigernut flour, arrowroot flour, baking powder, baking soda, cinnamon, and walnuts. Mix with your hands until well combined.

Line the baking pan with parchment paper and grease it with olive oil. Transfer the flour mixture to the baking pan and bake for 50 minutes or until a toothpick inserted in the center comes out clean.

Keeps well in an airtight container, at room temperature, for up to 5 days. If freezing, slice the bread and wrap each slice in parchment paper. Keep frozen for no longer than 3 months.

1½ tablespoons psyllium husk flakes (not powder)

⅔ cup hot water

3 medium-size ripe bananas, peeled and cut into chunks

⅓ cup melted coconut oil

1 tablespoon pure vanilla extract

Freshly grated peel of 1 orange

2 tablespoons freshly squeezed orange juice

½ teaspoon sea salt

2 cups tigernut flour

1 cup arrowroot flour

1 teaspoon baking powder

1 teaspoon baking soda

½ tablespoon ground cinnamon

½ cup chopped raw walnuts (optional)

Seed Bread with Figs

Liver detoxing, estrogen balancing, progesterone boosting

Unrefined grains and whole nuts and seeds create a hearty, wholesome bread. Pumpkin seeds and flaxseeds help rebalance estrogen levels, and the sesame and sunflower seeds support progesterone production, so it's a particularly good idea to eat this bread to rebalance your cycle or your estrogen levels if you are going through perimenopause or menopause.

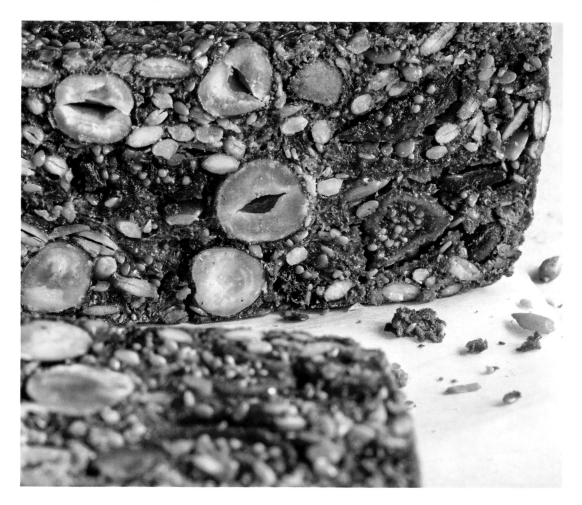

Preheat the oven to 325°F.

Line the loaf pan with parchment paper.

In a large bowl, combine all of the ingredients. The batter will be very liquid.

Pour the batter into the loaf pan. Bake for 45 minutes, or until the top of the loaf is slightly firm.

Remove the bread loaf from the oven. Lifting the parchment paper from the sides, remove the loaf from the pan and transfer it to the baking tray, with the top down on the baking tray. Bake for another 45 minutes or until the bread loaf sounds hollow when tapped. Cool on a wire rack.

Slice and serve with your favorite toppings. It's best when toasted.

The bread keeps well in the refrigerator for up to 10 days. Slice it before freezing. It keeps well for up to 6 months in the freezer.

ANTI-CANDIDA *Avoid for the first 4 weeks of the anti-Candida diet. Omit the figs and the molasses. Limit to one slice per day.*

LOW FODMAP *Replace the molasses with maple syrup. Omit the figs. If you have SIBO, limit to one slice every other day or omit.*

MAKES 1 loaf of 10 to 12 slices

PREP TIME 20 minutes

COOKING TIME 1 hour 15 minutes

EQUIPMENT 9 × 5-inch loaf pan, parchment paper, baking tray

1½ cups rolled oats

1½ cups filtered water

½ cup sunflower seeds

½ cup sesame seeds

½ cup pumpkin seeds

½ cup dried figs, coarsely chopped

½ cup whole hazelnuts

⅓ cup teff flour or brown rice flour

¼ cup chia seeds

4 tablespoons whole psyllium husk

3 tablespoons ghee or lard, melted

1 tablespoon blackstrap molasses

1 teaspoon sea salt

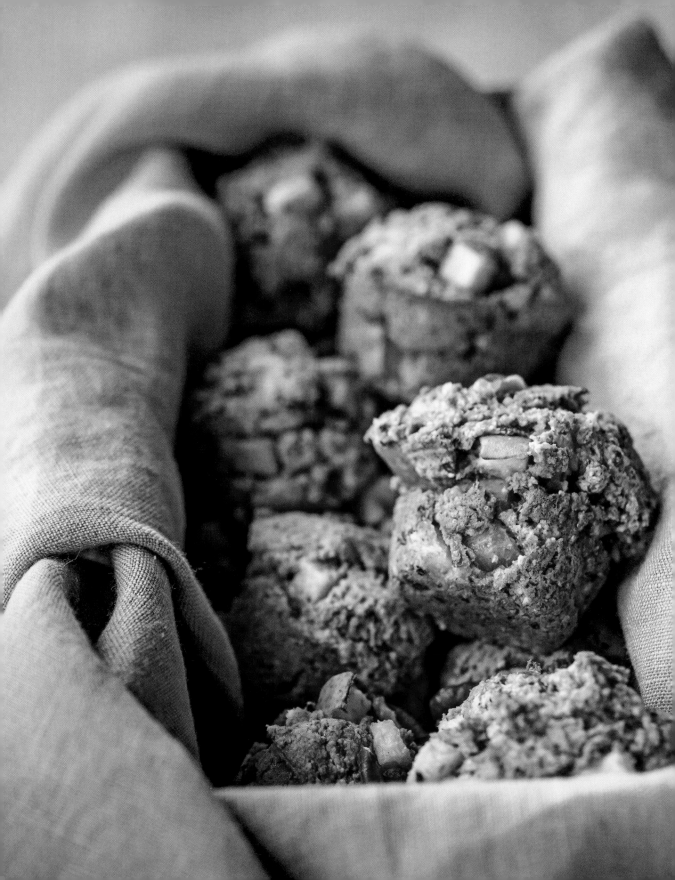

Rosemary Pear Muffins

Low in sugar, rich in fiber and prebiotics

The Spice Bible by Jane Lawson is one of my favorite culinary books, and I turn to it again and again when I'm developing new recipes and flavor combinations. Her book inspired me to pair pears with rosemary and orange. Tigernut flour is high in prebiotics and fiber. Even though tigernuts are called nuts, they are a tuber, so people with nut allergies can safely eat them. You can replace tigernut flour with the same amount of almond flour, plus add 2 tablespoons maple syrup.

Preheat the oven to 350°F.

In a small bowl, whisk together the ground flaxseeds and water and set aside.

In a medium bowl, mix together the tigernut flour, salt, baking soda, and rosemary.

In another medium bowl, whisk together the olive oil, grated orange peel, and orange juice. Mix in the flaxseed slurry.

Add the wet ingredients to the dry ingredients and stir to combine.

Fold in the pears and pecans.

Grease each muffin cup with a small amount of olive oil and fill it with about 1½ tablespoons batter.

Bake for 25 minutes or until the muffin tops are firm and brown.

Store in an airtight container at room temperature or the refrigerator for up to 3 days.

MAKES 20 mini-muffins
PREP TIME 15 minutes
COOKING TIME 20 minutes
EQUIPMENT 24-cup mini-muffin pan

3 tablespoons ground flaxseeds

½ cup hot water

2 cups tigernut flour

½ teaspoon sea salt

½ teaspoon baking soda

2 teaspoons finely chopped fresh rosemary or ¾ teaspoon finely chopped dried rosemary

¼ cup plus 1 tablespoon unrefined extra virgin olive oil

Freshly grated peel of ½ orange

2 tablespoons freshly squeezed orange juice

1 ripe green Anjou pear, cored and finely chopped

¼ cup chopped raw pecans

PALEO

Red Velvet Grain-Free Brownies

Liver detoxing, low in sugar, rich in magnesium

These moist brownies are packed with nutrients from the grated beets. It might seem odd to be adding beets to a brownie recipe, but trust me, you won't taste them and they will turn the brownies into a rich, velvety treat. Everyone will love them and ask for seconds. Be sure to grate the beets finely so you don't notice them when devouring the brownies.

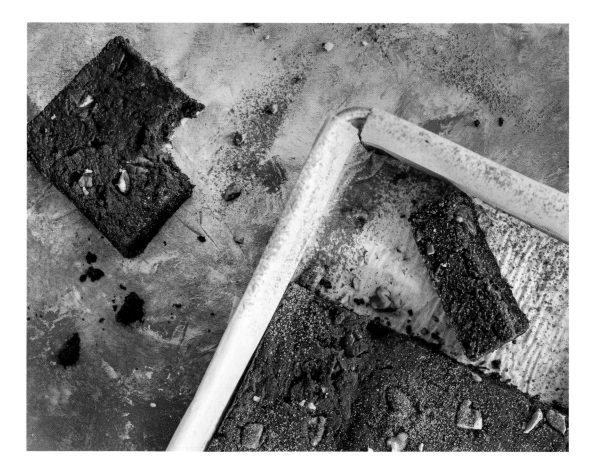

Preheat the oven to 350°F.

Whisk the flaxseeds and water in a small bowl and set aside.

Grease the baking pan with a small amount of coconut oil. If using an aluminum pan, line the baking pan with parchment paper.

In a large bowl, combine the flour, cacao powder, baking powder, and salt.

In another large bowl, add the beets, coconut oil, sugar, applesauce, vanilla extract, and flaxseed slurry and whisk until well combined.

Add the wet ingredients to the dry ingredients and stir, using your hands to combine. Fold in the pecans.

Spread the batter in the baking pan and bake until a toothpick inserted in the center comes out clean, 45 to 50 minutes. Cool completely in the pan before removing.

Store the brownies in an airtight container at room temperature for up to 4 days.

MAKES 16 squares

PREP TIME 25 minutes

COOKING TIME 45 minutes

EQUIPMENT 9 × 12 × 2-inch baking pan, whisk

¼ cup ground flaxseeds

⅔ cup hot filtered water

2 cups cassava flour

1⅓ cups raw unsweetened cacao powder

2 teaspoons baking powder

1 teaspoon fine sea salt

1 cup firmly packed peeled and finely grated red beets

1 cup coconut oil, melted

1 cup brown coconut sugar

1⅓ cups applesauce

2 tablespoons organic vanilla extract

½ cup chopped raw pecans

PALEO

AIP If you are sensitive to even a small amount of flaxseed, do not eat these brownies. Each square contains less than a teaspoon of flaxseed, which some people can tolerate. Replace the cacao powder with the same amount of carob powder. Replace the baking powder with an AIP baking powder (page 143).

LOW FODMAP Replace the applesauce with the same amount of pumpkin puree. Limit to one square per day.

Raspberry and Green Tea Lime Melties

Low in sugar, antibacterial, high in good fats

Whether you need a satisfying snack in the evening or a quick dessert for a dinner party, these melties have a good chance of becoming a staple in your house, as they are in mine. Make the meltie base and then choose the raspberry or green tea option.

MAKES 10 melties

PREP TIME 15 minutes

CHILLING TIME 20 minutes

EQUIPMENT Mini-muffin baking cups or molds, whisk

MELTIE BASE

¾ cup coconut butter

1 teaspoon freshly grated lime peel, plus extra to garnish

2 tablespoons freshly squeezed lime juice

1 tablespoon raw honey or coconut syrup

½ teaspoon vanilla extract

3 tablespoons hot melted coconut oil

Pinch of sea salt

10 fresh raspberries (for Raspberry Melties)

1 teaspoon green matcha tea powder (for Green Tea Lime Melties)

In a medium bowl, combine the coconut butter, grated lime peel, lime juice, honey, vanilla extract, coconut oil, and salt and whisk until well combined. The hot coconut oil should soften the coconut butter, but if the coconut butter remains lumpy, microwave the mixture for 20 seconds and whisk again until a smooth paste is formed.

For Raspberry Melties, place one raspberry in each mini-muffin cup and then cover it with slightly less than 1 tablespoon of the meltie base.

For Green Tea Lime Melties, whisk the green tea powder into the meltie base mixture and scoop slightly less than 1 tablespoon into each mini-muffin cup.

Garnish the melties (both kinds) with grated lime peel.

Place in the freezer for 20 minutes or until hardened. Serve chilled.

Keep in an airtight container in the refrigerator for up to 10 days.

PALEO

AIP

ANTI-CANDIDA *Replace the honey with six drops of stevia.*

LOW FODMAP *Replace the honey with coconut nectar or Grade B maple syrup.*

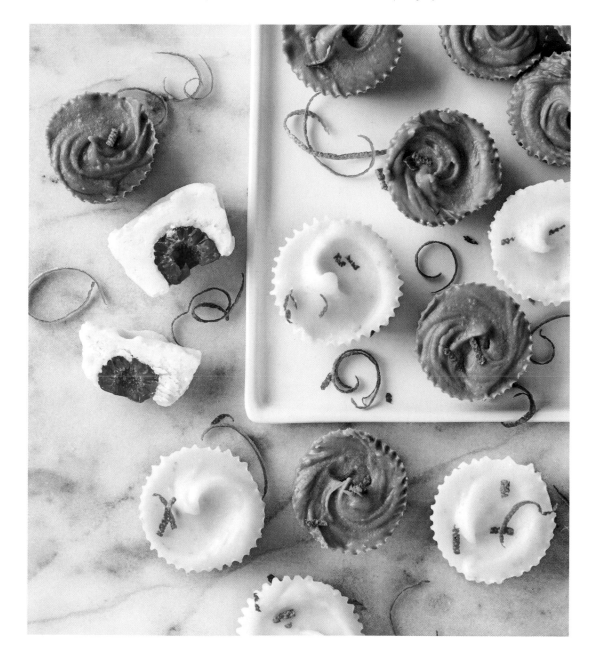

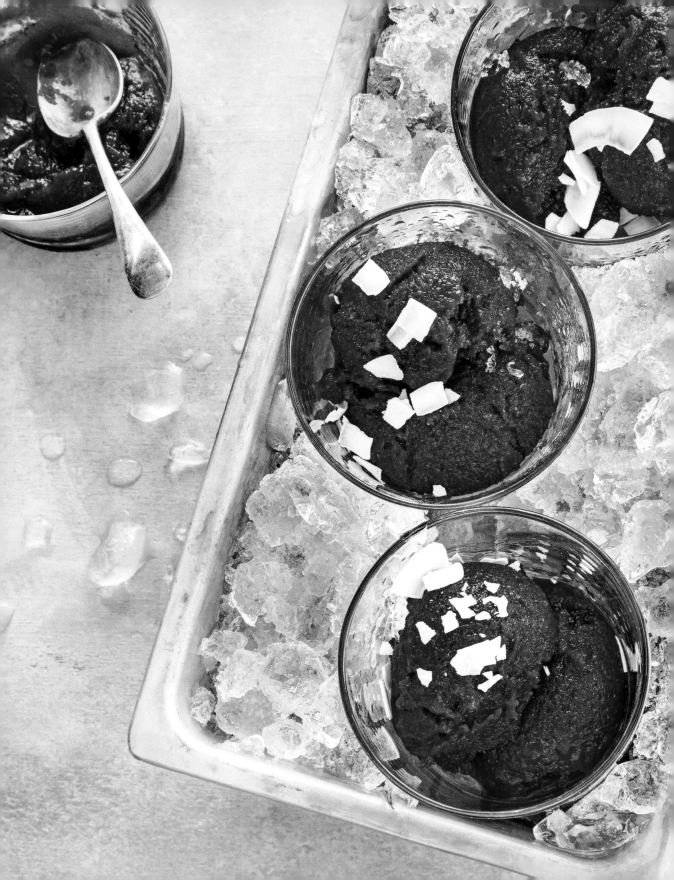

Tart Cherry Sorbet

Low in sugar, anti-inflammatory, high in antioxidants ⏲ Less than 30 minutes

This is a great dessert to cool things down on a hot summer day. I've also made it many times when dessert was an afterthought and managed to impress friends each time. Cherries are high in anthocyanins, which reduce inflammation and can help reduce pain, PMS, and menopause symptoms. Sour cherries (not sweet) are also high in antioxidants such as lutein, zeaxanthin, and beta-carotene.

This sorbet doesn't require an ice cream maker and contains no added sugar. I used star anise, which is an unusual spice, but it pairs well with cherries. Feel free to experiment with any other low-glycemic frozen fruit such as raspberries or blueberries and ground spices such as allspice, nutmeg, or aniseed.

Place the cherries, coconut butter, star anise, and salt in the blender. Blend on high until the sorbet reaches a creamy consistency. Add ¼ cup cold water, or more, if the blades are not blending the fruit.

Ladle into individual ramekins and sprinkle with coconut flakes. Serve immediately.

PALEO

AIP Replace star anise with ½ teaspoon ground cinnamon.

ANTI-CANDIDA Limit to ¼ cup per serving no more than twice per week, or replace the cherries with frozen blueberries.

SERVES 4

PREP TIME 15 minutes

EQUIPMENT High-speed electric blender

3 cups frozen sour cherries (sweet cherries will do as well)

¼ cup coconut butter

1 teaspoon ground star anise

Pinch of sea salt

Roasted unsweetened coconut flakes, to garnish

Creamy Lime Pudding

Sugar-free, rich in copper, magnesium, and zinc

It is very easy to get addicted to this decadent dessert, but it's best to exercise moderation, as cashews can strain the digestive system when consumed too often. Soaking the nuts helps to achieve a creamy consistency, and the salt brings out the sweetness of the cashews and the coconut butter. I encourage you to add rose water and rose petals for a uniquely Middle Eastern accent. This pudding is very rich; the serving sizes are small but highly satisfying.

SERVES 4

SOAKING TIME 15 minutes

PREP TIME 15 minutes

SETTING TIME 1 hour

EQUIPMENT High-speed electric blender, four small dessert bowls or cups

2 cups raw cashews

1 quart boiling filtered water

⅔ cup filtered water, lukewarm, or more if needed

⅓ cup coconut butter

Freshly grated peel of 2 limes

1½ tablespoons freshly squeezed lime juice

2 teaspoons vanilla extract

10 drops liquid stevia

Dash of sea salt

¾ teaspoon rose water (optional)

Rose petals, optional, for garnish

In a large glass bowl, cover the cashews with the hot water and soak for 15 minutes. Strain the cashews and discard the water.

Add the cashews and all of the remaining ingredients to the blender. Blend for 2 minutes or until the mixture reaches a creamy and silky consistency. If the mixture is too thick, add 2 tablespoons water at a time and process until the desired consistency is reached.

Pour into the serving bowls and place in the refrigerator until set, about 1 hour. Serve chilled. Garnish with rose petals.

PALEO
ANTI-CANDIDA

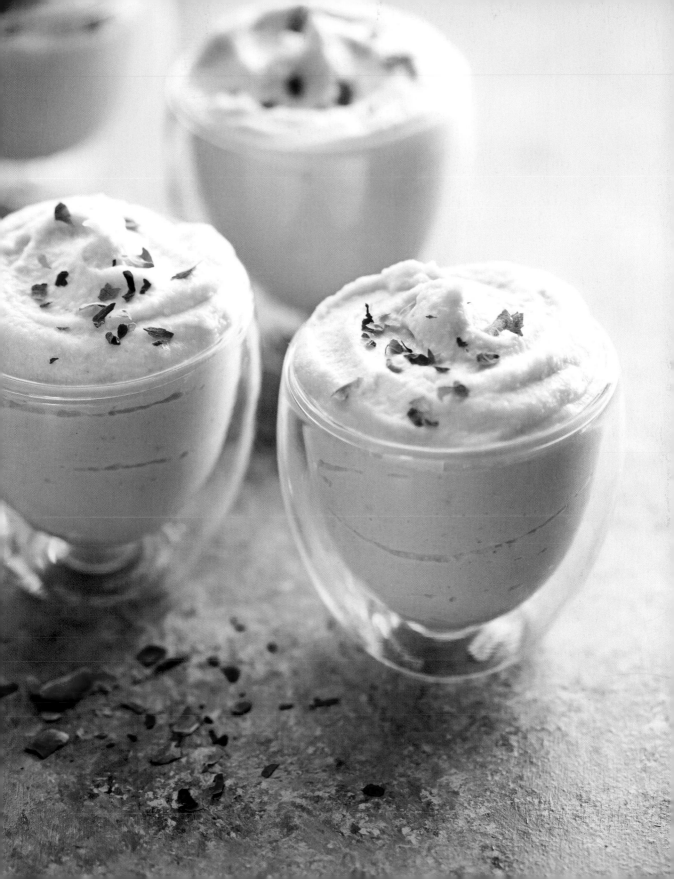

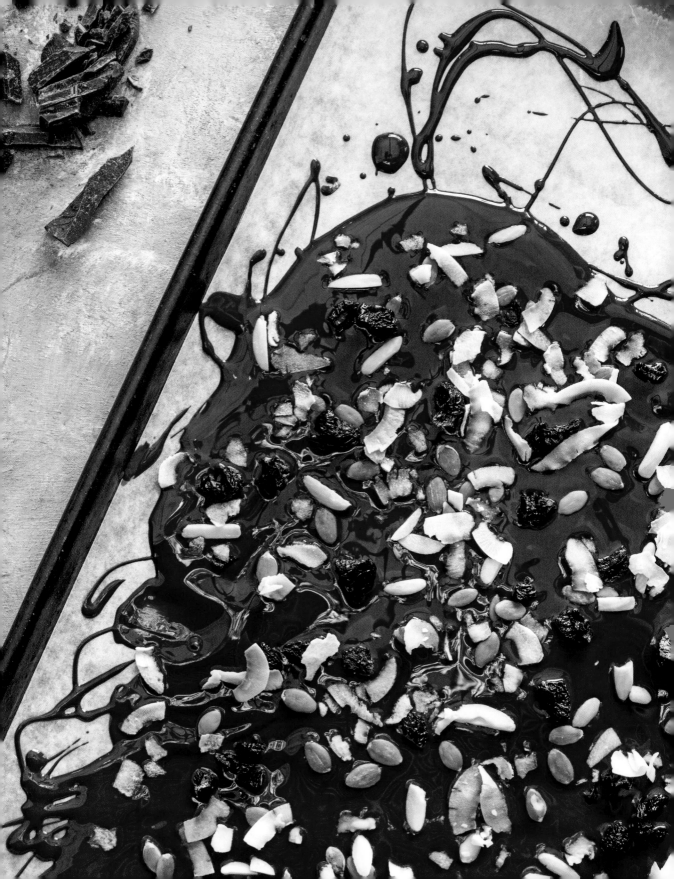

Crunchy Chocolate Cherry Bark

Rich in magnesium, fiber, and antioxidants

Turn the nutritional goodness of dark chocolate into a crunchy snack by adding your favorite dried fruit, nuts, and berries.

Line the baking tray with the parchment paper.

Melt the chocolate and macadamia oil in a double boiler, stirring frequently. Or, if using a microwave, set the timer for 20 seconds and then remove and stir. Repeat until fully melted (this will prevent the chocolate from burning), about two more times.

Pour the chocolate mixture onto the parchment paper and spread in a ⅛-inch-thick layer.

Immediately sprinkle with the cherries, coconut chips, almonds, pumpkin seeds, and salt flakes.

Chill in the refrigerator until hardened, about 30 minutes.

To serve, break into rough pieces.

Keeps well in an airtight container in the refrigerator for up to 2 months.

MAKES 10 pieces

PREP TIME 15 minutes

CHILLING TIME 30 minutes

EQUIPMENT Baking tray, parchment paper

1 cup shredded 85 percent dark chocolate, about 3½ ounces

1 teaspoon macadamia oil or coconut oil

2 tablespoons chopped dried unsweetened cherries

2 tablespoons unsweetened coconut chips

1 tablespoon raw or toasted almond slivers

1 tablespoon raw pumpkin seeds

Sea salt flakes

PALEO

AIP Replace the chocolate by combining ¾ cup melted cacao butter with ¼ cup carob powder. Replace the almonds and pumpkin seeds with the same amount of AIP-compliant dried fruit such as bananas, strawberries, or apricots.

LOW FODMAP Replace the cherries with dried blueberries.

Dinner-Stealing Pear and Orange Cobbler

Rich in fiber, antioxidant, anti-inflammatory

My good friend Sukaynah threw a big dinner party and told me afterwards that nobody commented on any of her dishes except for this cobbler. This recipe is versatile—use fruit that you like, that is in season, or that is in abundance in your garden or at the farmers' market. I often make this cobbler using 1 to 1½ pounds of any of these combinations: mixed berries, peaches and apricots, persimmons and pomegranate, or strawberry and mint. If using frozen fruit, let it thaw before baking. Create a signature cobbler that steals the show at your next dinner party!

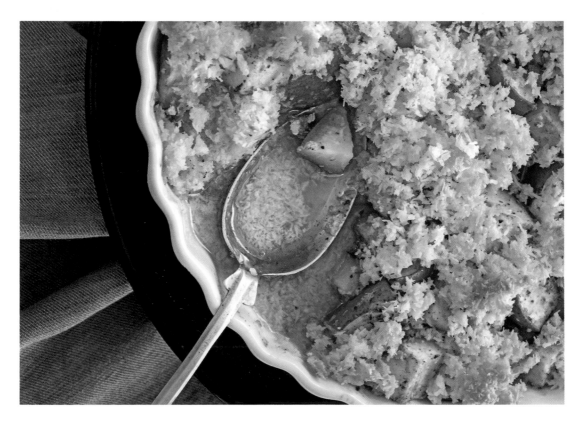

Preheat the oven to 350°F.

Grease the baking pie dish with coconut oil.

In a large bowl, toss all of the filling ingredients until well combined. Transfer to the baking dish and distribute evenly.

In a spice grinder, pulse the shredded coconut until it has the consistency of flour.

In a medium bowl, mix all the topping ingredients using your hands until a crumble is formed.

Spread the crumble evenly on top of the fruit.

Bake for 35 to 40 minutes or until the topping is brown.

Ladle onto individual plates and top with chilled coconut cream.

If using the cast iron skillet, transfer any leftovers to a glass container within 2 hours of baking. (Cast iron can leach iron into the food.)

Keeps well in the refrigerator for up to 4 days.

PALEO

AIP Replace star anise with 2 teaspoons ground cinnamon.

LOW FODMAP Replace the pears with 1 to 1½ pounds strawberries and/or blueberries.

SERVES 4 to 6

PREP TIME 20 minutes

COOKING TIME 40 minutes

EQUIPMENT 9½-inch baking pie dish or 10-inch cast iron skillet, spice grinder or high-speed electric blender

FILLING

4 ripe Anjou or Bosc pears, finely chopped

Freshly grated peel of 1 orange

2 tablespoons freshly squeezed orange juice

½ tablespoon vanilla extract or powder

2 teaspoons ground star anise

2 teaspoons arrowroot flour

Dash of sea salt

TOPPING

1 cup unsweetened shredded coconut flakes

½ cup ghee or coconut oil, melted

½ cup arrowroot flour

1 tablespoon Grade B maple syrup

½ tablespoon vanilla extract

Dash of sea salt

Whipped Coconut Cream (page 166) (optional)

Kudzu Calming Pudding

Sugar balancing, mitigates menopause symptoms ⏱ Less than 30 minutes

One of the reasons we wake in the middle of the night is because of fluctuating blood sugar levels. Kudzu, a root used in Chinese medicine as a calming and sleeping aid, balances blood sugar levels. It is also high in quercetin (which reduces inflammation and histamine release) and isoflavones (which reduce symptoms of perimenopause and menopause). Kudzu is available in most health stores or online. Rebecca Katz, a fabulous chef who also uses food as medicine, inspired this recipe.

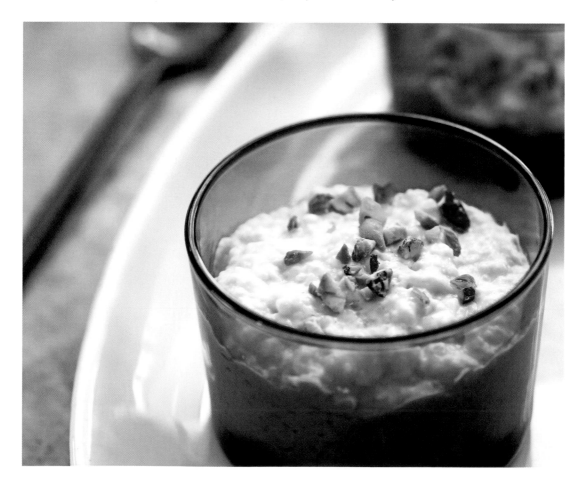

Crush the kudzu powder in a mortar and pestle, or use a bowl and spoon to remove all of the lumps.

In a small bowl, whisk the kudzu into ½ cup coconut milk and set it aside. Whisk the mixture once in a while.

Pour the rest of the coconut milk into a heavy-bottomed saucepan, and mix in the maple syrup, grated lime peel, lime juice, vanilla extract, stevia, rose water, and salt. Bring to a simmer over medium heat.

Whisk in the kudzu mixture and continue simmering until the pudding thickens, about 3 minutes, stirring constantly.

Pour into individual ramekins and let cool. The pudding will continue to thicken as it cools. If not serving the pudding right away, cover the ramekins with plastic wrap, pressing it down to the surface of the pudding before refrigerating.

To serve, garnish with pistachios.

Keeps well in the refrigerator for up to 3 days.

PALEO

AIP Omit the pistachios.

ANTI-CANDIDA Replace the maple syrup with six to ten drops of liquid stevia.

LOW FODMAP Replace the pistachios with pecans or pumpkin seeds.

SERVES 2 to 4

PREP TIME 10 minutes

COOKING TIME 5 minutes

EQUIPMENT Heavy-bottomed saucepan, mortar and pestle or bowl and spoon, whisk

3 tablespoons kudzu powder

1 13.66-ounce can full-fat coconut milk

2 tablespoons Grade B maple syrup

1 tablespoon freshly grated lime peel

2 tablespoons freshly squeezed lime juice

1 teaspoon vanilla extract

4 drops stevia

½ teaspoon rose water (optional)

¼ teaspoon sea salt

Raw pistachio nuts, crushed, for garnish

Strawberry and Lime Jelly Mousse

Gut healing, low in sugar, rich in potassium

This is a delightfully refreshing dessert with no added sugar that kids devour in no time. An added benefit: Gelatin helps gut healing, skin elasticity, and nail and hair growth. Create your own signature creamy jellies using your favorite fruit. I've had lots of success in creating a banana, coconut milk, and chocolate jelly mousse or an orange and mandarin jelly made with freshly squeezed juice. Fruits that won't set are kiwi, pineapple, papaya, and figs. If your strawberries are very tart, add a few more drops of stevia to sweeten the mousse.

SERVES 4 to 6

PREP TIME 20 minutes

CHILLING TIME 4 hours

EQUIPMENT High-speed electric blender or food processor, whisk

1 pound fresh strawberries, stemmed

1 ripe banana, peeled and chopped

½ cup full-fat coconut milk

1 tablespoon freshly grated ginger root

Freshly grated peel of 1 lime

20 drops liquid stevia (optional)

½ cup hot filtered water

1¾ tablespoons unflavored gelatin

PALEO

AIP

ANTI-CANDIDA *Replace the banana with an extra ½ cup chopped strawberries and limit to one serving per week.*

LOW FODMAP

Add the strawberries, banana, coconut milk, ginger, grated lime peel, and stevia to the blender and puree until silky smooth, about 1 minute.

Transfer to a saucepan and heat the mixture until very warm but not yet boiling.

In a small saucepan, bring the water to a boil. Remove from the heat and gradually whisk in the gelatin until fully dissolved.

Slowly whisk the gelatin mixture into the strawberry mixture. If lumps are formed, transfer to the blender and puree until well combined.

Pour into individual ramekins and transfer to the refrigerator until set, about 4 hours.

Keeps well in the refrigerator for up to 4 days. If not serving the mousse soon after chilling, cover the ramekins with plastic wrap.

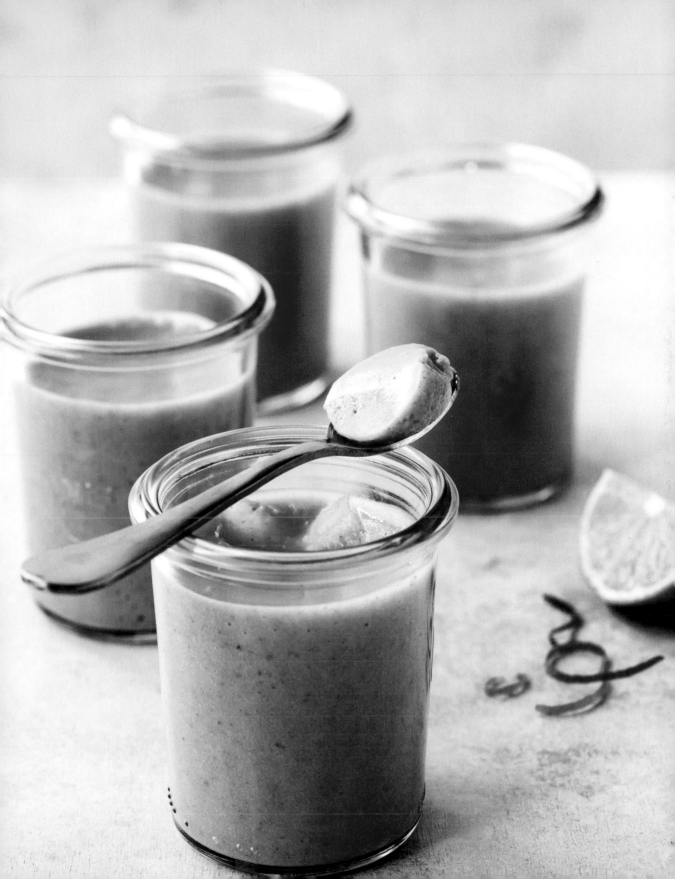

Stuffed Baked Apples

Gut healing, rich in prebiotics, rich in fiber

Living in a communist country during the 1980s meant limited food options, and many cooks had to get creative to satisfy a sweet tooth. My mom would carve out the core of an apple and bake the apple with a touch of honey for dessert. During Christmas in Poland, it is a tradition to add nuts and poppy seeds to baked apples. Those flavors are my inspiration for this recipe. Golden Delicious apples are my favorite as they become custard-like when baked.

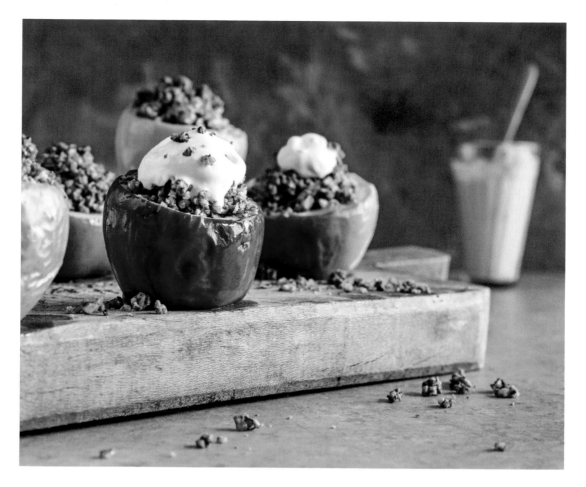

Preheat the oven to 375°F.

Scoop out the core of each apple, creating a cavity, without cutting to the bottom.

Place the pecans, poppy seeds, coconut oil, maple syrup, cinnamon, orange peel, and salt in the blender and pulse until a runny paste forms and the pecans are still in chunks.

Grease each apple with a small amount of coconut oil and place in the muffin pan indents. Place the muffin pan on top of a baking tray to catch the oozing juices when baking. If not using a muffin pan, line the baking tray with parchment paper and slice the bottom of each apple to ensure that it stands firmly on the baking tray.

Fill each apple with the nut and seed mixture.

Bake for 20 to 25 minutes or until the apple skins start to break open. (Granny Smith apples might need as long as 35 minutes.)

Cool for 15 minutes. Serve with a dollop of coconut cream on the side.

Keeps well covered in the refrigerator for up to 5 days.

PALEO

ANTI-CANDIDA *Use Granny Smith apples. Replace the maple syrup with twenty drops of stevia.*

MAKES 6 apples

PREP TIME 30 minutes

COOKING TIME 25 minutes

EQUIPMENT High-speed electric blender or food processor, muffin pan, baking tray, parchment paper

6 Granny Smith, Honey Crisp, or Golden Delicious raw apples

1 cup whole raw pecans or walnuts

½ cup poppy seeds

¼ cup melted coconut oil

2 tablespoons Grade B maple syrup

1 tablespoon ground cinnamon

1 tablespoon orange peel powder or freshly grated peel of 1 orange

¼ teaspoon sea salt

Whipped Coconut Cream (page 166) (optional)

Digestive Truffles—Two Ways

Gut healing, liver detoxing, rich in fiber

Have you gone to an Indian restaurant and been offered fennel seed, aniseed, or cumin seed after a meal? These herbs are wonderful digestive aids. Serving them in this bite-size dessert is the perfect way to end a dinner party and leave your guests with happy tummies. If you prefer stronger flavors, double the amount of spices used in these recipes. You can make orange peel powder by saving, drying, and grinding orange skins. Otherwise, get it online.

MAKES 16 truffles per recipe

PREP TIME 20 minutes

CHILLING TIME 1 hour

EQUIPMENT Food processor

Place all of the truffle mixture ingredients in the food processor and blend until smooth. Add 1 tablespoon more of coconut oil at a time if the mixture is not smooth.

Scatter the coating ingredient on a flat plate.

Scoop out 1 tablespoon truffle mixture, roll it in your hands to form a ball, and then roll it in the coating.

Place in the refrigerator for 1 hour to harden.

Keeps well in an airtight container in the refrigerator for up to 1 month.

PALEO

LOW FODMAP Replace cherries with dried blueberries.

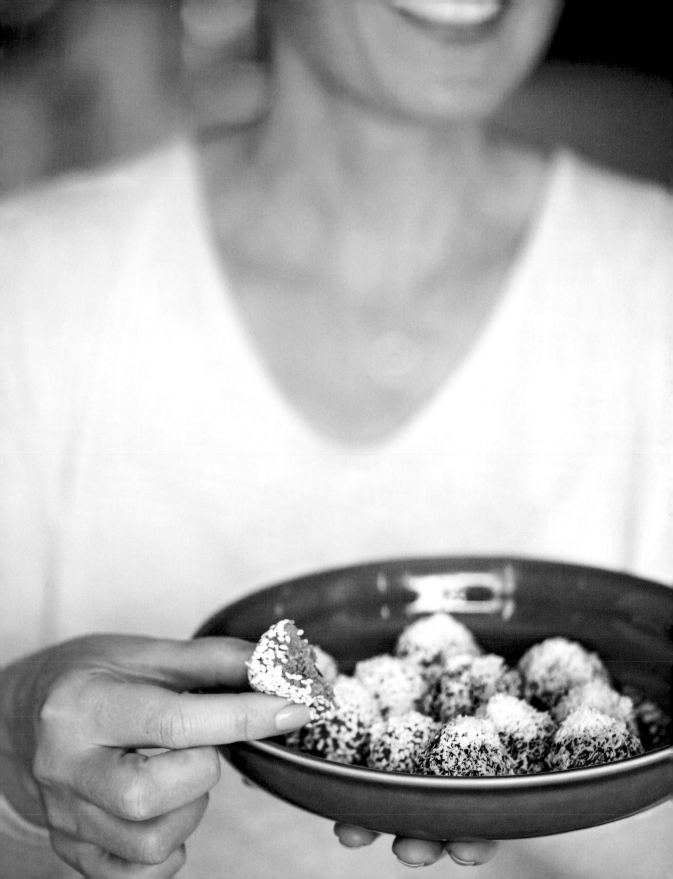

Ginger Orange Truffles

TRUFFLE MIXTURE

¾ cup coarsely chopped candied ginger

¾ cup raw tahini (ground sesame paste)

2 tablespoons coconut oil

2 tablespoons whole fennel seed, ground

2 tablespoons whole aniseed, ground

3 tablespoons orange peel powder

Dash of fine sea salt

COATING

⅓ cup white or black sesame seeds

Cherry Chocolate Truffles

TRUFFLE MIXTURE

⅔ cup sweetened dried cherries, coarsely chopped

¼ cup raw unsweetened cacao powder

⅔ cup coconut butter

2 tablespoons whole fennel seed, ground

2 tablespoons whole aniseed, ground

2 tablespoons melted coconut oil, or more if needed

2 tablespoons Grade B maple syrup

2 tablespoons vanilla extract

Dash of fine sea salt

COATING

⅓ cup unsweetened shredded coconut flakes

Notes

CHAPTER 1

25 *Synthetic estrogen, like Premarin and progestin . . .* Leif Bergkvist, Hans-Olov Adami, Ingemar Persson, et al., "The Risk of Breast Cancer after Estrogen and Estrogen–Progestin Replacement," *New England Journal of Medicine* 321 (1989): 293–97; Rowan T. Chlebowski, Garnet L. Anderson, Margery Gass, et al., "Estrogen Plus Progestin and Breast Cancer Incidence and Mortality in Postmenopausal Women," *JAMA* 304, no. 15 (2010): 1684–92.

26 *According to Dr. Michael Breus . . .* Michael J. Breus, "Why a Woman's Sleep Is Different from a Man's," Huffpost, June 13, 2011, http://www.huffingtonpost.com/dr-michael-j-breus/woman-sleep-different-than-man_b_875285.html.

27 *Research shows that sleep-deprived people . . .* Stephanie M. Greer, Andrea N. Goldstein, and Matthew P. Walker, "The Impact of Sleep Deprivation on Food Desire in the Human Brain," *Nature Communications* 4 (August 6, 2013), https://www.nature.com/articles/ncomms3259.

CHAPTER 2

32 *People who suffer from chronic digestive issues . . .* Lance M. Siegel, Peter D. Stevens, Charles J. Lightdale, et al., "Combined Magnification Endoscopy with Chromoendoscopy in the Evaluation of Patients with Suspected Malabsorption," *Gastrointest Endosc* 46, no. 3 (1995): 226–30.

33 *The latest medical research connects the health of these little bugs . . .* M. Kwa, C. S. Plottel, M. J. Blaser, and S. Adams, "The Intestinal Microbiome and Estrogen Receptor-Positive Female Breast Cancer," *J Natl Cancer Inst* 108, no. 8 (2016), doi: 10.1093/jnci/djw029.

33 *High estrogen levels can also be the cause . . .* Kwa, Plottel, Blaser, and Adams, *J Natl Cancer Inst* 108, no. 8 (2016).

36 *"When we carefully test people over age forty . . .* Jonathan V. Wright, *Why Stomach Acid Is Good for You: Natural Relief from Heartburn, Indigestion, Reflux & GERD*, 4th ed. (M. Evans, 2001), 76.

38 *Estrogen dominance (including birth control pills) can . . .* X. Zhang, M. Essmann, E. T. Burt, and B. Larsen, "Estrogen Effects on Candida Albicans:

A Potential Virulence-Regulating Mechanism," *Journal of Infectious Diseases* 181, no. 4 (2000): 1441–46.

40 *If you suffer from chronic digestive, skin, and mental issues* . . . Digestive issues: Yurdagül Zopf, Eckhart G. Hahn, Martin Raithel, et al., "The Differential Diagnosis of Food Intolerance," *Deutsches Ärzteblatt International* 106, no. 21 (2009): 359–70; skin and mental issues: J. P. Webster, P. H. Lamberton, C. A. Donnelly, and E. F. Torrey, "Parasites as Causative Agents of Human Affective Disorders? The Impact of Anti-Psychotic, Mood-Stabilizer and Anti-Parasite Medication on Toxoplasma gondii's Ability to Alter Host Behaviour," *Proc Biol Sci* 273, no. 1589 (2006): 1023–30.

40 *the Bristol Stool Chart* . . . K. W. Heaton and S. J. Lewis, "Stool Form Scale as a Useful Guide to Intestinal Transit Time," *Scandinavian Journal of Gastroenterology* 32, no. 9 (1997): 920–24.

44 *Many of my clients, especially those who embarked* . . . Serena Tonstad, Karen Jaceldo-Siegl, Mark Messina, et al., "The Association Between Soya Consumption and Serum Thyroid-Stimulating Hormone Concentrations in the Adventist Health Study-2," *Public Health Nutrition* 19, no. 8 (2016): 1464–70.

CHAPTER 3

56 *In 2006, the* Chicago Tribune *published an investigative* . . . Patricia Callahan, Jeremy Manier, and Delroy Alexander, "Where There's Smoke, There Might Be Food Research, Too," *Chicago Tribune*, January 29, 2006, http://www.chicago tribune.com/chi-0601290254jan29-story.html.

57 *According to the Centers for Disease Control and Prevention* . . . "Usual Daily Intake of Added Sugars" (table), National Cancer Institute, Division of Cancer Control and Population, Epidemiology and Genomics Research Program, last updated November 10, 2016, https://epi.grants.cancer .gov/diet/usualintakes/pop/2007-10/table_a40 .html.

58 *Scientists have found that sugar stimulates the same* . . . Nicole M. Avena, Pedro Rada, and Bartley G. Hoebel, "Evidence for Sugar Addiction: Behavioral and Neurochemical Effects of Intermittent, Excessive Sugar Intake," *Neurosci Biobehav Rev* 32, no. 1 (2008): 20–39.

58 *Neuroscientists at Connecticut College* . . . "Oreos May Be as Addictive as Cocaine, Morphine," *Bioscience Technology*, October 16, 2013, http://www.biosciencetechnology.com /news/2013/10/oreos-may-be-addictive-cocaine -morphine#.UtWl3fRDudI.

59 *High blood sugar levels are the leading cause of high testosterone in women* . . . Jennifer L. Phy, Ali M. Pohlmeier, Jamie A. Cooper, et al., "Low Starch/Low Dairy Diet Results in Successful Treatment of Obesity and Co-Morbidities Linked to Polycystic Ovary Syndrome (PCOS)," *Journal of Obesity and Weight Loss Therapy* 5, no. 2 (2015): 259; Nina Lass, Michaela Kleber, Katrin Winkel, et al., "Effect of Lifestyle Intervention on Features of Polycystic Ovarian Syndrome, Metabolic Syndrome, and Intima-Media Thickness in Obese Adolescent Girls," *Journal of Clinical Endocrinology and Metabolism* 96, no. 11 (2011): 3533–40.

59 *and low testosterone in men* . . . Mathis Grossmann, "Low Testosterone in Men with Type 2 Diabetes: Significance and Treatment," *Journal of Clinical Endocrinology and Metabolism* 96, no. 8 (2011): 2341–53.

59 *Therefore the first recommended dietary step for women with PCOS* . . . S. E. Kasim-Karakas, W. M. Cunningham, and A. Tsodikov, "Relation of Nutrients and Hormones in Polycystic Ovary Syndrome," *American Journal of Clinical Nutrition* 85, no. 3 (2007): 688–94.

59 *According to researchers at the University of Washington* . . . G. N. Ioannou, C. L. Bryson, and E. J. Boyko, "Prevalence and Trends of Insulin Resistance, Impaired Fasting Glucose, and Diabetes," *Journal of Diabetes and Its Complications* 21, no. 6 (2007): 363–70.

60 *Today, numerous scientific studies show* . . . Insulin resistance: Heather Basciano, Lisa Federico, and

Khosrow Adeli, "Fructose, Insulin Resistance, and Metabolic Dyslipidemia," *Nutrition and Metabolism* 2005, 2:5, https://nutritionandmetabolism.biomedcentral.com/articles/10.1186/1743-7075-2-5; leptin resistance: Alexandra Shapiro, Wei Mu, Carlos Roncal, et al., "Fructose-Induced Leptin Resistance Exacerbates Weight Gain in Response to Subsequent High-Fat Feeding," *American Journal of Physiology: Regulatory, Integrative and Comparative Physiology* 295, no. 5 (2008), http://ajpregu.physiology.org/content/295/5/R1370.short.

61 *It is no surprise, then, that many former drug, gambling, and sex addicts* . . . Nicole M. Avena, Pedro Rada, and Bartley G. Hoebel, "Evidence for Sugar Addiction: Behavioral and Neurochemical Effects of Intermittent, Excessive Sugar Intake," *Neuroscience and Biobehavioral Reviews* 32, no. 1 (2008): 20–39.

61 *A diet high in sugar has been linked to poor mental health* . . . David M. Sack, "4 Ways Sugar Could Be Harming Your Mental Health," *Psychology Today,* September 2, 2013, https://www.psychologytoday.com/blog/where-science-meets-the-steps/201309/4-ways-sugar-could-be-harming-your-mental-health; Carolyn Gregoire, "This Is What Sugar Does to Your Brain," Huffpost, Healthy Living, April 6, 2015, http://www.huffingtonpost.com/2015/04/06/sugar-brain-mental-health_n_6904778.html.

61 *Fructose, according to research, inhibits* . . . Veronique Douard, Abbas Asgerally, Yves Sabbagh, et al., "Dietary Fructose Inhibits Intestinal Calcium Absorption and Induces Vitamin D Insufficiency in CKD," *J Am Soc Nephrol* 21, no. 2 (2010): 261–71.

61 *Researchers at the Stanford University School of Medicine* . . . Susan Young, "Study Identifies Potential Anti-Cancer Therapy That Starves Cancer Cells of Glucose," Stanford Medicine News Center, August 3, 2011, https://med.stanford.edu/news/all-news/2011/08/study-identifies-potential-anti-cancer-therapy-that-starves-cancer-cells-of-glucose.html.

61 *It is not a surprise to learn that women with high sugar levels* . . . Paola Muti, Teresa Quattrin, Brydon J. B. Grant, et al., "Fasting Glucose Is a Risk Factor for Breast Cancer," *Cancer Epidemiology, Biomarkers and Prevention* 11, no. 11 (2002), http://cebp.aacrjournals.org/content/11/11/1361.short.

62 *According to the U.S. Census Bureau* . . . U.S. Census Bureau, "Per Capita Consumption of Major Food Commodities" (table), April 18, 2015, https://www.census.gov/search-results.html?q=sugar%2Bconsumption%2Bper%2Bcapita&search.x=0&search.y=0&search=submit&page=1&stateGeo=none&searchtype=web&cssp=SERP'.

64 *Studies have linked artificial sweeteners to changes* . . . S. P. Fowler, "Low-Calorie Sweetener Use and Energy Balance: Results from Experimental Studies in Animals, and Large-Scale Prospective Studies in Humans," *Physiol Behav* 164, pt. B (2016): 517–23; Jodi E. Nettletona, Raylene A. Reimera, and Jane Shearera, "Reshaping the Gut Microbiota: Impact of Low Calorie Sweeteners and the Link to Insulin Resistance?" *Physiol Behav* 164, pt. B (2016): 488–93.

65 *Studies show that berberine has the same efficacy* . . . Jun Yin, Huili Xing, and Jianping Ye, "Efficacy of Berberine in Patients with Type 2 Diabetes," *Metabolism* 57, no. 5 (2008): 712–17, https://www.ncbi.nlm.nih.gov/pmc/articles/PMC2410097/.

CHAPTER 4

70 *When the liver is overburdened* . . . S. G. Genes, "[Role of the Liver in Hormone Metabolism and in the Regulation of Their Content in the Blood]" (in Russian), *Arkh Patol* 39, no. 6 (1977): 74–80.

70 *Some practitioners believe that round brown spots* . . . Thomas P. Habif, "Light-Related Diseases and Disorders of Pigmentation," in Habif, ed., *Clinical Dermatology: A Color Guide to Diagnosis and Therapy,* 5th ed. (Philadelphia: Elsevier Mosby, 2009), chap 19.

71 *the bile also helps evacuate steroid hormones* . . . Richard A. Bowen. "Hormone Chemistry, Synthesis and Elimination," VIVO Pathophysiology, http://www.vivo.colostate.edu/hbooks/pathphys/endocrine/basics/chem.html.

74 *According to the Environmental Working Group* . . . "Exposures Add Up—Survey Results," EWG's Skin Deep Cosmetics Database, http://www.ewg.org/skindeep/2004/06/15/exposures-add-up-survey-results/.

CHAPTER 6

126 *Herbs such as berberine, turmeric* . . . Zeinab Ghorbani, Azita Hekmatdoost, and Parvin Mirmiran, "Anti-Hyperglycemic and Insulin Sensitizer Effects of Turmeric and Its Principal Constituent Curcumin," *International Journal of Endocrinology and Metabolism* 12(4), October 2014, https://www.ncbi.nlm.nih.gov/pmc/articles/PMC4338652/.

126 *Studies show that berberine* . . . Yin, et al. "Efficacy of Berberine," *Metabolism* 57, no. 5 (2008), https://www.ncbi.nlm.nih.gov/pmc/articles/PMC2410097/.

CHAPTER 8

148 *In their book* The Good Gut, *Justin and Erica Sonnenburg* . . . Justin Sonnenburg and Erica Sonnenburg, *The Good Gut: Taking Control of Your Weight, Your Mood, and Your Long-Term Health* (New York: Penguin, 2016).

149 *according to the U.S. Department of Agriculture National Nutrient Database* . . . U.S. Department of Agriculture, Agricultural Research Service, "Basic Report: 05661, Chicken, Liver, All Classes, Cooked, Pan-Fried," revised May 2016, https://ndb.nal.usda.gov/ndb/foods/show/1117?manu=&fgcd=&ds=; and "Basic Report: 05060, Chicken, Broilers or Fryers, Breast, Meat and Skin, Cooked, Roasted," revised May 2016, https://ndb.nal.usda.gov/ndb/foods/show/883?manu=&fgcd=&ds=.

KITCHEN BASICS

155 *The fat tissue in bone marrow is a significant source* . . . University of Michigan Health System, "Bone Marrow Fat Tissue Secretes Hormone That Helps Body Stay Healthy," *ScienceDaily,* July 3, 2014, https://www.sciencedaily.com/releases/2014/07/140703125216.htm.

163 *Medical research has shown* . . . Yanyan Li, Tao Zhang, Hasan Korkaya, et al., "Sulforaphane, a Dietary Component of Broccoli/Broccoli Sprouts, Inhibits Breast Cancer Stem Cells," *Clinical Cancer Research* 16(9), May 1, 2010: 2580–90, https://www.ncbi.nlm.nih.gov/pmc/articles/PMC2862133/.

DRINKS, TEAS, AND TONICS

308 *Research has shown that both cinnamon* . . . A. Gupta, R. Gupta, and B. Lal, "Effect of Trigonella Foenum-Graecum (Fenugreek) Seeds on Glycaemic Control and Insulin Resistance in Type 2 Diabetes Mellitus: A Double Blind Placebo Controlled Study," *Journal of the Association of Physicians of India* 49, November 2001: 1057–61; and https://www.ncbi.nlm.nih.gov/pubmed/11868855 and Hamid Nasri, Yahya Madihi, and Alireza Marikhi, "Commentary on Effects of Cinnamon Consumption on Glycemic Status, Lipid Profile, and Body Composition in Type 2 Diabetic Patients," *International Journal of Preventive Medicine* 4(5), May 2013: 618–19, https://www.ncbi.nlm.nih.gov/pmc/articles/PMC3733197/.

Recipe Index by Protocol

KEY

Elim = Elimination Diet (without the Big 7)
P = Paleo
AIP = AIP
AC = Anti-Candida
LowF = Low FODMAP
TH = Thyroid and Hashimoto's
ED = Estrogen Dominance and Low Progesterone
LE = Low Estrogen and Menopause

AH = Adrenal Health
HT = PCOS and High Testosterone
LT = Low Testosterone
30 = Less than 30 Minutes

✔ = Complies
✔ = Avoid during the first four weeks
✔ = Omit the kelp or dulse

	Elim	P	AIP	AC	LowF	TH	ED	LE	AH	HT	LT	30
Kitchen Basics												
Immune-Boosting Chicken Broth	✔	✔	✔	✔	✔	✔	✔	✔	✔	✔	✔	
Mineral Vegetable Broth	✔	✔	✔	✔	✔	✔	✔	✔	✔	✔	✔	
Healing Bone Broth	✔	✔	✔	✔	✔	✔	✔	✔	✔	✔	✔	
Life-Giving Sprouts	✔	✔	✔	✔	✔	✔	✔	✔	✔	✔	✔	
Coconut Yogurt	✔	✔	✔	✔	✔	✔	✔	✔	✔	✔	✔	
Whipped Coconut Cream	✔	✔	✔	✔	✔	✔	✔	✔	✔	✔	✔	✔
Homemade Applesauce	✔	✔	✔		✔	✔	✔	✔	✔		✔	✔

	Elim	P	AIP	AC	LowF	TH	ED	LE	AH	HT	LT	30
Creamy Egg-Free Mayo—Four Ways	✔	✔		✔		✔	✔	✔	✔	✔	✔	✔
Preserved Lemon	✔	✔	✔	✔	✔	✔	✔	✔	✔	✔	✔	
Whipped Herbal Butter—Two Ways	✔	✔	✔	✔	✔	✔	✔	✔	✔	✔	✔	✔
Fabulous Spice Mixes	✔	✔	✔	✔	✔	✔	✔	✔	✔	✔	✔	✔
Salt Brine for Cultured Vegetables	✔	✔	✔	✔	✔	✔	✔	✔	✔	✔	✔	✔

Breakfasts

	Elim	P	AIP	AC	LowF	TH	ED	LE	AH	HT	LT	30
Sweet Potato and Sage Pancakes	✔			✔	✔	✔	✔	✔	✔	✔	✔	
Farmer's Wife's Breakfast	✔	✔	✔	✔	✔	✔	✔	✔	✔	✔	✔	
Coconut Kefir Chia Pudding	✔	✔			✔	✔	✔	✔	✔	✔	✔	
Seed Rotation Porridge—Two Ways	✔	✔			✔	✔	✔	✔				✔
Breakfast Casserole One: Salmon and Broccoli	✔	✔	✔	✔	✔	✔	✔	✔	✔	✔	✔	✔
Energizing Matcha Lime Smoothie	✔	✔		✔	✔	✔	✔	✔		✔	✔	✔
Grain-Free Sunday Brunch Pancakes with Mixed Berries	✔	✔	✔		✔	✔	✔	✔	✔	✔	✔	
Breakfast Casserole Two: Pork Chops and Apples	✔	✔	✔	✔	✔	✔	✔	✔	✔	✔	✔	✔
Deep Green Spirulina Smoothie	✔	✔		✔	✔		✔	✔	✔	✔	✔	✔
Teff and Cherry Porridge	✔			✔	✔	✔	✔	✔	✔	✔	✔	✔
Parsnip Dill Pancake with Arugula and Smoked Salmon	✔	✔	✔	✔	✔	✔	✔	✔	✔	✔	✔	✔
Carrot and Beet Smoothie	✔	✔			✔	✔	✔	✔				✔
Bacon, Oysters, and Collard Greens Stir Fry	✔	✔	✔	✔	✔	✔	✔	✔	✔	✔	✔	✔
Zucchini Olive Muffins	✔	✔		✔	✔	✔	✔	✔	✔		✔	

	Elim	P	AIP	AC	LowF	TH	ED	LE	AH	HT	LT	30
Decadent Chocolate Cherry Smoothie	✔	✔		✔	✔	✔	✔	✔		✔	✔	✔
Perfect French Crepes	✔	✔	✔		✔	✔	✔	✔	✔		✔	

Soups and Stews

	Elim	P	AIP	AC	LowF	TH	ED	LE	AH	HT	LT	30
Hearty Beet Stew (Borscht)	✔	✔	✔			✔	✔	✔	✔	✔	✔	
Easy Chicken Curry Stew	✔	✔	✔	✔	✔	✔	✔	✔	✔	✔	✔	
Icelandic Fish Stew	✔	✔	✔	✔	✔	✔	✔	✔	✔	✔	✔	
Seriously Mushroom Soup	✔	✔	✔			✔	✔	✔	✔	✔	✔	✔
Quick Detoxifying Soup	✔	✔	✔	✔	✔	✔	✔	✔	✔	✔	✔	✔
Cauliflower and Sweet Potato Soup	✔	✔	✔			✔	✔	✔	✔		✔	
Quick Miso Soup					✔		✔	✔	✔	✔	✔	✔
Squash, Apple, and Turmeric Soup	✔	✔	✔	✔		✔	✔	✔	✔	✔	✔	
Porcini Mushroom Beef Stew	✔	✔	✔			✔	✔	✔	✔	✔	✔	

Entrees

	Elim	P	AIP	AC	LowF	TH	ED	LE	AH	HT	LT	30
Honey Glazed Tarragon Chicken	✔	✔	✔	✔	✔	✔	✔	✔	✔	✔	✔	
Grain-Free Pizza—Two Ways	✔	✔	✔	✔		✔	✔	✔	✔	✔		
Nutritious Quick Bowls—Two Ways	✔	✔	✔	✔	✔	✔	✔	✔	✔	✔	✔	✔
Lamb with Collard Greens and Radishes	✔	✔	✔	✔	✔	✔	✔	✔	✔	✔	✔	✔
Nomad's Kebabs (Liver and Bacon)	✔	✔	✔	✔	✔	✔	✔	✔	✔	✔	✔	✔

	Elim	P	AIP	AC	LowF	TH	ED	LE	AH	HT	LT	30
Butter Cod with Gremolata	✓	✓	✓	✓	✓	✓	✓	✓	✓	✓	✓	✓
Sticky Spare Ribs Casserole	✓	✓	✓		✓	✓	✓	✓	✓		✓	
Walnut Crusted Salmon	✓	✓			✓	✓	✓	✓	✓	✓	✓	
Fennel and Coriander Crusted Liver	✓	✓		✓	✓	✓	✓	✓	✓	✓	✓	
Creamy Rosemary Chicken	✓	✓	✓	✓	✓	✓	✓	✓	✓	✓	✓	
Rosemary and Garlic Stuffed Lamb Roast	✓	✓	✓	✓	✓	✓	✓	✓	✓	✓	✓	

Salads and Vegetables

	Elim	P	AIP	AC	LowF	TH	ED	LE	AH	HT	LT	30
Detoxing Beet and Carrot Salad	✓	✓	✓			✓	✓	✓	✓		✓	✓
Quick Salads—Four Ways	✓	✓	✓	✓	✓	✓	✓	✓	✓	✓	✓	✓
Steam 'n Toss Veggies and Proteins on the Run	✓	✓	✓	✓	✓	✓	✓	✓	✓	✓	✓	✓
Zesty and Creamy Collard Greens	✓	✓	✓	✓	✓	✓	✓	✓	✓	✓	✓	✓
Tuscan Shredded Fennel and Orange Salad	✓	✓	✓	✓		✓	✓	✓	✓	✓	✓	✓
Sauerkraut Carrot Salad	✓	✓	✓	✓		✓	✓	✓	✓	✓	✓	✓
Creamy Celeriac and Cauliflower Mash	✓	✓	✓	✓	✓	✓	✓	✓	✓	✓	✓	✓
Jicama and Pomegranate Slaw	✓	✓	✓	✓		✓	✓	✓	✓	✓	✓	✓
Fries Baked in Duck Fat	✓	✓	✓	✓	✓	✓	✓	✓	✓	✓	✓	
Japanese Seaweed and Cucumber Salad	✓	✓	✓	✓	✓		✓	✓	✓	✓	✓	✓
Kohlrabi Kraut	✓	✓	✓	✓	✓	✓	✓	✓	✓	✓	✓	
Cultured Vegetable Medley—Four Ways	✓	✓	✓	✓	✓	✓	✓	✓	✓	✓		

	Elim	P	AIP	AC	LowF	TH	ED	LE	AH	HT	LT	30
Dollops, Dressings, and Spreads												
Homemade Seed Butter (for Seed Rotation)—Two Ways	✔	✔		✔	✔	✔	✔	✔	✔	✔	✔	✔
Salad Dressing—Five Ways	✔	✔	✔	✔	✔	✔	✔	✔	✔	✔	✔	✔
Herbal Pesto		✔	✔	✔	✔	✔	✔	✔	✔	✔	✔	✔
Easy French Pate	✔	✔	✔	✔	✔	✔	✔	✔	✔	✔	✔	✔
Olive and Preserved Lemon Tapenade	✔	✔	✔	✔	✔	✔	✔	✔	✔	✔	✔	✔
Spiced Nut Butter—Two Ways	✔	✔		✔	✔	✔	✔	✔	✔	✔	✔	✔
Silky Chocolate Hazelnut Butter	✔	✔			✔	✔	✔	✔	✔	✔	✔	✔
Salmon and Avocado in Nori Sheets	✔	✔	✔	✔	✔	✔	✔	✔	✔	✔	✔	✔
Drinks, Teas, and Tonics												
Matcha Frappe	✔	✔	✔	✔	✔	✔	✔	✔		✔	✔	✔
Nut and Seed Milks	✔	✔	✔	✔	✔	✔	✔	✔	✔	✔	✔	✔
Healing Tea Infusions and Decoctions	✔	✔	✔	✔	✔	✔	✔	✔	✔	✔	✔	
Nourishing Lattes	✔	✔	✔	✔	✔	✔	✔	✔	✔	✔	✔	
Better Than Coffee Latte	✔	✔	✔	✔		✔	✔	✔	✔	✔	✔	✔
Hot Chocolate with Pink Roses	✔	✔	✔	✔	✔	✔	✔	✔	✔	✔	✔	✔
Ginger Beet Kvass	✔	✔	✔			✔	✔	✔	✔	✔	✔	
Strawberry Ginger Ale	✔	✔	✔		✔	✔	✔	✔	✔		✔	
Fizzy Orange, Carrot, and Beet Soda	✔	✔	✔			✔	✔	✔	✔		✔	

	Elim	P	AIP	AC	LowF	TH	ED	LE	AH	HT	LT	30
Breads, Muffins, and Crackers												
Rustic Olive Bread	✔			✔	✔	✔	✔	✔	✔		✔	
Pomegranate Crackers (Progesterone Boosters)	✔	✔			✔	✔	✔	✔	✔	✔	✔	
Flaxseed Crackers (Estrogen Boosters)	✔	✔		✔	✔	✔	✔	✔	✔	✔	✔	
Grain-Free Sourdough Flatbread	✔					✔	✔	✔	✔		✔	
Coconut Banana Bread (Grain-Free)	✔	✔			✔	✔	✔	✔	✔		✔	
Seed Bread with Figs	✔			✔	✔	✔	✔	✔	✔		✔	
Rosemary Pear Muffins	✔	✔			✔	✔	✔	✔	✔	✔	✔	
Desserts												
Red Velvet Grain-Free Brownies	✔	✔	✔		✔	✔	✔	✔	✔		✔	
Raspberry and Green Tea Lime Melties	✔	✔	✔	✔	✔	✔	✔	✔	✔	✔	✔	
Tart Cherry Sorbet	✔	✔	✔	✔	✔	✔	✔	✔	✔		✔	✔
Creamy Lime Pudding	✔	✔		✔		✔	✔	✔	✔	✔	✔	
Crunchy Chocolate Cherry Bark	✔	✔	✔		✔	✔	✔	✔	✔		✔	
Dinner Stealing Pear and Orange Cobbler	✔	✔	✔		✔	✔	✔	✔	✔		✔	
Kudzu Calming Pudding	✔	✔	✔	✔	✔	✔	✔	✔	✔	✔	✔	✔
Strawberry and Lime Jelly Mousse	✔	✔	✔	✔	✔	✔	✔	✔	✔	✔	✔	
Stuffed Baked Apples	✔	✔		✔		✔	✔	✔	✔	✔	✔	
Digestive Truffles—Two Ways	✔	✔			✔	✔	✔	✔	✔	✔	✔	

Index

Tart Cherry Sorbet
recipe, 340–341
tea infusions and decoctions
recipes, 302–308
Teff and Cherry Porridge
recipe, 198
testosterone: androgen
dominance and high levels
of, 21; bile helps evacuate,
71; body fat distribution
and levels of, 23; converted
to estradiol, 11, 13, 20,
105; description of, 11,
12–13; estrogen dominance
and, 59; Lowering High
Testosterone Levels and
Treating PCOS Food Guide,
21, 126–131; low levels of,
21, 24; PCOS (polycystic
ovary syndrome) and, 21, 22;
Raising Low Testosterone
Levels Food Guide, 127–131;
stomach acid and, 37; sugar
levels and, 59; zinc role in
conversion to estrogen, 127
Thick and Cheesy Salad
Dressing recipe, 286
thyroid disorders: Hashimoto's
disease, 5, 21–22, 48,
112–115; hyperthyroidism,
5; hypothyroidism, 21–22;
Restoring Thyroid Health and
Treating Hashimoto's Food
Guide and Meal Plan, 110–115
thyroid gland, 10–11
thyroxine (T4) hormone,
13, 71, 111

toxins: detoxing liver from, 30,
70–77; everyday sources of,
25, 74–75, 77, 105–106, 111,
128; filtered by the liver, 149;
The In-Out Guide to Reducing
Toxins in Your Life, 73–74
TPO antibodies, 71, 111, 112
triiodothyronine (T3)
hormone, 13, 71, 111
turmeric, 76, 104, 111,
126, 137, 152
Tuscan Shredded Fennel and
Orange Salad recipe, 262–263
type 2 diabetes, 58

uterus fibroids, 15, 24, 33

Vanilla and Rose Macadamia
Butter recipe, 295
vegan or vegetarian diet, 44
vegetables: AIP food List, 97;
Anti-Candida Food List,
82; bitter greens, 42, 75,
101; buying and prepping
tips and tricks, 141–142;
cruciferous vegetables, 72,
75, 103, 111, 150; to keep or
throw out of the kitchen, 136;
Low-FODMAP Food List,
88; nightshade, 35, 36, 47;
Paleo Food List, 93; sea, 76
vinegars (Anti-Candida
Food List), 82
Vitamin A, 42, 71, 112
Vitamin B, 75, 112, 116
Vitamin B1, 112
Vitamin B6, 71, 109, 112

Vitamin B12, 71, 112
Vitamin C, 76, 116
Vitamin D, 71, 111
Vitamin E, 71, 116
Vitamin K, 71
vitamins, 61, 71, 112
vitex/chasteberry, 110, 121

Walnut Crusted Salmon
recipe, 244–245
Warming Chai Latte recipe, 310
weight gain, 22–23, 38
weight loss, 45, 127
weight training, 126
Whipped Coconut
Cream recipe, 166
Whipped Herbal Butter—Two
Ways recipe, 172–173
Why Stomach Acid Is Good
for You (Wright), 36
Wright, Jonathan V., 36
www.HormonesBalance.com/
book: detoxification pathways,
71–72; gallbladder, 72; Gut-
Healing Guide download
on, 42; PCOS Balance Kit,
126; 16 Hacks to Better
Sleep, 117; sleep disorders,
27; Soaking and Sprouting
Guide, 147; Sugar Balance
Kit, 65; uterus fibroids, 24

Zesty and Creamy Collard
Greens recipe, 261
zinc, 25, 32, 37, 110, 111, 112,
121, 127, 149, 150, 214, 252
Zucchini Olive Muffins recipe, 205